THE
Migraine Relief
PLAN

An 8-Week Transition to Better Eating,
Fewer Headaches, and Optimal Health

STEPHANIE WEAVER, MPH, CWHC

FOREWORD BY IAN PURCELL, MD, PHD

S

**SURREY
BOOKS**

AN AGATE IMPRINT

CHICAGO

Printed in the United States

The Migraine Relief Plan
ISBN 13: 978-1-57284-209-0
ISBN 10: 1-57284-209-1
ebook ISBN 13: 978-1-57284-789-7
ebook ISBN 10: 1-57284-789-1
First printing: February 2017

10 9 8 7 6 5 4 3 2 1   17 18 19 20 21

Surrey is an imprint of Agate Publishing. Agate books are available in
bulk at discount prices.

agatepublishing.com

For everyone who suffers from migraine, chronic headaches, vertigo, and Meniere's disease

———— ••• ————

table of contents

———— ••• ————

foreword

———— ••• ————

I've been treating people with migraine, Meniere's disease, and balance disorders for more than twenty years. In working with them, I have come to believe that these disorders often have an autoimmune component that greatly benefits from diets that are anti-inflammatory, free of known headache triggers, and reduced in sodium. I have always recommended this approach in general, but was not able to offer my patients any specific resources beyond a three-page handout. Until now.

I've seen over and over again that it's extremely difficult for people to make these modifications on their own. Many don't stick with them long-term because they can't make the changes or don't see results.

What impressed me about this book was the author's thorough, thoughtful, and tested approach to each of these factors. She took the low-tyramine diet sheet many doctors use, researched it, and decided it wasn't good enough. She took her own experience with migraine and became a wellness advocate. After creating and testing this eight-week plan to help people ease into the diet, she expanded it to include additional useful lifestyle information about regular sleep, eating, gentle exercise, and how to reintroduce possible trigger foods, and then added an entire cookbook full of recipes to ensure their success.

Now I can give this book to the people I treat and know they will get a thorough grounding in both the why and the how.

I would recommend anyone suffering from headaches, dizziness, migraine, or Meniere's disease to read this book and follow the Plan.

And I would encourage all physicians who work with migraine, Meniere's disease, and balance issues to read this book and recommend it in their practice.

IAN PURCELL, MD, PHD, *is developing the world-class Balance Institute at San Diego's Senta Clinic. He currently practices clinical Neurology with an additional focus in otoneurology and headache management. He conducts extensive research in balance disorders, and heads the Division of Balance Research at the Center for Neurological Studies.*

introduction

———— ••• ————

WHY I WROTE THIS BOOK

———— • ————

Hi, I'm Stephanie. In early 2014, I found myself in a neurologist's office after three scary bouts of vertigo. I had no idea that migraine attacks could cause vertigo. At the time, what I knew about migraine I had learned from coworkers: headaches so bad that people miss work for three days while they lie miserable in a dark room. Now I know that migraine attacks are far more complex, with symptoms and triggers unique to each person.

Over the course of a few weeks that winter, I saw two different doctors to address my vertigo. Each gave me a different diet-related handout and a different prescription medication. I received a diagnosis of migraine with Meniere's variant from the second doctor. I gladly took their medication and their advice, as I desperately wanted the room to stop spinning.

Once I started feeling a little better, I wanted to learn more. Looking over the two diet handouts (one low-sodium, one low-tyramine), I had no idea that so many foods could cause or contribute to migraine attacks. Since I write a food blog, have a degree in nutrition education, and am a health coach, exploring how diet could help me was a priority. What I thought was a relatively simple task—combining two guides into a single sheet—set me on a path that was part detective story and part medical education.

Like any good researcher I began online, ordering just about every migraine book available in print and in the Kindle store. As I delved deeper into Meniere's disease and migraine research, I ended up at the local university's medical library. After reading dozens of books and hundreds of medical studies and research papers, I developed an eating plan that worked for me and gained some understanding of why it was helping—and I started feeling better.

I became determined to create a plan to help others. I was lucky that my body responded so quickly, that my symptoms weren't more severe, and that I had such great resources available to me, in addition to a unique skill set that allowed me to pull it all together. Most people don't have the time or the resources to do this—especially when they are in pain. I wanted to share my findings with other people so they could start feeling better, too.

That's why I wrote this book: to make it all available to you. All the research, all the trial and error. I spent months creating recipes and testing out this Plan with other migraine sufferers so you don't have to do all that work. I've broken all the information down into tiny little bite-sized nuggets spread out over a few months, so that you can successfully incorporate it into your life without too much work or additional stress. Think of me as your personal wellness coach! I walk beside you each week, encouraging you to gradually make small changes that will make a big difference in your overall health.

I'm a strong believer in taking the lead on your own health, and utilizing excellent physicians and other healthcare providers as trusted allies and resources. I do my best to think of long-term health challenges as health opportunities. This book gathers together so many facets of my life and experience: utilizing my background in public health and nutrition, more than two decades of educational technical writing, 30 years of recipe renovation, six years of food blogging, and my doggedness to figure out this migraine problem. I hope you'll find a lot here to put into practice, and that doing so will help you feel significantly better, empowered about taking charge of your own health.

IS THIS BOOK FOR YOU?

People who don't get migraine or Meniere's attacks don't understand. They have probably never thrown up in front of their chiropractors. They've probably never returned from an appointment only to throw up on the neighbor's lawn in front of a bunch of construction workers. They might never have had a vertigo attack so bad that it felt like the car was doing doughnuts. I have. I know how embarrassing and frustrating migraine attacks are and how out of control they can make you feel. I know what it feels like to worry before every airplane flight whether I'm going to get sick—when should I time my pill, and will drinking lots of water help? I know what it's like to dread super-bright days, and I sometimes live like a mole woman to try to prevent an attack.

If you are sick and tired of migraine pain or vertigo derailing your life, this book is for you. If you are tired of thinking of yourself as a "patient" and having migraine threaten to define your life, this book is for you. If you worry about taking too much migraine medication, or if you're rationing out your migraine meds during the month, this book can empower you to step off the rebound-headache rollercoaster without fear. If you have daily headaches, sinus headaches, tension headaches, or headaches that seem to be weather-related, this book is for you.

My approach may even help those of you who don't have a migraine diagnosis, too. The symptoms related to migraine, Meniere's, and vertigo all overlap; it's still not clear to researchers if all these illnesses are separate. My Plan is as comprehensive as possible to help cover all the recommendations. If your doctor has ruled out benign paroxysmal positional vertigo (BPPV) or another illness as a cause of your vertigo, it's possible my Plan will help you.

If you have ever gotten a headache from eating cheese or Chinese food, or from drinking alcohol or diet soda, it's possible that foods contribute to your migraine and headaches, and this book is for you. I've always been sensitive to light, alcohol, some cheeses, diet soda, caffeine, and MSG. Before my diagnosis, I had never made the connection between these sensitivities and migraine.

But perhaps you have tried making a few dietary changes in the past and didn't think they worked. This book is still for you, because my step-by-step approach to migraine relief is based on nutritious eating *and* lifestyle. All the recipes are free of known migraine triggers, completely sugar-free[1], and gluten-free. My Plan focuses on whole, unprocessed foods and utilizes information from the most current nutrition research to provide a balanced diet that should help reduce the frequency and severity of your attacks. But my approach also includes guidance on digestion, sleep, hydration, regular gentle movement, meditation, alternative treatment options, and environmental factors.

I created this Plan to help support you if you are ready to try a food- and lifestyle-based approach. Even if you're not quite ready, reading this book will help you think about migraine or Meniere's differently, and it will be there for you when you are ready to make a change.

My philosophy about health is rooted in my own experience and mindset. I have seen—both in myself and in others close to me—the positive impact that excellent nutrition and attitude can have on problems considered impossible to solve. I truly believe that the way we think about ourselves, the language we use, and the intention we put behind our efforts to regain our health are powerful. I believe that our body's core desire is to heal, and that we have innate wisdom about what can heal us. I believe I am creative, capable, and unbroken.

As your health and wellness coach, I believe this is true for you as well.

Welcome!

HELPFUL DEFINITIONS

CLUSTER HEADACHES: Considered the most painful headaches, also called suicide headaches. Attacks of severe pain on one side of the head (often described as a hot poker through the eye or temple). Each headache can last 15 to 180 minutes, with attacks ranging from once every other day to eight or more times a day. Clusters can be seasonal. Nearly three-quarters of cluster headache sufferers are men.

HEADACHE: Pain in the head, usually caused by muscle tension or stress. Pain is mild to moderate, usually on both sides of the head, may feel like a band tightening, is not worsened by physical exertion, and does not have a pulsating quality. Can include either light or noise sensitivity, but not both.

MENIERE'S DISEASE: Once thought to be a separate illness, Meniere's disease is now believed by many doctors to be a unique manifestation of migraine. Symptoms include dizziness, vertigo, and tinnitus (ringing or roaring in the ears). Meniere's disease can only be formally diagnosed once a patient has lost hearing in one ear. In Meniere's disease, excess fluid in the inner ear puts pressure on the tiny hairs and bones that make up the vestibular system, which regulates our balance. Too much pressure for too long causes permanent damage, leading to hearing loss and loss of balance. Meniere's is complex, and little research has been conducted on the condition. Causes could include viruses, genetics, allergies, and/or autoimmune disruptions.[2]

MIGRAINE: A complex neurobiological disorder with genetic, vascular, and biochemical components. Some doctors believe that migraine has an autoimmune component, indicating the body's natural immune response may be working incorrectly. Migraine attacks can include four phases (see page 6). Less common types include abdominal (usually occurring in children), hemiplegic (genetic), basilar-type, and retinal migraine. Colic in babies may be the first sign of migraine. Not all migraine attacks include head pain, but if they do, pain is usually on one side of the head and is moderate to severe. Migraine attacks are worsened by physical exertion and have a pulsating quality. Attacks can include nausea, vomiting, and extreme sensitivities to light, sound, and/or touch. Nearly three-quarters of migraine attack sufferers are women.

MIGRAINE TRIGGER: A variety of stimuli, both external and internal, can trigger a migraine. It's believed that people prone to migraine attacks are far more sensitive to these stimuli than everyone else. Triggers are not the underlying cause of migraine, which is still unknown. Triggers are always cumulative (that is, one trigger will rarely be enough to set off a migraine attack). People with migraine seem to have a threshold. Stay below the threshold and you won't have an attack. Go above it and you will. Triggers may include food, light, sound, odors, barometric pressure changes, hormones, stress, lack of sleep, irregular meals, and too little or too intense exercise. Every person's triggers are different.

> Following *The Migraine Relief Plan* will reduce as many triggers as possible so you can live far below your threshold.

MEDICATION OVERUSE HEADACHES (MOH, FORMERLY KNOWN AS REBOUND HEADACHES): Headaches and migraine attacks caused by the overuse of either over-the-counter (OTC) or prescription medications. Doctors' opinions vary about how much medication is "too much" (see page 119 for more guidelines). Doctors agree that the following can all cause MOH: antihistamines, decongestants, caffeine-containing medications (especially those with more than one painkiller), ergotamines, triptans, and codeine-, barbiturate-, or narcotic-containing prescriptions. Note that self-medicating by using caffeine-containing beverages plus OTC painkillers can also cause MOH.

SINUS HEADACHE: Now considered an incorrect diagnosis, as 90 percent of sinus headaches are undiagnosed migraine attacks. True sinus headaches are from a serious sinus infection and include infected nasal discharge, fever, chills, and other symptoms of infection. See a headache specialist or neurologist to learn more.

VERTIGO: A sensation of rotating or spinning in space while not moving, which can cause nausea and balance issues. Vertigo is a symptom of migraine attacks in 25 to 35 percent of people with migraine. People who get motion sickness may be more likely to have migraine attacks. Vertigo attacks caused by tiny crystals coming loose in the ear are called benign paroxysmal positional vertigo (BPPV); these are diagnosed using a specific set of head and neck motions called the Epley maneuver. Crystals can be repositioned and the vertigo can go away fairly quickly. BPPV is unrelated to migraine.

WEATHER HEADACHE: Headaches that regularly accompany specific changes in weather (such as thunderstorms or hot, dry winds) are likely undiagnosed migraine attacks. I had these for 30 years before getting diagnosed; my mother has had them her whole life. See a headache specialist or neurologist to learn more.

MIGRAINE PHASES:

PRODROME:
Premonitory phase (experienced by 30 to 40 percent of people with migraine):
TIME FRAME: 4 to 48 hours before the attack
SYMPTOMS: fatigue, urge to sleep or sleep issues, mood shifts including depression, food cravings, dizziness, gastrointestinal upset, problems concentrating, reading, or speaking, hyper- or hypoactivity, increased thirst or urination, nausea, light or sound sensitivity, repetitive yawning, stiff neck[3]

Aura (experienced by 20 percent of people with migraine, with a genetic component):
TIME FRAME: 20 to 45 minutes before the attack
SYMPTOMS: visual disturbances, numbness, tingling, difficulty with speech. Caused by cortical spreading depression[4]

ATTACK:
TIME FRAME: 4 to 72 hours
SYMPTOMS: moderate to severe pulsing pain (usually on one side but can be bilateral), nausea, vomiting, sensitivities to light/sound/touch

POSTDROME:
TIME FRAME: a few hours to a day following the attack (if experienced)
SYMPTOMS: fatigue, brain fog, continued sensitivities to light/sound/touch

PART I
CREATING
THE PLAN

————— ··· —————

The story of how I came to write this book is interwoven into my own medical history and a surprising diagnosis I got later in life. It's part medical mystery, part detective novel. It underscores how important it is for us all to be active participants in our own health stories, working with our doctors and healthcare providers to determine what works best for us. In Part I, you'll see how this unfolded for me, how I researched this Plan, and how I came to write this book using my unique skill set.

my story

Let me tell you a little about me. In my mid-30s, I had some issues with fatigue and headaches that baffled my doctors, as I was otherwise very healthy and active.

I ate low-fat meals full of whole grains, beans, fruits, and vegetables, mostly home-cooked, with very little meat. I ate this way because I believed it was the healthiest possible diet, because I had been taught in my master's program in public health that fat was bad, butter was evil, whole grains were much healthier than white flour, and fatty meats would eventually kill me. Since I had never loved meat anyway, it was easy to eat vegetarian, and I dutifully replaced butter with heart-healthy margarine and real cheese with fat-free, lite, or low-fat versions. I didn't drink or smoke, I exercised fairly often, I wasn't overweight, and I was good at cooking for myself.

Despite my super-healthy lifestyle, I had weird bouts of fatigue, headaches, and flu-like symptoms. I was tested for a range of conditions by many specialists over the years with no conclusive results, leaving us all frustrated when they couldn't help me. At one point in my late 30s, my weather-related headaches were bad enough that my doctor prescribed Imitrex and an anti-nausea medication. I don't remember being told even then that I was having migraine attacks, despite episodes of vomiting, light sensitivity, and terrible head and neck pain.

As I got into my 40s, I experienced a year of deep fatigue and body aches that did not line up with any known disease. I took months off work, had two back surgeries to fuse a stress fracture, and made three significant changes to my diet to try to feel better: (1) I gave up sugar and processed food, (2) I gave up gluten, and (3) I went plant-based.[5]

I occasionally ate gluten, sugar, or animal products, usually when traveling. When I did, the next morning my fingers would be swollen like pork sausages, my joints would ache, and I would feel either fatigue or flu-like symptoms. I always returned to my gluten- and sugar-free, plant-based diet pretty quickly. I continued to have piercing headaches when the weather changed, and usually had a mild to moderate headache every day, which I just tried to ignore. My mother is a stoic German woman who prides herself on never crying, so I learned early on to suck it up and not complain about aches and pains. (At 89 she underwent chemotherapy and was a total warrior.) It didn't occur to me to go to the doctor for my headaches; they were just a part of my life, along with a funky back.

I learned how to make grateable vegan cheese from cashews and agar agar, a white powder made from seaweed. I brewed probiotic kombucha tea, fermented my own sauerkraut, and perfected cashew yogurt. I experimented with gluten-free, vegan baking until I could make reduced-sugar vegan cookies, cakes, and pies that were amazing. I shared my recipes on my new food blog, RecipeRenovator.com.

A NEW, SCARY SYMPTOM

I would have been happy to follow that diet for the rest of my life, but in the fall of 2013, I had my first two bouts of vertigo. I was riding home from Los Angeles with a friend, about a two-and-a-half-hour drive. I had a pounding headache. The headache had started in LA on the left side of my head, feeling like an iron band that got tighter and tighter, with a little spike through my left temple for good measure. The bright sun bouncing off the cars, the strobe effect of the light as we went under overpasses, everything made it worse. I got headaches a lot, but nothing like this.

When the car pulled into a parking lot, I felt the sensation of it spinning around like a whip-pan camera shot, a full 360 degrees, and I thought I would be sick. I went into the restroom at Starbucks, certain I needed to throw up and having no idea what was going on.

When this happened a second time, I scheduled an appointment with my general practitioner. He didn't find anything wrong but did a thorough ear cleaning, just in case it was wax in my ear. That seemed to help, so I forgot about it. My daily headaches continued; I was so used to them that I didn't notice. On bad days I would take ibuprofen. On really bad days, like those when I experienced headaches that aligned with changes in the weather, I would take a generic Fioricet, a mixture of caffeine, acetaminophen, and butalbital that my doctor had prescribed for what he called my "tension headaches." It usually worked, but seemed to be less effective each time I took it. (I now know that this medication is no longer recommended, as it can cause rebound headaches.)

In January 2014, the vertigo happened a third time, minus the long car trip. I woke up with a headache that worsened throughout the morning. At lunch that day, my friend Ellen was telling us about her crazy vertigo attack that happened over the holidays; she was terrified she had a brain tumor. As she talked, I could feel the blood pulsing in my head, and I hoped I wouldn't have to go to the bathroom to throw up.

Ellen didn't have a brain tumor as she feared; she had something called benign paroxysmal positional vertigo (BPPV). BPPV is caused by tiny crystals coming loose within the ear's balance mechanism and messing up your equilibrium, and it's relatively easy to fix. She suggested I make an appointment with her doctor. My nausea was so bad by the time I got home that I vomited, which I could not remember doing in more than 10 years. I lay in the dark bedroom with a cold pack on my head, wondering what was happening to me. I vowed to call Ellen's doctor as soon as I was able.

THE FIRST OPINION (OF TWO)

I went to see the ear, nose, and throat doctor Ellen recommended, whom I will call Dr. X. He was professional and welcoming, and I felt confident that he was competent and would take good care of me, especially after Ellen's great experience. I was certain mine would be an easy fix like Ellen's. He asked me a ton of questions about my hearing, my balance, my headaches.

"OK, now I'm going to have you do a test. I want you to stand over there, close your eyes, and put your hands over your ears. I want you to march in place, really raising your knees as high as you can each time, like you're in a marching band. Try your hardest to stay in the same position and keep your eyes closed. Keep going until I tell you to stop. Ready?"

I nodded, my eyes closed, hands over my ears. I started marching, feeling this was an odd and obviously easy test.[6] After a lot of marching, I heard him say, "Stop! Now, don't open your eyes. Do you think you are in the same place as you started?"

Confused, I said yes. Hadn't he told me to stay in place?

"OK, open your eyes."

I did, instantly becoming disoriented. Despite doing as I was told and feeling I was exactly where I started in the middle of the room, I had marched five feet to the left and turned nearly 90 degrees, almost running into his white laminate countertop.

He had me sit back down.

"Unfortunately, you don't have BPPV. That's a shame, because that's a pretty easy fix. I think you have a balance disorder called Meniere's disease."

I was not expecting this and tried to absorb what he was telling me.

"It's a disease we don't know much about. It causes your body to hold sodium. The sodium retention increases the fluid level in the chambers of your inner ears, affecting your balance. Some people lose their hearing, usually in one ear." He didn't mention anything about my headaches.

Instead of loose crystals, I have something I've never heard of, and I could go deaf?

He sent me to the hearing test booth. I instantly remembered sitting in one of these in grade school. It smelled and felt exactly the same, musty and oddly still, with schlubby beige fabric walls. The technician put heavy earphones on me and instructed me to listen for the tones and signal with my hand each time I heard one.

I tried desperately not to fail the test. *How bad is it? Am I going deaf already? How had I not noticed this?* I fought back the tears that were welling up as I listened as hard as I could for the tones, concentrating with every fiber of my being, willing myself not to fail. *Was I hearing enough of them? Was that one? Did I miss one?*

Afterwards, he took a look at the results.

"Your results aren't definitive. You have some minor hearing loss in the lower register on your right side. It's not unusual for a woman your age. Our best course of action is to put you on a diuretic, which will help remove the sodium from your body. Have you been feeling bloated at all?"

Truthfully, I have felt bloated off and on my whole life, watching my weight as most women do. I didn't know how to answer, so I just said no, embarrassed.

"If you lose a bit of weight the first week on the diuretic, that will help tell us whether it's Meniere's. Call us in a week and let us know. This medication will probably make you feel pretty tired. And it will make you pee like a racehorse. I want you to cut back on your sodium, too. We'll give you a sheet."

I went home, my brain spinning along with my equilibrium.

THE PATH TOWARD A LOW-SODIUM DIET

My instinct for the next week or two was to hold myself as still as I could, as if that would help stop the world from spinning. Even sitting still, I had the sensation of floating, rotating slowly forward, as if I were an astronaut in zero gravity. It made me borderline nauseated much of the time. I soon realized that I couldn't live like that, and that stillness might well kill me before anything else.

I lost five pounds in five days on the diuretic, so that seemed to indicate that I had, in fact, been bloated. While the lifelong dieter in me was thrilled with the easy weight drop, my rational brain was concerned. How long had this been going on? How had I not noticed how bloated I truly was? I had been mentally flogging myself for being puffy and putting on a little weight, blaming menopause, and it turned out it wasn't my fault.

Dr. X had cautioned me to be careful how much I read on the Internet about

Meniere's, as there was "a lot of depressing stuff. Stick with WebMD or other reputable sites." Despite his warning, I did go on the Internet, where 10 minutes of surfing on forums completely freaked me out. People with Meniere's lost their jobs, couldn't function, and were so dizzy during the unpredictable attacks they had to crawl to the bathroom. They had loud ringing in one or both ears, which didn't necessarily stop once they had gone deaf in one ear.[7] I had occasional ringing and buzzing; sometimes it sounded a little like being underwater. Sometimes I lost my balance a little, which before my diagnosis I had attributed to not paying enough attention and multitasking.

I deputized my husband to do some research and tell me what he thought would be helpful. Meanwhile, I focused on what I could control: my diet. Ten minutes of research revealed that the low-sodium handout from Dr. X was outdated, so I set out to follow the current American Heart Association guidelines: 1,500 milligrams of sodium per day.

I had recently started using a fitness and dieting app, so I had some hard data about what I had been eating.[8] I ate a few plant-based processed foods: shredded vegan cheese, gluten-free pizza crust, and gluten-free bread. Being processed foods, all are shockingly high in sodium. We ate out once or twice a week as well, which made those days sodium-heavy. Once I started reading labels, I learned that my beloved Bragg's Liquid Aminos, a gluten-free, natural soy sauce, is crazy-high in sodium, as are miso paste, Thai curry paste, Dijon mustard, ketchup, and Worcestershire sauce. So are Japanese, Chinese, Thai, and Indian foods. All my go-to snacks, take-out items—everything needed to be rethought.

I felt so lost and frustrated, as everything that was prohibited seemed to be key to my previously "healthy" diet. And despite being gluten-free and vegan and eating very little processed and fast foods, I still had been piling on the salt. While I didn't use white table salt, I was using Himalayan pink salt throughout my cooking process and Maldon sea salt to finish. I had a huge gourmet salt collection in the pantry: ochre kiawe-smoked salt from Hawaii, chocolate salt from Portland, hefty zip-top bags of beautiful pink and blue crystals from our trip to France.

Since I didn't eat a lot of processed foods, I had been averaging between 1,800 and 2,300 milligrams of salt per day, not terribly high and well within the range of Dr. X's recommendations. I wondered how much more I could change and how much it would make a difference.

Despite being a great cook for more than 30 years, writing a blog that specialized in recipe renovations, and having a public health degree in nutrition education, I had no idea where to begin with low-sodium cooking. The sheet from Dr. X listed no resources.

I ordered some books from Amazon and asked my food blogging friends for ideas, finding wonderful information from Jessica Goldman Foung of Sodium Girl[9] and Donald Gazzaniga of MegaHeart.[10] They were generous, lovely, and supportive, and I felt less alone.

I began learning about sodium, salt, and aspects of low-sodium diets. I learned about a salt-free diet from Jess and Donald, which provides around 500 milligrams of sodium per day. While not yet well studied by researchers, some people who followed this diet reported healing themselves of kidney disease,[11] chronic heart failure, and even Meniere's. This salt-free diet had the stamp of approval from a cardiologist at Stanford.[12] Besides the challenge of *following* the diet, there were no negative side effects and lots of possible positives. I was slightly skeptical but excited to try it; maybe I could heal from this.

I realized that I could write my own story. Other people's stories were their stories, not mine.

I learned that 90 percent of Americans are expected to develop hypertension in their lifetimes, in part due to sodium content in their diet.[13] That is plain crazy, as blood pressure normally falls when we age; it shouldn't rise.

I learned that going cold turkey on the salt-free diet was awful. Food tasted terrible for seven weeks until my palate adjusted. Food, one of the great loves of my life, was simply depressing during that time. I remember standing at the refrigerator looking inside, trying to figure out what I could eat, and not being excited about any of it. I simply ate for fuel. There were no happy dances at the dinner table. I lost weight. And then finally, there was the moment when I bit into an orange cherry tomato, warm from the garden, and tasted the flavorful sweet-tart sugar explosion. I nearly cried when I realized that food could be a pleasure for me again. Because my experience was so poor, I designed the Plan in this book to be a far gentler transition.

Being the good researcher that I am, I also wondered if I should find another doctor, one who specializes in vertigo, balance, and Meniere's disease. I was referred to one of the top specialists on balance disorders in the country, who happens to practice in San Diego. I made an appointment for a second opinion about my diagnosis.

THE SECOND OPINION

I was feeling so poorly on the day of my appointment that my husband drove me to see the specialist, about three weeks after meeting Doctor X. This office was very different than the first, with a high-energy vibe emanating from the specialist, who I'll call Dr. Y.

The appointment started at 10:30 a.m. with a young physician's assistant asking me a ton of questions and typing the information into my medical chart displayed on a huge screen on the wall. We went over the same ground as I had with Dr. X: three bouts of vertigo with nausea and the circumstances surrounding them.

Dr. Y came in and immediately began talking to me. The PA added notes to my chart while Dr. Y talked nearly nonstop.

"Dr. X is a great doctor. He's a really nice guy," said Dr. Y. "My experience is that Meniere's is really, really hard to diagnose. I need more data points. I can't say from one hearing test that you have Meniere's."

I felt validated that he respected the previous doctor, but even though I had come for a second opinion, I found myself surprised to learn that a diagnosis one doctor had seemed so certain about could be in question—at the time, I didn't understand how complex both migraine and Meniere's are.

"I don't know that you do have it. I want to see you a bunch of times, whenever you are having symptoms," said Dr. Y. "I want you to come in when you're feeling really lousy. That's the best time for us to get data. We can't tell much when you're feeling OK. Alright?"

I nodded, but inside I thought, *I'm supposed to get in the car when I'm all dizzy and come here? That sucks.* I understand now that it's most helpful for him to be able to see me when I'm having symptoms, but it was hard to hear at the time.

"We want to get you in The Chair and make sure we rule out BPPV. We'll do a hearing test each time you come in, so we can see progression."

I kept nodding, trying to keep up.

"The hearing loss is an issue, of course. But it's a $100,000 disability. The balance issue is much more critical. That's a million-dollar disability."

Caught off guard, I could only blink. *What did he just say?* I hadn't come in to this appointment thinking I would hear the word *disability*.

"You are a complex patient. You need to have your own copy of your medical chart and bring it with you to every appointment," Dr. Y continued. "You need to keep on top of it. Doctors don't know enough about this stuff."

Until that point, it had never occurred to me that a doctor wouldn't have all the answers, or that I might have a condition that still needs years of research.

"You'll need to advocate for yourself. We'll send you for an MRI. You should pay extra to get the DVD afterwards. You want the DVD in your chart. The MRI will rule out a benign tumor."

Wait, I could have a tumor?

"Without more data, I can't say for certain yet, but I think you have what's called Meniere's with migraine variant. MMV if you want to search for it on the Internet."

I'm having migraine attacks?

"Migraine attacks are crazy. Some people come in here and they look like they are having a stroke; half of their face is slack. That can be a migraine," he said. "You can have all kinds of symptoms, because it's an inflammation that spreads across your brain. Depending on what functions it hits, those are your symptoms. Some people have migraine with auras, where they have visual disturbances like halos around lights, or they hear weird sounds, or they have numbness in an arm. Others, like you, don't have aura, so they don't have that warning period. People don't necessarily have head pain during a migraine attack. We want to be aggressive about treating your symptoms."

That makes sense, but what does he mean by aggressive?

"I'm not happy with this diuretic," he said, flipping through my chart. "Put her on the potassium-sparing diuretic and the potassium supplement, too."

Did he just switch my medication? I think he did. By this point, I was wishing that I had brought my husband into the exam room with me, as a second set of ears. I knew I wouldn't be able to remember all these details later. I could tell that Dr. Y was trying to pack as much information as possible into the short time he had with me.

"You want to be as anti-inflammatory as possible. You're gluten-free? That's great. You're a step ahead. Get her the low-tyramine diet sheet."[14]

I realized Dr. Y was talking half to me and half to the PA, who was still typing notes into my chart. *What's tyramine?*

"It's another name for a migraine diet," he added. "You'll want to follow it as closely as you can. It removes foods that can trigger migraine, like wine, chocolate, nuts and seeds, fermented foods, stuff like that."

Wait, no nuts? *I can't have nuts?* At this point, my brain raced off, and I didn't hear much else. I thought of my refrigerator, which was full of cashew yogurt, cashew cheese, homemade kefir, cacao nibs, and sauerkraut—basically, everything on the freaking list. I felt my lower lip starting to quiver as he directed the PA to take me to The Chair.[15]

I asked to stop at the bathroom and sat on the toilet. *What is happening to me? I don't feel that bad, and suddenly I could have a tumor or go deaf?* I cried as quietly as I could for several minutes. While I rarely cry in my regular life, it happens more often than I'd like in doctors' offices, where I must drop my veneer of "everything is fine" and tell them what's going on, leaving me feeling acutely vulnerable. But I pulled myself together, determined to hold it together in front of the PA, who looked so very young to me despite wearing scrubs.

The Chair looks like a sci-fi apparatus, with straps and clips to lock you in and high-tech goggles to cover your eyes. It spins you rapidly and abruptly upside down and backwards, then you're told to open your eyes and hold them open while it films your eye movement. Then it spins again, abruptly leaving you in another odd position.

The goggles were tight and hurt my head. My test was not definitive, so I went three rounds in the chair while the doctor and the PA conferred. The straps were heavy and dug into my shoulders. By that point, I was emotionally and physically exhausted. I was also starving, as it was now after noon.

They still had a hearing test and blood work to do, but I asked if we could have a lunch break. I didn't feel like I could even talk coherently, and I had no idea what I was supposed to eat. My husband and I went to a nearby Lebanese place to regroup. I started looking at the new diet sheet the doctor gave me.

It said: "Tyramine (TIER-ah-meen) is a compound produced in foods from the natural breakdown of the amino acid tyrosine. Tyramine is not added to foods. Tyramine levels increase in foods when they are aged, fermented, stored for long periods of time, or are not fresh."

According to the sheet, three-quarters of my—seemingly healthy—plant-based diet were now out: no nuts, soy, fermented foods, vinegar, or aged foods. A few key favorite fruits and vegetables were also out, like bananas, avocados, dates, red plums, and broad beans. No citrus at all. About half of the dried beans I depended upon for protein, along with all lentils, were also out.

It seemed like a list someone created by throwing darts at a dartboard. Thwack! Raspberries are out, but all the other berries are OK! Thwack! Lima beans are out, but black beans are OK!

We had recently planted red plum and Meyer lemon trees in our yard, and our avocado and orange trees were full of fruit. Trees of fruit I may never be able to eat. I couldn't comprehend how I was going to do it, but it was clear that, with almost all my plant-based protein sources axed, I could no longer eat vegan. That much was for sure.

We got home nearly six hours after we left. I sat down to study the sheet the doctor gave me, labeled "The Low-Tyramine Headache Diet." The three-page sheet had colored boxes with columns that said "Allowed," "Use with Caution," and "Avoid If on an MAOI."

I assumed, although the doctor had not told me so, that the "Avoid" column applied to me even though I didn't think I was on an MAOI. (I later learned MAOI stands for *monoamine oxidase inhibitor*, a class of drugs used to treat depression and Parkinson's disease. And no, I wasn't prescribed an MAOI; the same diet is also recommended for people with migraine.)

Despite having kept up with the latest nutrition research over the years since grad school, I had never heard of tyramine. So my first question was, *What is tyramine and how is it related to migraine?*

That seemingly simple question and the process of investigating it led me to write this book. I learned that advocating for myself within the healthcare system is critical. I learned that there is way too little research being done on migraine and Meniere's, considering they affect at least 36 million people and cost an estimated $13 *billion* every year in the U.S. alone.[16] And I learned that looking at the whole picture, from a wellness perspective versus an illness perspective, was critical in my recovery.

I found out that the list of foods my doctor gave me wasn't the most comprehensive list for migraine, and I learned how relatively little even the top researchers and doctors currently know about Meniere's, vertigo, migraine, and headaches. I learned that, while I found several books on the subject, there is virtually no useful research about dietary approaches to managing these illnesses. I learned that every list was frustratingly different.

Reading the list and looking at the food in my kitchen told me that I had a huge challenge ahead of me. About 75 percent of my daily foods were on the "Avoid" list. I was going to have to rethink my entire diet, my entire lifestyle. This was going to be big.

At first I was gamely carrying on, but after a few days it hit me. Why me? I had already done so much, worked so hard to feel well. I, an annoyingly optimistic person who rarely cries, spent the weekend in tears. Every time I felt like I was pulling myself together, the wailing started again. How was I going to manage this?

My husband, who hates it when I cry more than anything in the world, kept trying to cheer me up, which did not help. I finally told him, "Look, I need the weekend. I need to cry this out. If I'm still crying on Monday, then you can kick my ass. But today I need to feel sorry for myself."

On Monday, I started the work that became this book.

searching for the answer

———— ••• ————

Here is how my brain works: I looked at the low-sodium sheet from Dr. X and the low-tyramine sheet from Dr. Y, and I knew that I could never make sense of the information without visually combining them. At the time I wasn't thinking that I was going to write a book. I was dizzy and nauseated and my head hurt constantly. I was simply trying to make sense of what both doctors had recommended.

My first step was to create a Word document that I could work from, so I searched online for the tyramine sheet Dr. Y gave me, hoping I could cut and paste that sheet into a new document and then cross-reference all the low-sodium foods, ending up with one sheet.

I found the tyramine sheet on a website, downloaded it, and started to work on it. But something was off. The sheet looked like mine, but the wording was a little different. Some foods were in different columns. The recommendations had changed. In fact, it was less strict than the one he had given me. Why?

Further searching turned up the original version given to me by Dr. Y, which was originally posted by a headache organization in July 2010.[17] It was updated between July and December of 2010 with slightly relaxed guidelines.

I called the headache organization's office to learn more: Why had the sheet changed? What were the changes based upon? I called three times and emailed more than five times over a period of weeks, but no one ever responded. It was a dead end.

I found varying versions of the sheet everywhere on the web, from Northwestern University to Johns Hopkins Medical Center. Yet no one was accessible who could tell me where the information came from, who compiled it, or where you could find the data about foods containing tyramine, this mysterious compound that lurked in nearly all my favorite foods. Tyramine content wasn't listed in the USDA database, so how did they figure out which foods contained it?

Since following the sheet would effectively prohibit me from continuing to eat a solely plant-based diet—which at the time I still believed was my healthiest choice—I wanted to be certain of the information and why it was recommended.

Following the handout to the letter would mean I could eat things that are cooked fresh, and leftovers the next day only.[18] I would need to buy only a few days' worth of fresh vegetables at a time, only what I could cook and eat fresh. I could freeze foods and reheat them later. This would completely change how I shopped, cooked, and stored food, as I normally shopped for at least an entire week's worth of food at a time. My freezer was fairly empty; my refrigerator was packed with produce. And yes, in the past I would miss vegetables pushed to the back of the drawer, and they would spoil or be cooked far past their prime. Making this change was doable but would involve a ton more work—especially if the low-tyramine guidelines were combined with the low-sodium guidelines. The few canned beans that the low-tyramine sheet allowed, like pintos, garbanzos, and black beans, wouldn't work for me unless I could find salt-free versions, so I would have to cook those beans from scratch.

I realized that I was going to have to be flexible about what I was willing to eat as I learned this new diet. I picked up some salt-free canned tuna and salmon, got some low-sodium goat cheese, and asked my neighbors who kept chickens for a few eggs. I read a lot of labels. Trips to the grocery store took at least an hour. I frequently came home discouraged.

I had to take three months off from writing my food blog, as I had no idea how to feed myself for the first few weeks, let alone develop recipes. At that moment I couldn't envision what my food blog might become in the future: a low-sodium and migraine-friendly haven.

After weeks of trying to get information about the low-tyramine sheet, I finally decided that I should talk to Dr. Y. He had given me the sheet; I hoped he would be able to explain why he gave me that particular sheet and not the newer, less restrictive one. The thought crossed my mind that he might not know the sheet was outdated. I really hoped that wasn't true, as I knew that meant he wouldn't have an answer for me. While I knew he was the best doctor for me, and completely trusted his clinical skills, he had already told me that he didn't have time to research nutrition.

After talking with his physician's assistant, I learned that Dr. Y wasn't aware the sheet had been updated. I know from consulting with doctors professionally in the past that they are all crazy pressed for time; the health care system is so broken that they don't have time for the patient care they all want to do. However, just because he couldn't research the topic more thoroughly didn't mean I couldn't. During one appointment, Dr. Y deputized me to learn as much as I could and report back to him what I was learning. He was (and continues to be) completely supportive of my work. It was at that point that something in me shifted and I stepped into an advocacy role, both for myself and for others.

Most people in the patient role are not me; they wouldn't have turned their lives upside down to try to follow handouts. It was also becoming clear that the information from various legitimate resources on the Internet is contradictory, which is enormously frustrating if you're looking for The Answer. My final realization was both disquieting and empowering: I may know more about the migraine diet, or I *will* know more about the migraine diet, than my doctor and his staff do.

At that moment, as frustrated as I felt that I didn't have The Answer, I knew there had to be a better way. Regular people, people who are dizzy or puking or in chronic pain and don't have my skill set, who aren't a freaking terrier-with-a-bone like I am, would just give up on the diet sheets. These people would be categorized by doctors as "noncompliant." Not because they don't want to feel better, but because when you feel crappy, trying to make diet and lifestyle changes is often too hard and too confusing. Especially when the resource, even one given to you by a great doctor, stinks.

If there were answers, they weren't going to be easy to find. But the terrier in me was now on the case. I *would* find the answers, or I would make my own.

WHAT ARE FOOD TRIGGERS AND HOW MIGHT THEY CAUSE HEADACHES?

Chemical compounds in foods can set off migraine attacks in some people. Many of these chemical compounds are breakdown products from amino acids that occur naturally in foods. Some are known as *pressor amines* (also called *biogenic* or *vasoactive amines*). Pressor amines act upon the vascular system, either by dilating (widening) or constricting (narrowing) blood vessels. Many pressor amines are also neurotransmitters, carrying electrical or chemical signals within the body. People prone to migraine attacks seem to be more sensitive to the action of these pressor amines and other dietary compounds, although it's not yet known why. Here are the current theories regarding how these compounds may contribute to migraine:

1. Any compound that dilates vessels in turn causes inflammation, which generates anti-inflammatory chemicals to address that inflammation and heal those vessels.

2. Pressor amines interact with other neurotransmitters—such as serotonin and norepinephrine—causing a chemical chain reaction that could trigger pain pathways.[19]

3. Dietary triggers may stimulate the migraine control center, combining with other non-dietary triggers like stress (which generates particular chemicals and neurotransmitters in our bodies), hormones (also chemicals), and barometric pressure changes (which physically affect our blood vessels).[20]

4. Dietary triggers might make the brain cells more reactive in general.

5. Food allergies may play a role by creating a pro-inflammatory condition that encourages migraine when other triggers are added to the mix.[21] Dr. David Perlmutter believes that many people have developed food sensitivities through leaky gut syndrome (see page 81). In people prone to migraine, these food sensitivities could be a trigger.[22] When inflammation is present in the body, the body generates anti-inflammatory compounds to address it.

6. The common thread in all migraine triggers may be oxidative stress. A 2015 study theorized that migraine triggers (food and others) all cause oxidative stress in the brain, which may explain how so many different types of triggers, from weather to food to stress, can all have the same outcome: a migraine attack.[23]

7. Not all researchers agree that food elements trigger migraine. We may learn in the future that what seem to be food triggers are food cravings that appear in the premonitory stage of migraine, before people are aware that an attack has already begun.[24]

When I interviewed cutting-edge pain researchers at the University of California San Diego, they said it may be years before they know for certain what is happening inside our heads when a migraine is triggered.

Pressor amines and other dietary compounds that may trigger migraine

Now that you know a little bit about how pressor amines might be involved in migraine, here's what is understood about the two most important ones:

*   **HISTAMINE**. This one is likely familiar to you, as it causes our allergy response; treatment is an *anti*histamine that blocks this inflammatory response. Histamine is formed from the amino acid histidine and is a neurotransmitter released by our bodies during the normal process of digestion. For some, the act of eating *anything* triggers a migraine, because their bodies don't produce enough of the digestive enzyme diamine oxidase (DAO). In these people, taking a DAO supplement can

be extremely helpful.[25] One small study found that 90 percent of the migraine sufferers studied were deficient in this enzyme. In this study, taking the DAO supplement reduced the number and length of attacks but didn't reduce pain.[26] Eating coconut and/or palm oil increases DAO activity and may be helpful for people with histamine intolerance.[27]

- **TYRAMINE**. This pressor compound is formed when the amino acid tyrosine breaks down in the body. Tyrosine and tyramine are naturally occurring in foods; they aren't additives. There is a well-documented response to tyramine-containing foods—which tend to be aged, cured, or fermented—if someone is taking a monoamine-oxidase inhibitor (MAOI). MAOIs are the original class of antidepressants, still used occasionally for depression and as a treatment for Parkinson's disease. If someone on an MAOI eats foods containing tyramine, their blood pressure can shoot dangerously high; some have died.[28] For this reason, low-tyramine diet sheets are distributed by hospitals and medical centers as well as by many migraine doctors. While these sheets may be widely available, the science is still frustratingly inconclusive as to the role tyramine plays in migraine, and focusing solely on tyramine is too limited a view.

Besides histamine and tyramine, there are many other forms of pressor amines in food—cadaverine, putrescine, spermidine, and spermine, among others—that could play a role in migraine but haven't yet been studied. Citrus fruits contain octopamine and synephrine. Chocolate contains beta-phenylethylamine, as well as flavonoid phenols and theobromine.[29] Food also contains neurotransmitters like acetylcholine, catecholamines, and serotonin.[30] Any of these could be a migraine trigger for a particular individual.

What else can trigger migraine attacks?

Although many people with migraine are advised to avoid tyramine, it's important to note that pressor amines may not be the only dietary triggers. Other chemical compounds found in foods may also trigger migraine attacks:

- **Caffeine**
- **Monosodium glutamate (MSG)** (and other naturally occurring **glutamates** such as those in celery)
- **Nitrites** and **nitrates**
- **Alcohols**
- **Aspartame**[31]

As I delved deeper into the published research on migraine triggers, I realized two things: (1) Many of these lists were created without chemical assays to determine whether the foods actually contain tyramine, and (2) there are many migraine triggers besides tyramine that we may need to avoid—everyone is different.

I found very limited research—from Toronto,[32] Spain,[33] Portugal,[34] and Korea[35]—reporting on chemical assays to determine tyramine content in foods. In fact, the most updated tyramine sheet from the group in Toronto, based on their chemical assays, has a very short list of foods to avoid if you're solely concerned about tyramine. They found that many foods thought to contain tyramine (which may still contain migraine triggers) did not contain it.[36]

In other words, identifying dietary migraine triggers and how they cause migraine attacks is still murky territory. Since everyone is different, and triggers are known to be cumulative, my approach is to remove as many of them as possible during the initial portion of the Plan, until you can test each for yourself.

HOW THE PLAN EVOLVED

After getting nowhere with the origin of the low-tyramine diet sheet, I finally tracked down the group of researchers in Toronto who had tested foods for tyramine to learn more. Their research showed some of the foods on my original handout don't actually contain tyramine, or at least didn't when they tested that food.

Around this same time, I found an article in *The Lancet* from 1965 describing one person's hypertensive crisis after eating green bananas stewed in their skins.[37] Surely this couldn't be the sole reason why bananas were on the list?

Yes.

No.

Maybe?

Many of the medical journal articles I found described migraine or hypertensive reactions that seemed to implicate certain foods. Those foods may not have been chemically tested for tyramine (an expensive endeavor requiring specialized equipment). They might have just been added to the "no" list, perhaps due to a mention in a single journal article referencing a single occurrence. Since none of the lists include explanations of how they were compiled, we'll never know. Some of the articles described studies with very small groups of people: 6, 11, some up to 60. It's difficult to extrapolate results to large groups of people from such small studies, and yet it appears that some people may have done just that.

I started to wonder if there *was* a reliable list I could follow and decided to see what kind of diet studies had been done on migraine. It turns out that, despite the fact that migraine affects an estimated 36 million people in the United States alone, very little diet research has been done.

The trouble with scientific studies

Nearly all diet-related studies rely on *self-reports*, meaning that people are given a diary and asked to keep track of what they eat during the study period: anywhere from a few days to a few weeks. Some studies are retroactive, meaning they ask people days, weeks, or months later to recall what they ate in general. I remember from working on a Northwestern University cholesterol study how notoriously unreliable those self-reports are. People tend to forget, embellish, or rose-color reports of what they eat. They have no idea about portion size, so they might note they ate something, but guess they had eaten half as much as they had actually consumed. Having them weigh all their food isn't realistic. Changing people's habits—by asking them to weigh all their food, for example—adds bias to any study. People also act differently when they know they are being watched.

If people are using a tracking app with a bar code scanner, their reports may be more accurate, but getting an accurate idea of their portion size is still an issue, especially when dealing with whole foods that don't have bar codes, such as meat, vegetables, grains, and fruits. Some newer dietary studies are experimenting with people wearing cameras that snap photos of what they are eating.

I did find some bright spots. In one small but encouraging study from Turkey, 30 migraine patients were tested for food allergies and then went through two six-week periods of diet intervention. During the elimination diet period (when foods to which they were sensitive were removed from their diets), their migraine attacks dropped by about half. Neither the clients nor the researchers knew their allergy test results during the study.[38]

While it's ideal to have scientifically valid studies, dietary studies are incredibly expensive and difficult to run. To truly test a migraine diet, for example, you would have to find a large number of people, split them into two groups that are as evenly matched as possible (age, severity of symptoms, gender, etc.), control for all other factors (such as activity level, stress, weather, and medications), and then have one group eat only from the migraine diet list and the other eat foods with triggers. And then the groups would have to switch. The only way you could be certain they were eating only foods from the list would be to provide 100 percent of their food. Even doing this for two weeks would be insanely expensive, and two weeks isn't enough time to determine if the diet is helping. Since every person who gets migraine is different and has different triggers, even this hypothetical study might not be enough to test whether a dietary intervention can help.

Finding a starting point

During my literature review, I found two popular migraine books that reported their results from clinical practice: *The Migraine Miracle*, by Dr. Josh Turknett, and *Heal Your Headache*, by Dr. David Buchholz. It's important to distinguish these results from those bolstered by anecdotal evidence. Anecdotal evidence is one person who tells you (or writes on the Internet) that they cured themselves of migraine attacks by drinking cayenne–pepper water, salt water, or some other "cure." Clinical practice results are when a doctor's practice prescribes a set treatment and sees a long-term reduction in symptoms in many, many people. A doctor is unlikely to continue to prescribe that treatment if he or she is not seeing results.

Because the medical literature was unclear, sometimes conflicting, and the lists on handouts were unsubstantiated, I decided to base my Plan on a diet that was refined in a clinical practice. Dr. Turknett's clinical experience with the ancestral approach (which I discuss on page 162) is currently just a few years old, and the recipes in his book include migraine triggers like bananas, almonds, and onions. (In his experience, following an ancestral diet—sugar-, grain-, and bean-free with almost no dairy—negates the effect of migraine triggers.) While I think it has immense value, the ancestral approach to eating is difficult for many people to follow and is so far from what most people currently eat that it didn't seem like a realistic starting point for my Plan.

In contrast, Dr. Buchholz created the unique list found in *Heal Your Headache*[39] during three decades of work in his neurology practice, so I decided to use his list as my starting point. He explains in his book why the foods are on the list and why it's so extensive. His 12 recipes do not include any known migraine triggers. I got in touch with him and was able to refine my Plan based on his experience.

HOW THIS PLAN IS DIFFERENT

In addition to Dr. Buchholz's diet list, I have taken the best concepts from the available literature to build this Plan, utilizing more than three dozen books and more than 100 medical journal articles. The Plan eliminates all known triggers, which I outline below, and every recipe is trigger free. Most migraine diet books either include triggers in the recipes or use a list that may be unsubstantiated.

You might wonder why I spent so much time focused on food. First, it's my area of expertise. Second, I wanted to learn as much as possible about how food contributes to migraine attacks. Food is something we can control, and in the past I had seen very positive effects when I changed my diet for health reasons. Outside of the medical literature, I found many self-reports—anecdotal evidence—of people who greatly improved their symptoms by making diet changes. Finally, we eat at least three times every day; food is a powerful part of our well-being. It made sense to me that food should be part of my solution.

Sugar-free and gluten-free

Since many experts, including my neurologist, believe that migraine is an inflammatory process, I incorporated gluten-free and sugar-free recommendations into my Plan. There are strong correlations between migraine and celiac disease, non-celiac gluten sensitivity, and irritable bowel syndrome (IBS). Some researchers believe that these correlations have to do with inflammation in the gut-brain axis.[40] Noted neurologist Dr. David Perlmutter, author of *Grain Brain* and *Brain Maker*, believes that both sugar and gluten are enormously impactful in brain health and brain-related diseases by triggering inflammation in the brain. After you've completed six months on the Plan, you can experiment with both sugar and gluten-containing foods to see how they affect you. While neither Dr. Perlmutter nor I recommend adding sugar and gluten back into your life, you might find an occasional treat will work for you. I like Dr. Mark Hyman's quote about sugar: "I like sugar. I just think of it as a recreational drug."

Low-sodium

After reading about sodium and the strong connection between migraine and balance disorders like Meniere's, my recommendations are to eat as salt-free as possible, saving sea salt for the table only. As previously mentioned, there is a strong correlation between people who get Meniere's disease and people who have migraine. Several doctors I've spoken with believe that Meniere's disease is part of the migraine spectrum and isn't a separate illness at all.[41] Balance specialist Dr. Ian Purcell, who wrote the foreword for this book, believes that Meniere's disease and migraine are both autoimmune conditions;

Dr. Buchholz believes they are very closely related and that Meniere's is a form of migraine disease. Meniere's is distinguished by its low-frequency hearing loss as well as ringing in the ears (tinnitus).[42] There are also a lot of people who get balance-related symptoms and dizziness with their migraine attacks.[43]

Too much sodium in your body or in your diet may contribute to these issues. Your body holds onto water to keep sodium in proper solution at all times. The balance structures of your inner ear contain fluid, and when your body is too full of fluid, that increases the pressure in your inner ears. Too much constant pressure over a period of time presses on the tiny hairs that control your balance and can destroy them over time, causing hearing loss and balance issues. Note that there is little information about the cause of Meniere's and vestibular migraine (also called migraine-associated vertigo) and not many treatment options.

There is also a great deal of evidence that we eat far too much sodium, and reducing or eliminating added white salt from our diets can help heal and prevent a host of diseases.

Additional diet and lifestyle guidance

After reading *The Migraine Miracle*,[44] *Good Calories, Bad Calories*,[45] *The Primal Blueprint*,[46] and *The Wahls Protocol*,[47] I incorporated ancestral (Paleo) suggestions into Month 7 (page 156). My Plan emphasizes sustainably produced protein as well as healthy saturated fats. Shifting away from processed foods to a lower-carbohydrate diet made up of whole foods can have many positive effects on other health conditions that often show up with migraine, such as obesity, diabetes, and gut imbalances.

While not everyone is sensitive to food triggers, everyone has potential lifestyle triggers. I incorporated key lifestyle factors into the Plan that should help every migraine and headache sufferer: gentle exercise, regular sleep patterns, relaxation, hydration, regular meals, and the intention to have a positive attitude despite chronic pain.

You may be surprised by some of the elements in the Plan, but trust that I have based my recommendations on the latest, most current research about what constitutes a healthy diet, applying that specifically to headaches, migraine, and Meniere's disease. The Plan offers a balanced diet composed of whole foods as well as lifestyle changes. Even if you were to receive no migraine-specific benefit, you'll greatly improve your overall nutrition and health by following it.

I encourage you to think of the foods on the Plan as your allies, wanting the absolute best for you, and filling your plate with love.[48] Once you've been on the Plan for six months (two months' transition, four months on the Plan itself), you'll be able to test and add back foods that you are missing. So if you're concerned that the diet is too restrictive, know that the restrictions are for a relatively short period. My goal is to help you get back as many whole foods into your life as possible.

A realistic transition with proven results

Yes, six months sounds like a long time, but in my experience as a wellness and health coach, it's the best path to success. I'd love to be able to give you a 10-day miracle or a 21-day magic bullet. Migraine doesn't respond to a quick fix, and there is no cure. Instead, I've built in the changes gradually over the first two months to make them as painless as possible. I started seeing results after seven weeks on the Plan, when I woke up to discover that my head didn't hurt for the first time in years. I've gone from three to five migraine days a week (often with vertigo and vomiting) and a daily headache to very infrequent headaches and one to two migraine days per month.

The Plan was tested by two groups of migraine sufferers; all saw improvement in their migraine frequency and severity. All testers were having migraine: from one to five migraine days per week. Some testers were single, some had kids, some lived in big cities, and some lived in rural areas. Some were adventurous eaters with lots of cooking experience, others were self-described picky eaters with little kitchen time in the past. All the testers were able to follow the program and learn more about their unique triggers. One found that dairy was a problem for her, another high-sodium foods, and for another it was sugar. One Plan tester named Sarah had called in sick to work on a weekly basis because her migraine attacks were so severe. She was worried about losing her job. A few months after she started the Plan, I got an email from Sarah telling me that she hadn't called out sick in over a month. That's when I knew I had to share this with others.

The six months you will spend trying the Plan is going to pass either way. Don't you want to see how much better you might feel? I'd love to hear your success story.

how the book is organized

―――――― ••• ――――――

Because I am nice, I do not expect you to go cold turkey and give up all of your favorite foods overnight. Instead, I have created an easy way to ease into the Plan over a period of eight weeks. Each week you have one assignment, designed to fit into your busy life. In addition, you might not be feeling well some days, so the assignments are simple and achievable. After the first eight weeks, your assignments will come in month-long increments. Through the whole six months, you'll be tracking your diet, symptoms, movement, and more. You'll find deeper dives into special topics throughout the Plan sections. Here's a brief overview of the first eight weeks of the Plan:

- **WEEK 1 (PAGE 38)**. Your sole assignment is to get organized and start tracking your food, symptoms, and how many steps you take per day. You'll need a pedometer or a fitness-tracking device, plus a tracking program. You don't make any dietary changes in the first three weeks; it's enough to begin tracking, including choosing how you're going to count your steps, and to remember to enter all your foods into the tracking program you choose, whether that's an online app like MyFitnessPal or a table like the one I provide in this book. The reason we focus on step count is simple: Regular, gentle movement is universally recommended for migraine prevention. These fitness-tracking devices are easy to use; pedometers cost as little as $10.

- **WEEK 2 (PAGE 48)**. Prepare your home environment to support the Plan by cleaning out your freezer. You'll be comparing your freezer contents with the trigger-free foods on the list, and organizing your freezer for success. You are still eating the way you've always eaten, but now you have an organized freezer and have been tracking for nearly two weeks.

- **WEEK 3 (PAGE 53)**. Tackle your pantry items in the same manner as your freezer.

- **WEEK 4 (PAGE 61)**. Clean out and organize your refrigerator as you have for your freezer and pantry. You also have a second assignment: switch over all your snacks to trigger-free foods on the Plan. This is the first week you'll be making any changes to what you're eating, but it's non-threatening and fun: snacks!

- **WEEK 5 (PAGE 71)**. Switch over your regular breakfasts to food on the Plan.

- **WEEK 6 (PAGE 76)**. Switch over your regular lunches to food on the Plan.

- **WEEK 7 (PAGE 83)**. Switch over your dinners to food on the Plan.

- **WEEK 8 (PAGE 93)**. Learn and practice strategies for eating out in restaurants, at work, and at parties.

For best results, I recommend you stay on the Plan for four solid months once you have switched over—a total of six months before you begin testing foods. I've provided ideas for each of those months to further improve your health habits to support your wellness:

- **MONTH 3 (PAGE 106)**. We'll take a look at self-care methods, adding relaxation practices and types of bodywork that may be most helpful for you.

- **MONTH 4 (PAGE 117)**. I'll help you detox your body, home, and work space, allowing you to remove potential hidden triggers.

- **MONTH 5 (PAGE 128)**. I've found this is the toughest month: you're starting to feel better, the diet feels restrictive, and you start to lose steam. I'll give you a plan to "fail"—which is the best way to be successful long term—and help remind you of why you're doing this in the first place. I include my three-day reboot, which I use to get myself back on track when I stray too far off the Plan.

- **MONTH 6 (PAGE 143)**. We'll talk more about sleep and movement.

Next, Part IV (page 155) will give you all the information you need about testing your favorite foods once you've completed the full six months on the Plan, and also some possibilities for further food tweaks if you aren't seeing the results you want. For a detailed look at the Plan in table form, check out Appendix C (page 302).

And then come the recipes! The last section of this book is packed with easy, tested recipes that are delicious and completely trigger-free. My recipe testers—nearly 30 people in four countries—put the recipes through their paces in their own home kitchens. There are more than 75 recipes in all, starting with a 14-day meal plan and then following the order of the program: Snacks; Breakfast; Lunch; Dinner; Desserts, Drinks, and Treats; Sauces, Condiments, and Salad Dressings; and Recipes That Use Leftovers.

I mention some of my source material throughout. You'll find a list of books I recommend in the Resources section (page 304). You may find that certain books intrigue you, and I encourage you to read those for yourself. My online membership program includes detailed book summaries each week in addition to other bonus materials, support, and recipes not found in this book. Learn more at MigraineReliefPlan.com.

Thanks for coming along on this journey with me. I hope you feel better soon!

WHY EIGHT WEEKS?

- Habits are formed over time. It takes eight weeks for your body to adjust to the taste of low-sodium, unprocessed foods made without sugar.[49] If you are currently eating processed, fast, and/or restaurant foods on a regular basis, it may take as many as three months for your palate to adjust.[50] But since you'll be gradually shifting over, food will still taste good as you transition.

- It takes a few weeks to stop craving sugar and processed foods.

- It takes two to eight months to instill a new habit (estimates range from 66 to 180 days), so you'll have the foundation built once you finish the eight-week program.[51]

- Gradual adjustment means that you are more likely to be able to integrate the changes into your lifestyle and stay on the Plan long term.

- There is a *lot* of change to absorb and new behaviors to learn, so doing a little each week is easiest, and is how I adjusted.

    You will likely be having migraine or headaches throughout this period, so I've made the assignments small each week so you'll be more likely to complete them.

WHY TRACK?

If you don't track what you're eating, your symptoms, and other factors, you'll have no idea what is triggering your migraine attacks and you can't improve your situation. While a recent study shows a correlation between keeping a migraine journal and fewer headache days, only 44.2 percent of the people in the study were actively keeping one.[52]

Keeping my tracking sheets for six months was the number-one thing that helped me improve, and my Plan members agree as well. You can use a fitness or nutrition tracking app (many are free, and often are accessible without a smart phone) or download a tracking sheet from my website: MigraineReliefPlan.com.

the migraine relief plan
food list

————— ••• —————

Grains

Approved

Amaranth	Gluten-free bread (choose whole-grain and low-sodium where possible)	Millet	Sorghum
Corn (tortillas, tortilla chips, polenta)		Oats (certified gluten-free)	Tapioca (pearls and flour)
Garbanzo bean (chickpea) flour	Gluten-free pasta	Quinoa	Teff
		Rice	

Excluded *Wheat berries; couscous; cracked wheat; rye; barley; spelt; triticale; einkorn; farro; white, wheat, or all-purpose flour; garfava flour*

Veggies and beans

Approved

Adzuki beans	Chickpeas	Jerusalem artichokes (sunchokes)	Salsify
Artichokes	Chile peppers	Jicama	Shallots
Arugula	Chives	Kale	Spinach
Asparagus	Cilantro	Kidney beans	Split peas
Bamboo shoots	Corn	Kohlrabi	Squash (all, including summer squash and zucchini)
Beet greens	Cucumbers	Leeks	
Beets	Daikon	Lettuce	Sweet potatoes
Bell peppers	Eggplant	Lotus root	Swiss chard
Bitter melon	Fennel	Mung beans	Taro
Bok choy	Galangal root	Mushrooms	Tomatillos
Broccoli	Garlic	Parsley	Tomatoes
Brussels sprouts	Gingerroot	Parsnips	Truffles
Cabbage	Green beans (haricot verts)	Peas	Turnips
Cactus leaves (nopales)	Green onions (scallions, spring onions)	Perilla	Wax beans
Cardoni		Pinto beans	White beans
Carrots		Potatoes	Yams
Cauliflower	Greens (such as mustard, dandelion, collard)	Pumpkins	Yucca
Celery		Radishes	
Celery root	Horseradish (fresh)	Rutabagas	

Excluded *Broad beans, fava beans, Italian beans, lentils, lima beans, navy beans, onions, pea pods, sauerkraut, snow pea pods*

Notes
- Fresh sprouts are OK if from approved list.
- Fresh vegetables on the list may be dried in a home dehydrator.
- Home-canned sauces, made from fresh ingredients, are fine.
- Dried chiles and mushrooms are OK without sulfites.

THE MIGRAINE RELIEF PLAN FOOD LIST *(continued)*

Fruits

Approved			
Apples	Dragon fruit	Mangoes	Purple plums
Apricots	Gooseberries	Mangosteens	Quince
Blackberries	Grapes	Melons (all)	Rambutans
Blueberries	Guavas	Nectarines	Rhubarb
Cactus pears (prickly pear fruit)	Jujubes (the fruit, not the candy)	Peaches	Sapotes
		Pears	Starfruit
Cherimoyas	Kiwis	Persimmons	Tamarind (without sugar or sulfites if dried/paste)
Cherries	Longans	Plumcots	
Coconuts	Loquats	Pluots	
Cranberries	Lychees	Pomegranates	Tejocotes

Excluded *Avocados, bananas, citrus or citrus zest, dates, figs, pineapple, papayas, passion fruit, raspberries, raisins, red plums*

Notes
- Dried fruits (except raisins) are OK as long as they do not contain sulfites.
- Fresh fruits on the list may be dried in a home dehydrator.

Sweetener

Approved Stevia (without any additives, even raw sugar)

Excluded *Sugar, honey, maple or other syrups, artificial sweeteners, sugar alcohols like xylitol or maltitol*

Protein (should be fresh and freshly cooked)

Approved			
Beans (except exclusions)	Fish (fresh or frozen without coatings or seasonings)	Salmon (if canned, Wild Alaskan with no salt or other additives)	Shellfish (no salt, sodium, or other additives)
Beef (grass-fed/pastured)	Pork (pastured)		Tuna (if canned, no salt or other additives)
Eggs (local, free-range)	Poultry (free-range)	Seeds (sunflower, flax, chia, sesame, hemp)	

Excluded *Dried or smoked fish, smoked or preserved meats (like sausage), favas, limas, navy beans, soybeans, lentils*

Notes
- Uncured reduced-sodium pastured bacon can be tested after four months.

Dairy

Approved			
American cheese	Cottage cheese	Cream cheese	Milk
Chèvre (fresh goat cheese)	Cream	Mascarpone	Ricotta

Excluded *Hard, aged cheeses, processed cheese*

Notes
- If you can find American cheese that is organic and soy-free, most lists include it as OK. It's not recommended for Meniere's because of its high sodium content. The plastic-wrapped "singles" are not OK.

THE MIGRAINE RELIEF PLAN FOOD LIST *(continued)*

Fats and oils (organic extra virgin if possible)

Approved	Butter (organic, grass-fed, and unsalted)	Lard or rendered bacon fat (from pastured pigs)	Sesame oil (regular and toasted in small amounts)	Tallow (beef fat from grass-fed cows)
	Coconut oil	Olive oil	Sunflower seed oil (in small amounts)	

Excluded	*Trans fats; corn, cottonseed, canola, rapeseed, soybean, peanut, nut oils*

Herbs, spices, and condiments

Approved	All herbs (except exclusions)	All spices (except exclusions)	Clear, white vinegar (limited to ½ teaspoon per recipe)

Excluded	*Spice blends containing MSG, salt, seaweed or seaweed extracts (including kombu, nori, hijiki, carrageenan, and agar agar), "flavorings," onion powder, yeast, nutritional yeast, store-bought condiments, salad dressings, and vinegar other than organic white vinegar*
Notes	• Some people may be sensitive to paprika, smoked paprika, chili powder, and curry powders containing chili powder. • Even white vinegar can be a trigger, so limit consumption. • After four months on the diet, you can test apple cider vinegar, rice wine vinegar, white balsamic, and white wine vinegar. • Use the smallest amount possible in recipes, unless you are positive that vinegar isn't a trigger.

Drinks

Approved	Coconut milk	Hemp milk (page 255)	Infused water (page 258)	Vodka (small amounts)
	Coconut water	Herbal teas (except exclusions)	Milk	White wine[53] (small amounts)
	Filtered or spring water		Sparkling water (without citrus flavoring)	

Excluded	*Nut milks; boxed milks that include carrageenan or gums; soy milk; red wine; hard liquors; beer; soda (regular or diet); caffeinated tea; herbal tea containing citrus, raspberry, or hibiscus; caffeinated coffee*
Notes	• Do not use wine in cooking for the first four months, then test it for yourself. • Besides being a powerful migraine trigger, coffee also raises cortisol levels for up to six hours. Elevated cortisol levels can lead to an overactive immune system, sleep disruptions and impairment, and depression.[54] • Decaf coffee is OK but might still be a trigger

AT A GLANCE: THE NO LIST

Common triggers

Aged foods and cheeses	Condiments	Nutritional yeast	Soy products
Avocados	Cured meats	Nuts	Soy sauce
Bananas	Dried fish	Salad dressings	Vinegars
Citrus and most tropical fruits	Fermented foods (sauerkraut, miso, kombucha, kefir)	Seaweed	

Additives that are triggers[55]

Autolyzed yeast	Glutamic acid	Natural flavors/flavorings	Textured vegetable protein
Calcium caseinate	Hydrolyzed protein	Protein-fortified items	Ultra-pasteurized items
Carrageenan	Kombu (seaweed extract)	Sodium caseinate	Whey protein and any protein powder
Enzyme-modified items	Malt extract	Soy protein concentrate/isolate	Yeast extract
Fermented or cultured items	Malted barley	Store-bought broth, stock, bouillon	
Gelatin (grass-fed gelatin is OK)	Maltodextrin		
	MSG		

Notes • Visit truthinlabeling.org to find a longer list of potential names for soy and sugar additives.

Hidden sugars

Agave nectar or syrup	Crystalline fructose	Inulin	Sorbitol
Barley malt or syrup	Date sugar	Jaggery	Sorghum molasses or syrup
Beet sugar	Dextrin	Lactitol, lactose	Sucrose
Brown rice, rice bran syrup	Dextrose	Malt or malted syrup	Sugar or syrup (brown, demerara, invert, muscovado, palm, rapidura, raw cane, sucanat, turbinado)
Cane crystals, juice, or syrup (dehydrated/evaporated)	Ethyl maltitol	Maltodextrin	
	Fructose	Maltose	
Coconut (sugar)	Fruit juice concentrate	Mannitol	Treacle
Corn (sugar, syrup, solids)	Galactose	Maple syrup, sugar	Yacon
Corn syrup (solids), high-fructose corn syrup	Glucose (syrup, solids)	Molasses	
	Golden syrup	Monk fruit (luo han guo)	
	Honey	Mono- or Oligosaccharide	
	Hydrogenated or hydrolyzed starch	Panela, panocha	
		Saccharose	

Notes • Watch out for anything with the words *sugar, granulated, syrup, saccharide,* and *crystal,* and any ingredients with an –ose at the end of them.

PART II
THE PLAN

———— ··· ————

In the first month of the Plan, you'll have one assignment per week to help you get ready to change how you eat to improve your migraine, headaches, and Meniere's symptoms. If you've read everything thus far, you know that I am going to ease you into the program. If you're impatient, you might be starting on this page, and that's OK. You're excited to begin the program, and you want to feel better *now*. I will caution you to be as patient as possible, as this isn't a miracle cure, nor is it effortless or magical. Some days it might feel hard. It is *doable*, though. The people who have gone through the program (myself included) have found the effort to be completely worth it, because for a lot of us it works. And because we deal with your entire lifestyle, not just food, the Plan should help even if food triggers aren't an issue for you.

In the second month, you'll be switching over your meals to the Plan. To make this easier, we focus on one meal of the day each week, starting with snacks. By Week 8, you'll be completely on the Plan and we'll talk about eating out and getting ready for the maintenance phase. You'll stay on the delicious maintenance phase for four months, then you can start testing foods and adding them back into your diet.

WEEK 1
your mindset and habits

————— ••• —————

The most important action you will take on this journey is not changing what you eat, how much you walk, or how well you sleep. It's deciding to take the first step. That's it. It's starting to wrap your brain around approaching your health differently. It's beginning to change your mindset as well as your habits.

Everything else is laid out for you step by step over the next few weeks and months. I'll show you how to get prepared. I'll walk you through the gradual changes in eating, drinking, moving, and sleeping. All you need to do today is begin. This week, your sole task is getting used to tracking your daily habits. You're not changing anything at all. You are simply learning to add tracking into your daily routine.

❶
②
③
④
⑤
⑥
⑦
⑧

WEEK 1 ASSIGNMENT: START TRACKING YOUR FOOD, SYMPTOMS, MOVEMENT, AND SLEEP

————— • —————

TOOLS NEEDED: *Pedometer or other wearable fitness device, fitness app, and/or tracking sheet*
WHAT I USE: *Fitbit One ($99), MyFitnessPal (free)*

Your Week 1 goal is to track everything you are eating and drinking, get a feel for the foods you regularly eat, track your symptoms (because we're looking for the correlation between what we choose to put in our mouths and how we feel over the following few days), and learn the average number of steps you take in a day. *You will not be changing anything that you eat or drink this week, nor will you be changing anything about your activity level.*

You might find that it takes you more than a week to complete this task. That's OK! Just wait until you have tracked at least five days consistently before moving on to Week 2. Trust me, you'll be more successful overall if you get the tracking under control and it becomes a habit for you. There's no rush here. Take another week if you need it.

DAILY TRACKING GOALS

- **Everything you eat and drink**.
- **Hours slept**.
- **Your symptoms**.
- **Step count**. Use a pedometer, smartphone app, or fitness device to measure the number of steps you take.
- **Sodium intake**.
- **Caffeine intake**.

Tracking your food and drink

This week, it's all about setting your baseline. What are you eating now, and what are your symptoms? I have found that creating a tracking system is *the* most effective thing I have done to change my health status. Maybe I have an anal-retentive bent, but I find it fun and satisfying to understand the relationship between what I eat and how I feel. According to Gretchen Rubin in *Better Than Before*, habits help people feel more in control and less anxious. She also recommends tying a new habit onto an existing one to create an external trigger, such as, "When I sit down to a meal I'm going to pull out my tracking app." We'll talk more about sodium and caffeine in the coming weeks. For now, just track them.

Tracking your sleep

Over time, the Plan will also help you set some sleep goals. The number of hours you sleep is not as critical as the consistency of your sleep pattern. I'll talk about sleep in detail in Month 6 (page 143).

Tracking your symptoms

Experts do not agree on how long it takes before food may trigger a migraine response. Estimates range between 2 and 96 hours (four days!). My approach is to remove all known triggers for at least four months, then try a phased reintroduction of your favorite foods. Find more on that process in Month 7 (page 156).

Since there are many triggers besides food, and everyone is different, part of the learning curve is tracking your own symptoms to see what affects you. Other triggers can be *chemical* (from within our body's normal chemistry), *electrolyte-based* (caused by stressful events, skipping meals, or exercise), *sensory* (strong odors, bright lights, sunlight, strobe-lighting effects from fans, or driving), and *hormonal* (especially due to menstrual cycles).[56]

①
②
③
④
⑤
⑥
⑦
⑧

Write down every symptom that you experience, even if you think it's odd or unimportant. You may learn that a suddenly stuffy nose or a fit of yawning is an indicator of an attack. After a while, you will begin to learn your pattern. You can use the symptoms on the Example Tracking Sheet (page 42) as a starting point, but be aware that you may have different ones. You'll begin to see patterns the longer you track. One thing I learned when I tracked was that an intense craving for pizza seemed to correlate with an attack the next day. At first I thought the pizza was the cause, but after a while I began to wonder if the craving for something salty and fatty was an indicator of a migraine coming on. Many people have unusual symptoms and may simply be unaware that what they are experiencing is part of their migraine pattern. For instance, I had never made the connection between my light sensitivity and migraine attacks. Now I'm extremely aware of it.

Tracking your movement

Why am I asking you to track your number of steps? I'll talk more about movement in Month 6 (page 143), but for now just know that research shows a relationship between regular movement and improvement in migraine attacks, an improvement equal to taking the prescription migraine preventive topiramate.[57] You don't have to overdo it though—just walking is great, especially on days when you don't feel well. Each week there will be an easy step target, and over time an "active minutes" target, which will gradually increase over the weeks. "Active minutes" refers to any type of exercise that gets your heart rate up and causes you to sweat. This might include activities like brisk walking, jogging, or any type of cardio workout.

Most of the fitness apps are free, and allow you to customize your profile and target goals. Most apps will tell you how many minutes you were active, how many steps you took, and how many calories you burned. When you set up your tracking app, do *not* tell it that you want to lose weight. Just input your current weight.

Why?

Even if you would like to lose weight, studies about behavior change show that we have a finite bank of willpower to spend each day. Once it's gone, it's gone.[58] So you don't want to expend your precious willpower energy on weight loss when you have other changes to make. Don't worry: You will most likely lose weight on this Plan if you are carrying excess pounds. But don't tell the app that, or it will restrict your calories. There is **no calorie restriction** on this eating Plan. I'll talk in more detail on pages 149 to 151 about why calorie restriction doesn't work for weight loss.

Our primary goal is to reduce the frequency and severity of our migraine attacks, not to lose weight.

Along the way, you'll start to see whether there is a relationship between calories eaten, calories burned, and your weight; which foods provide the most nutritional bang for the buck; and which macronutrients might be most impactful for you. We'll be targeting some specific nutrients later in the Plan, so using an app and getting in the habit of tracking will help you down the road. Most people on the Plan track for about six months. If you don't have a smartphone, you can download a blank tracking sheet from my website, MigraineReliefPlan.com. Dr. Elizabeth Seng, a health psychologist who specializes in migraine, also suggests tracking for the 30 days before each doctor visit so you can give your specialist useful data. Although some people may find tracking to be useful in the long term, Seng cautions against assuming that everyone should make tracking a lifelong habit. Particularly for people who are prone to anxiety, worry, and depression, habitual tracking may make you overly focused on illness and interfere with a more adaptive focus on wellness.[59]

❶
②
③
④
⑤
⑥
⑦
⑧

example tracking sheet

	S	M	Tu	W	Th	F	S	Weekly Averages
Tingly fingers								
Tingly feet								
Headache	slight, took Cambia last night and this a.m.		tender point lower jaw, vomited 11 a.m. (bad goat cheese?), mild diarrhea	neck still stiff	up at 1:40 a.m. with ringing head, finally took injectable at 4 a.m.	inter-mittent headache lunch-on, took ibuprofen	bit of a headache from last night, 800 mg ibu @ 7:30 a.m.	
Ringing in ears	slight, rt ear	slight	slight, fullness		yes			
Dizzy	some, afternoon	slight						
Vertigo								
Swollen fingers								
Tiredness	yes		2 hr nap after puking					
Lightheadedness								
Neckache	yes	yes	no	yes	yes	no	no	
Sinus pain								
Ear pain								
Dry mouth								
Light sensitivity								
Aura								
Spacy/foggy head								

① ② ③ ④ ⑤ ⑥ ⑦ ⑧

	S	M	Tu	W	Th	F	S	Weekly Averages
Headache scale: 0: pain-free 1: OTC meds 2: migraine meds 3: migraine meds & bed	2	0	3	1	2	1	1	1.428
Hours slept	7.5	7.25	7.75	7.25	5	7.5	8	7.18
Yoga/meditation	yes	20 min						
Breakfast	egg, kale, hot pepper sauce	2 eggs, 1 toast, butter	bite eggs, berry smoothie w goat cheese	2 eggs, hot sauce	oatmeal, coco milk	2 eggs, chili sauce	1.5 eggs, turkey, red pepper omelet	
Snack						avo, rice cake		
Lunch	bean soup, pasta, chèvre, ghee	6 oz salmon, cabbage, chips, guacamole	pasta, butter, salt, chix broth	2 bites tuna, potato salad, salad	potato salad, lentil soup, butter	6 oz chicken, 2 mini corn tortillas	chili, brown rice	
Snack	10 chips	avo rice cake		mango salsa, chips	mango salsa, chips		2 lemon bars	
Dinner	salmon cakes, hollandaise, salad, curried greens	2 sm salmon cakes, sm potato, ghee	potato salad, tuna salad, butter	tri-tip, rice, beans	chili, rice	turkey pho	turkey pho	
Snack			chips, hot sauce			brown rice, butter, chips, mango salsa	chips, sauce, strawberries	
Steps walked	5671	4763	4101	4726	2848	5242	4957	4615
Caffeinated bevs	0	0	0	0	0	0	0	0
Sugary snacks	0	0	0	0	0	0	0	0
Sodium total	435	625	520	1145	130	895	390	591
Carbs (grams)	I wasn't keeping carb data at this time, but I did after a while using MyFitnessPal.							

1
2
3
4
5
6
7
8

A closer look at: the "migraine brain"

Having read more than a dozen migraine books and more than 100 migraine research articles, and interviewed migraine researchers and doctors, I can safely say that they still have no *definitive* idea what causes migraine. The most current thinking is that migraine attacks are caused by an underlying neurobiological condition, with a hereditary component in at least some types. In the literature, migraine is described as everything from a "masochistic little glitch" to a neurological illness to a disability. But honestly, no one has The Answer yet. Far more research is needed. This is frustrating to people in pain, fascinating if you aren't suffering. Wanting The Answer is high on everyone's list.

I can tell you what I choose. I reject any label that includes the word *disability* or that refers to my brain as broken. I have an excellent brain. It's smart and quick and imaginative. My body has done a great job of getting me through 50+ years. I took some time to consider the effect this language had on me, in light of my personal experience with other health challenges.

I remember in 2003 when I was super sick with what doctors thought was chronic fatigue syndrome and fibromyalgia. My doctor finally convinced me to apply for a handicap placard. I had a love-hate relationship with that thing. I loved that it made my life easier. I worried that people would think I was misusing it, as I looked perfectly fine. I worried that I would need it forever, and that it could become a permanent part of my life. It was red plastic for "temporary," but it could become blue plastic for "permanent." Having it in my glove box challenged how I saw myself. While it was a useful tool at the time, I saw how just having it in the car, whether I used it or not, changed how I felt about myself. I felt it weakened my belief that I had the ability to heal.

I have found that when I accept a negative label, it changes me. It starts owning me. It robs me of my power to change, heal, and grow. It shifts my brain chemistry, and not in a good way.[60] This is especially challenging for me as a woman, as I believe women are taught to value other peoples' opinions of us intensely.

In addition, if I place the responsibility of my problems on something I can't control ("I have a neurological disability"), it feels impossible for me to do anything about it.[61] Feeling in control is a key component in how much pain we feel. In her book *Minding the Body, Mending the Mind*, Dr. Joan Borysenko talks at length about the dangers of chronic helplessness, which affect our immunity as well as our happiness level.[62]

Instead of falling into that mindset, after my diagnosis, I asked myself these questions: "Who am I? What would someone like me do in this situation? Am I the kind of person who can successfully take care of my body? Am I a healthful person? A logical person? A responsible person?"[63] Engaging my identity, seeing myself as a person who is healthful and capable, as a health learner,[64] is much more helpful to me.

> I started to wonder: Can I be an extraordinarily healthy person who happens to get migraine attacks?[65]

Of course I think it's important for people to get a proper diagnosis and see a doctor who specializes in migraine attacks, headaches, or balance issues. If you need a handicap placard to help you function in your life as I did, please understand that I'm not criticizing you in any way. You might have similar conflicting feelings about it. I would encourage you to consider whether terms like *patient* or *disability* are becoming a part of your identity, and if so, *whether that is helpful to you.*

SHOULD A DIAGNOSIS DEFINE YOU?

It's important to remember that a diagnosis simply means your symptoms fit with an average number of other people who have a similar constellation of symptoms, and that doctors have a particular way of treating that diagnosis based on (hopefully) the latest research and knowledge. That's how Western medicine works, and most of the time, it's a wonderful thing. The danger with a diagnosis is that it can start to define us. If I walk into a doctor's office and walk out an hour later with a diagnosis, does that suddenly mean I am "disabled"?

I have been greatly influenced by many personal stories of overcoming serious health crises. I was fascinated to discover psychologist Ellen Langer's work, described in her book *Counterclockwise*.[66] Langer is sometimes called the mother of positive psychology. Her scientific focus over 30 years has been to study how beliefs affect health status in measurable ways. She reminds us that a diagnosis is a useful label from a medical perspective, but that it represents an average experience of many people. She suggests taking doctors off a pedestal and thinking of them as consultants in our health experience. I have many friends who are doctors; I know how much they struggle with the limitations of the healthcare system. I know how much they care about the people they treat. And I know they're human, too.

It's understandable to want our doctors to know everything. Then *they* are in charge, they will fix us, and it's their fault if something goes wrong. But that's not realistic either. How can someone who sees you once a month for 10 minutes, no matter how amazing their training and experience, know more about what it feels like to be in your body than you?

Langer talks at length about the power of priming, as study after study shows that priming subjects with positive or negative words has a measurable effect on their health. In several intriguing studies, for example, young people who were primed to think of old age (by sorting photos of people into "young" and "old" categories or by solving anagrams with age-related words) walked more slowly to the elevator after the test than subjects of the same age who were given a similar assignment unrelated to age. Langer's work has led her to believe that if we accept labels as truths without thinking about them, then even words as seemingly innocuous as "patient" or "prescription" can be detrimental to our health.

I find Langer's work fascinating and challenging, as my personal experience has been that "having a positive attitude" has not prevented me from having symptoms, health challenges, and getting this diagnosis. I can have a positive attitude and still have chronic pain in my back nearly every day. I know that many people who suffer from migraine attacks are frustrated with anything that smacks of blaming the victim.[67]

However, I will say that my mental health is greatly improved when I focus on the positive, and that reframing my experience in positive ways helps me feel better emotionally. It doesn't mean that I can talk myself out of a migraine when the weather is a certain way, but overall it helps me. Dr. Robert Cowan of Stanford University, who also gets migraine attacks, prefers to see people with migraine as an evolved part of the species, rather than damaged.[68]

In my deliberate identity shift, I rejected the broken-brain/disability story and instead decided that I have a Maserati brain. I pictured it in my mind: candy-apple red. It costs $300,000. It runs on crazy-expensive high-octane fuel. It's beautiful, fast, and very, very finicky. It needs to be perfectly tuned and maintained. If I feed it unleaded gas, it may run for a short time, but it will be very unhappy.

I believe that's a helpful metaphor for my brain, one that gives me agency in maintaining it. What I eat and other lifestyle choices I make are absolutely critical to the performance of my high-octane brain. I don't know why I'm built that way, but I am. There are challenges *and* benefits.

If this metaphor is helpful to you, feel free to choose your own custom sports car, or another metaphor that feels empowering. At the very least, consider what kinds of words you use to describe yourself and whether those words are helping you.

①
②
③
④
⑤
⑥
⑦
⑧

WEEK 2

set up your environment to succeed

———— ••• ————

I have been fascinated by behavior change since graduate school, and I continue to read about it as new books and research come out. One book I loved was *Switch: How to Change Things When Change Is Hard,* by Chip and Dan Heath. They describe one key element of making changes: setting up your environment to mold the behavior you want.

We are highly influenced by our environment. Researchers wanting to influence health behaviors in a West Virginia community targeted something super-specific: buying skim or 1 percent milk instead of whole milk. They found that once they successfully changed buying behavior, people would drink whatever was in their fridge.[69] So if you want to choose foods that support your health goals, creating a successful environment is key. This week, you'll take your first step toward setting up your environment by taking a peek inside your freezer. Over the next three weeks, you'll gradually make some kitchen shifts to get you ready to change your eating, one meal at a time.

WEEK 2 ASSIGNMENT: CLEAN OUT YOUR FREEZER

———— • ————

TOOLS NEEDED: *masking tape, permanent marker, gentle cleanser, sponge*
WHAT I USE: *Snapware glass storage containers, 1-quart zip-top freezer bags, Simple Green to clean, regular masking tape, black Sharpie fine point marker*

Your Week 2 goal is to do an inventory of your freezer to see which foods you'll be able to eat on the Plan and which you won't. You have the option of getting rid of items (see page 57) or simply labeling and organizing what you can and cannot have. Ideally, create a space in your freezer where your food can be stored so that you can easily see what is available to you.

If you live alone, or if your housemates or family members will be eating exactly what you eat, you may wish to get rid of some items, or eat them up in the next couple of weeks.

DAILY TRACKING GOALS

- **Everything you eat and drink.**
- **Hours slept.**
- **Your symptoms.**
- **Step count.** If your step count last week averaged fewer than 4,000 steps per day, increase your number of steps to 4,000 per day. Otherwise, continue on at your current number.
- **Active minutes.** Increase "very active" minutes to 5 per day if your tracker shows that statistic. You don't have to sprint, just be breathing a little bit fast and sweat a little bit. If your tracker doesn't track this, use your watch or phone to keep time.

- **Sodium intake.** If your sodium intake was higher than 3,000 milligrams per day last week, reduce it to 3,000 milligrams per day.
- **Caffeine intake.** If you drank more than 2 cups (16 ounces) of caffeinated beverages per day last week, reduce your caffeine intake to 16 ounces per day this week. Replace any additional cups of coffee, caffeinated drinks, or caffeinated sodas with filtered or spring water. Since our brains are 85 percent water, it's especially important to keep your body from getting dehydrated.

① ❷ ③ ④ ⑤ ⑥ ⑦ ⑧

Food that is not expired can generally be returned to the store for store credit. Neighbors are also often happy to take foods you can no longer eat.

When you buy new freezer items, make sure they are on the Plan, and label them as you bring them home. Start looking for replacements for freezer foods that are not on the Plan. For example, if you eat frozen pizza one night a week, you'll need to figure out a replacement for it, such as gluten-free frozen pizza crusts topped with ricotta cheese, low-sodium spaghetti sauce (or just salt-free tomato sauce), herbs, veggies, and home-cooked meat.

Continue to track everything you are eating and drinking this week; track your symptoms, sodium, and steps, making some small adjustments as outlined in this week's tracking goals.

FREEZER CLEANOUT TIPS

This is a great week to scrub your freezer and check dates. Any food more than one year old should absolutely be tossed. Visit foodsafety.gov for specific guidelines on storing meats and leftovers. Unopened, unexpired packages of processed frozen foods might be able to be returned to the grocery store for store credit. See page 57 for more information.

As we go along, you will be cooking and storing foods in the freezer, so you will always have homemade options. You will need space in your freezer and freezer-safe containers in order do this. Label and date everything so you know what you have and how old it is.

Your fridge will likely start looking quite different. My refrigerator went from being packed with a fairly empty freezer to the reverse: only a few days' worth of fresh items and leftovers in the fridge and a completely loaded freezer compartment.

FREEZER STAPLES

- **GLUTEN-FREE BREAD**. Make sure it has a reasonable sodium content (80 milligrams or less per slice) and not too much sugar (2 grams per slice). One of my favorites is Trader Joe's Gluten Free Multigrain Brown Rice Bread. If you are sensitive to eggs or gums, be sure to read the label. Most gluten-free breads include egg whites unless they are labeled vegan.

- **UNBRINED MEAT, POULTRY, AND FISH**. Make sure it's the freshest, sustainably raised, pastured meat you can buy, and wild-caught fish if possible. Do what you can within your budget. I'll talk more about the quality of your protein on page 66. Ask at the meat counter if the meat is brined; they should know. Brining is a process of soaking meat in salted water to preserve freshness and plump it up. It can triple or quadruple the amount of sodium naturally found in meat. Usually meat in pre-sealed Tetra Paks *is* brined. Assume that rotisserie chickens and turkey breasts are brined. Check the labels on quick-frozen chicken and fresh value packs of chicken to see if they have added sodium.

- **FROZEN VEGETABLES**. Buy options with no added salt. Stay away from lima beans, broad beans, and blends that include onion.

- **FROZEN FRUIT**. Choose fruit blends that do not contain raspberries.

- **FRESH CORN TORTILLAS**. You can also freeze other types of gluten-free tortillas.

A closer look at: seafood and fish

Since you'll be adding protein and healthy fat to your diet, here is some helpful information about seafood and fish to help you shop and choose wisely. You can use high-sodium seafood in smaller quantities to flavor soups and stews, rather than as a full portion of protein. *Nutritional information is from the USDA database and is based on their recommended serving size of 3.5 ounces (100 grams).*[70]

Product (raw and untreated)	Sodium per serving	Notes
Calamari and octopus	230mg	Make sure it's unfrozen, unbrined, and unbreaded.
Clams	601mg	
Crab, Alaskan king	836mg	
Crab, Dungeness	285mg	
Lobster, northern	423mg	Also known as Canadian, true, and Maine lobster.
Lobster, spiny	177mg	
Mussels	286mg	
Oysters	106mg	If you can find fresh oysters, they are low in sodium. Some canned oysters are low as well. Read your labels and rinse well.
Scallops	392mg	Scallops are safe to order at restaurants, as they are usually not pre-salted or marinated. Just be sure to specify "no salt or citrus. Butter and olive oil are OK."
Shrimp	119mg	Sustainable brands to look for include Shrimper's Pride, Dominick's, and Wild Planet (canned). Look for the Seafood Watch logo on packages or signs at the seafood counter to help you choose.[71]

CANNED FISH: ANCHOVIES, SARDINES, TUNA, SALMON

Choose unsmoked canned fish with no added salt; fish and water or olive oil should be the only listed ingredients. (Use the olive oil in sauces, soups, or stews.) Fish canned with soy protein isolate or other glutamates can be headache triggers. If possible, choose wild-caught fish, such as the Wild Planet brand and some varieties at Trader Joe's. Some people might be sensitive to canned fish due to possible higher tyramine or histamine content. If you have been sensitive in the past, then avoid it. If you're not sure, try one can and see; it's possible you had problems with the additives, not the actual fish. These fatty types of fish are high in omega-3 fatty acids; diets higher in these fats (and lower in polyunsaturated omega-6s) are being researched to see if they impact chronic pain, and so far the results are encouraging.[72]

FRESH FISH

If you have access to fresh fish, all varieties are great. Fatty cold-water fish (salmon, sardines, herring, anchovies, mackerel) provide the highest levels of omega-3 fatty acids, which provide excellent support for migraine brains. Try to rotate the types of fish you eat—fresh, frozen, or canned—and choose wild-caught whenever possible. For example, eat tuna, salmon, cod, and tilapia in rotation, not just tuna day after day. This will lessen your risk from mercury or other contaminants.

Make sure you ask at the supermarket if the fish has been previously frozen. Much has and is often brined to help maintain freshness. Specifically ask if the item has been brined; providers are not required to label it as such. If the fish has been frozen, only buy it if it was thawed that day *and* you will cook it that day.

You may be able to find sustainably farmed yellowtail tuna from Baja, Mexico. Look for seals from the Monterey Bay Aquarium's Seafood Watch, Aquarium of the Pacific's Seafood for the Future, or NOAA FishWatch. Do not buy shark unless you can find green thresher shark from California waters, as it is the only sustainable shark presently available.

Avoid: fish or seafood farmed or caught in Southeast Asia, the South Pacific, China, and Japan. Raw fish, for sushi or sashimi, must be from reputable sources that can speak to the safety of the fish, where it was caught, and how it was handled.

FROZEN FISH

There are wonderful varieties of frozen fish available, and they may be less expensive than fresh. Usually wild-caught fish are flash-frozen onboard the ship, which means they are very fresh and usually not brined. For the best results, thaw the unopened package in the refrigerator overnight. (While you can quick-thaw fish packages in a bowl of cold water, that method is very hard on the flesh of the fish, making it flabby.) Firm fillets like tuna are easier to cut when slightly frozen. Open the package, drain, rinse the fish, and then pat it dry with towels. Grill, poach, sear, or pan fry.[73]

WEEK 3
take on the nonperishables

———— ⸬ ————

You might not have a formal walk-in pantry, but you likely have spaces where you store all nonperishable food items: canned goods, spices, pastas, and boxed foods. For some people, their pantry is one shelf or cupboard. My friend Carole has two huge walk-in spaces. If you have a large space or many spaces, this week's task could take several days. Take your time. Use this as an opportunity to clean cupboards, check spices for freshness, and potentially donate some food to a local food pantry or soup kitchen. In my 1,000-square-foot house, my pantry includes three large shelves under the kitchen island, one counter where my spices and dried beans are stored in jars, a smaller cabinet with lazy Susans to use that space efficiently, and two more shelves in the hall closet that I appropriated a few years ago for bulk items.

① ② ❸ ④ ⑤ ⑥ ⑦ ⑧

WEEK 3 ASSIGNMENT: CLEAN OUT YOUR PANTRY

———— • ————

TOOLS NEEDED: *tote bags, gentle cleanser, sponge*
WHAT I USE: *reusable tote bags, Simple Green to clean*

Your Week 3 goal is to do an inventory of your pantry to see which foods are OK for the Plan and which are not. You have the option of actually getting rid of items (see page 57) or just labeling what you can and cannot have. Stop buying pantry foods that you cannot eat, and find replacements for them that are on the Plan using the list that follows. Continue to track everything you are eating and drinking this week; track your symptoms, sodium, and steps.

PANTRY CLEANOUT TIPS

———— • ————

If you are just trying out the Plan and/or you live with other people, there is no need to get rid of foods at this point. Ideally, create an eye-level shelf in your pantry where your food can be stored, so that you can easily see what is available to you. This process can be an

DAILY TRACKING GOALS

- **Everything you eat and drink.** Do your best to eat six small meals (or 3 meals, 3 snacks) throughout the day to maintain even blood sugar levels.
- **Hours slept.**
- **Your symptoms.**
- **Step count.** Increase number of steps walked (via pedometer, smartphone app, or fitness device) to 5,000 per day (or add 500 steps to last week's average if that feels like too much for you).

- **Active minutes.** Increase very active minutes to 10 per day, 2 to 3 days per week.
- **Sodium intake.** Reduce your sodium intake to 2,500 milligrams per day; reduce the amount of salt you add to foods when eating or cooking.
- **Caffeine intake.** Reduce your caffeine intake to 1.5 cups/drinks per day; replace with water, infused water, and approved herbal teas.

① ② ❸ ④ ⑤ ⑥ ⑦ ⑧

emotional one and might feel overwhelming if you have a large pantry or multiple spaces to tackle; ask a supportive friend to help you, and don't feel you have to do it overnight.

Since my pantry encompasses multiple spaces, I did one shelf or cupboard each evening until I had gone through everything. This includes:

- Pasta and grains
- Spices
- Canned foods
- Seeds (I recommend storing in the refrigerator to maintain freshness)
- Cookies and crackers
- Dried beans

Check that spice blends do not contain salt (many do). You won't be using table salt or spice blends with salt any longer. (You may choose to use small amounts of sea salt at the table.) For example, you can use garlic powder but not garlic salt. Onion powder and onion salt are not recommended on the Plan because onions are strong triggers for many people.

To check if a spice is fresh, open the container and take a whiff. If it smells musty, stale, or dull, it will not do your food any good and you should toss the contents. (Compost them if you have a compost pile.)

You don't need to throw out the container. Just wash it out, let it dry thoroughly, and refill it with fresh spices you purchase in bulk. Many stores have bulk spice sections, allowing you to buy very small amounts so they don't go stale. Note that if you have food allergies or celiac disease, you should not purchase items in bulk because of possible cross-contamination. One favorite company of mine is Spicely Organics. Their packages contain the perfect amounts, they're organic and gluten-free, and their small plastic bags can be easily opened and poured into reusable jars.

My spice cabinet did not change much, nor did my grains or beans section, but there were lots of items I had to return because of the high sodium content. This area of my kitchen involved a lot of grocery store returns, as packages were unopened and I wanted to have the money to spend on my new foods.

PANTRY STAPLES

Choose organic items whenever your budget allows for three reasons: (1) It reduces your intake of GMOs, pesticides, and herbicides (which have unknown consequences for migraine but known negative effects on our microbiome), (2) It increases your intake of nutrients (important to feed your brain cells), and (3) It increases the demand for organic products, and their overall prices will go down as more companies produce them. It's especially important to choose products made with organic corn, as they are free of GMOs and the herbicide residue that comes with GMO corn. (This herbicide residue is damaging to the helpful bacteria in our guts.) I'll give you tips in Week 7 (page 91) on how to make organic affordable. The following chart outlines some items to make sure you keep on hand.

Cans (BPA-free) and Tetra Paks			
Canned beans, reduced sodium or no salt added	Fire-roasted tomatoes, no salt added	Low-sodium broth or stock (no onions)	Tomatoes, diced, no salt added
Coconut water	Light and regular canned coconut milk (ingredients are coconut and water only)	Tomato paste, no salt added	

Bottles and jars			
Chili pepper sauce (containing small amounts of distilled vinegar and sugar)	Red pepper spread with eggplant and garlic (may contain sugar)	Soy-free mayonnaise	Unsweetened applesauce

Bagged or bulk items

Amaranth	Dried beans (garbanzos, white beans, black beans, split peas, black-eyed peas, kidney beans, pinto beans, split mung beans)	Individually bagged potato chips	Teff
Arborio rice		Lightly salted rice cakes	Unsalted corn tortilla chips
Brown rice		Millet	
Buckwheat		Polenta	Unsalted microwave popcorn (if you really need it—seems to be the least noxious of the microwave popcorns)
Corn tortillas (store fresh corn tortillas in the freezer)	Gluten-free pasta, made with brown rice, corn, quinoa, Jerusalem artichoke, or blends	Quinoa	
		Rice noodles (Asian)	
	Gluten-free rolled oats or steel cut oats	Tapioca, pearls or flour/starch	White rice

Notes
- While I recommend buying certified gluten-free oats if you have celiac disease or gluten sensitivity, you can buy regular oats, preferably organic, and rinse them before using. Oats are naturally gluten-free, but they are easily cross-contaminated by wheat.
- For rice cakes, I only recommend Lundberg Farms in the United States; other brands taste like packing peanuts.
- Ideally, purchase organic popcorn in bulk and pop it in a brown paper bag with the top rolled down to eliminate potential chemicals found in the bags. If your microwave doesn't have a popcorn setting, use the same timing as you would for the packaged version.

Fats and oils

Coconut oil	Extra virgin coconut oil	Grass-fed ghee	Toasted sesame oil
Coconut oil spray	Extra virgin olive oil	Olive oil spray	

Notes
- Check oil spray ingredients to make sure it doesn't contain soybean oil or lecithin.
- Ghee is OK even if you are lactose-intolerant, as the milk proteins have been removed.
- Extra virgin olive oil goes rancid very quickly. If possible, buy from an olive oil store that can tell you when it was harvested, and store it in the refrigerator.

Miscellaneous and seeds

Chia seeds	Organic stevia packets	Sesame seeds	Stevia liquid
Hemp seeds	Pumpkin seeds	Sparkling water (without citrus or raspberry)	Sunflower seeds

Notes
- All seeds are best stored in the refrigerator.
- For stevia packets, I recommend Natvia, Wholesome Sweeteners, and Pyure.
- For stevia liquid, I recommend NuNaturals.

Teas

Chamomile	Mint	Rooibos

Notes
- Most of the teas in my pantry included potential triggers.
- Check to make sure your teas don't contain citrus peel, black or green tea, raspberries, or any other non-approved item like hibiscus.
- If you like Mexican food, note that the drink called "Jamaica" is made from hibiscus.

HOW TO RETURN FOOD

————————— • —————————

- Before you return food, check to make sure it isn't expired. If it is, you should simply toss or compost it. The store is not allowed to take it back. You can ask your local food pantry if they accept expired items.

- Choose one store at a time.

- Bring a receipt if you have it.

- Go at a time when the store is not busy.

- Go to the Customer Service desk, not a cashier (unless it's Trader Joe's in the United States; its cashiers will take care of you with no questions asked).

- Start by apologizing for the inconvenience. Smile.

- Ask if you can have store credit.

- Tell them you have been told to change your diet by your doctor, and you can no longer eat these foods.

- Say you understand if they can't give you credit without a receipt. Smile a lot.

- If you still end up with food you can't eat, donate it to a food pantry or pass it along to neighbors or friends.

A reminder

The reason I recommend gluten-free and sugar-free eating is to reduce inflammation. Migraine is an inflammatory process, so the less inflammation our bodies are dealing with, the better. We are constantly updating the approved food lists on MigraineReliefPlan.com, so please join us to see the most updated lists and submit other brand-name items you find. I use tiny amounts of maple syrup, coconut sugar, and molasses in a few recipes for flavor. Otherwise, I use only stevia.

A *closer look at:* sodium, migraine, and Meniere's disease

Without diet changes, 90 percent of all Americans will develop high blood pressure, also called hypertension, in their lifetimes. This is especially concerning because normally human blood pressure lowers with age.[74] Most experts agree that diets high in sodium contribute to this condition.

Most Americans eat far too much sodium. The standard American diet can range from 3,000 to 8,000 milligrams of sodium per day, and 80 percent of the sodium comes from processed foods[75] and added salt.[76] For example, one Happy Meal contains 810 milligrams of sodium. A Quarter Pounder with cheese and large fries contain 1,800 milligrams of sodium. Restaurants oversalt food to improve taste but also to create thirst and increase beverage sales.[77]

Those who live with migraine or Meniere's disease need to be particularly cautious when it comes to sodium. For one thing, a high-sodium meal may trigger headaches. People with chronic migraine have double the risk of developing hypertension.[78] A high-sodium diet can also contribute to generalized inflammation through the stimulation of Th17 cells.[79] The white salt found in processed foods and saltshakers, bleached and stripped of minerals, may be a contributor to autoimmune conditions.[80] One research study found that, while sodium levels in the blood may not be elevated, sodium levels within the lymphoid tissues may be, which might be generating the autoimmune response.[81]

We actually need only a small amount of sodium for our bodies to function properly, estimated to be around 500 milligrams per day, which is naturally occurring in the whole foods we eat. We do not need added salt to be healthy. Primitive tribes probably got between 400 and 800 milligrams of sodium per day in their diets, without any salt available on a daily basis.[82] Today, the American Heart Association recommends no more than 1,500 milligrams per day be consumed by everyone.

My recommendation is to live between 1,200 and 1,500 milligrams per day, although if you have Meniere's disease or any balance problems, experiment with maintaining a consistent average on the lower end of that range. Here are a couple of tips to keep in mind:

- **BE PATIENT**. Once you reduce your sodium intake, it takes two months, possibly three, for your palate to heal and get used to low-sodium foods. They do eventually taste great—I promise!

- **DON'T ELIMINATE ALL SALT**. If you eliminate processed foods and salt from your cooking, you can enjoy adding sea salt to your food at the table where you really taste it.

- **CHOOSE YOUR SALT CAREFULLY**. I recommend selecting natural sea salt with a tint to it, which contains many important trace minerals. For example, Himalayan pink sea salt contains more than 80 trace minerals, including iron, iodine, copper, zinc, selenium, and molybdenum, which are all important for people with autoimmune conditions.[83] Five twists of my salt grinder is the equivalent of 100 milligrams of sodium. While sea salt is more expensive than regular iodized table salt, it lasts a long time since you only use a small amount at the table. If you can't find sea salt at a local store, order it online. Look for iodized sea salt or take a multivitamin that contains iodine so you don't have to worry about thyroid conditions.

- **DON'T TRY TO CURE MIGRAINE WITH SALT**. You may have seen on the Internet that taking a large quantity of salt will instantly "cure" a migraine. I don't recommend that approach, nor does any reputable doctor.

Keep in mind that low-sodium diets can improve more than your migraine. They can also improve:

- Diabetes symptoms
- Carpal tunnel syndrome
- PMS symptoms
- Joint issues and joint pain
- Meniere's Disease–related dizziness and vertigo (It's important to maintain a daily average that's consistent, ideally around 1,000 milligrams per day.[84])

SALT-FREE FLAVOR INTENSIFIERS

When you start eating lower-sodium foods, it takes a while to adjust, and food doesn't have that zing. I found that these foods can help add that punch I used to get from salt. As you clean out your pantry, think about items you'll need to replace, like onion salt, and look for an alternative to try.

- Diced celery, frozen in one-cup servings
- Thinly sliced leeks, white and light green parts only, frozen in one-cup servings
- Roasted garlic, frozen in ice cube trays, then stored in a zip-top freezer bag
- Roasted red peppers, puréed and frozen in ice cube trays (You can use jarred peppers *if* they have no added salt, vinegar, or sodium bisulfite.)
- Oven-roasted tomatoes drizzled with olive oil, garlic, and black pepper
- Mushroom broth, reduce down (especially shiitake)
- Mushroom purée (cooked)
- Unsalted chicken broth, reduced down
- Tomato paste (no salt added)
- Truffle oil
- Infused olive oil, such as basil, garlic, chili pepper
- Roasted eggplant purée

Remember that tomatoes and mushrooms are naturally high in glutamates, which may be a migraine trigger for some people.

WEEK 4
clean out the fridge and start snacking

———···———

When I started the process of changing my diet, I didn't know any better, so I went cold turkey. I tried to change everything that I was eating overnight. I freaked out a lot. It was not enjoyable. When I designed the Plan, I made it as user-friendly as possible. It's intimidating to think about changing everything you eat all at once. Many popular diet programs take an all-or-nothing approach, but as a health coach, I find that for long-term lifestyle change, gradual works best.

That's why in Week 4—the first week you'll change something about your food— we're starting with snacks. While snacks aren't technically meals, they are an easy way to transition into a new way of eating. Plus, snacks are fun. Who doesn't love snacks? And one more thing: It's important to keep your blood sugar balanced throughout the day, so eating a small healthy snack between meals is ideal for people who get migraine attacks. If you find that you regularly wake up with a migraine, experiment with eating a small snack with protein just before bed.

①
②
③
❹
⑤
⑥
⑦
⑧

WEEK 4 ASSIGNMENT: CLEAN OUT THE FRIDGE AND REPLACE SNACKS

———·———

TOOLS NEEDED: *tote bags, gentle cleanser, sponge*
WHAT I USE: *reusable tote bags, Simple Green to clean*

Your Week 4 goal is to do an inventory and reorganization of your fridge to see which foods are OK for the Plan and which are not. You have the option of actually getting rid of items (see page 57) or just labeling what you can and cannot have. Continue to track everything you are eating and drinking this week; track your symptoms, sodium, and steps. Start buying fresh foods that you *can* eat, and continue to do so as you shop. This is the first week you'll be eating your snacks on the Plan.

DAILY TRACKING GOALS

- **Everything you eat and drink**. Do your best to eat 5 to 6 small meals (or 3 meals and 2 to 3 approved snacks) throughout the day. Have your last meal or snack three hours before bedtime if possible (unless you wake up with a migraine, see page 61).
- **Hours slept**.
- **Your symptoms**.
- **Step count**. Increase number of steps walked (via pedometer, smartphone app, or fitness device) to about 6,000 per day, or 500 more than last week's average.

- **Active minutes**. Increase very active minutes to 15 per day, 2 to 3 days per week.
- **Sodium intake**. Reduce your sodium intake to 2,000 milligrams per day; do not add salt to foods when cooking.
- **Caffeine intake**. Reduce your caffeine intake to 1 cup or drink per day; add another glass of filtered or spring water instead.
- **Sugary snacks**. If you regularly eat sugary snacks, start swapping them for Plan-approved snacks.

① ② ③ ❹ ⑤ ⑥ ⑦ ⑧

SNACK IDEAS

Purchased		
Organic, unsalted microwave popcorn	Individually bagged potato chips	Organic, unsalted tortilla chips topped with hot sauce or Chile Pepper Sauce (page 267)
Notes	• Popcorn and potato chips are transitional snacks. As you get used to the Plan, you'll need these less in the future.	

Homemade			
Smoothies Sunflower Seed Butter (page 195) on apples, pears, carrots, or celery Vanilla Ricotta Cream (page 263) with fruit, if you like	Gluten-free toast or high-quality rice cakes spread with: • Unsalted butter and Vietnamese cinnamon • Strawberries and mascarpone or cream cheese	• Sunflower Seed Butter (page 195) • Hummus made without lemon juice • Red pepper spread and mascarpone or cream cheese	• Herbed Cheese Spread (page 189) • Creamy Not-ella Carob Butter (page 188)
Notes	• Try not to eat fruit alone as it can spike your blood sugar. • Always add a saturated fat and/or protein like approved cheese or seed butter. • Red pepper spread is a transitional snack. As you get used to the Plan, you'll need it less in the future.		

FRIDGE CLEAN-OUT TIPS

Create several areas in your fridge where your food can be stored, so that you can easily see what is available to you. This is a great opportunity to clean out old condiments and all those random items that tend to multiply in your refrigerator. I took every shelf and drawer out and did a thorough scrubbing, which felt cathartic. Currently, in a drawer designated for my husband, there are just a few items that only he eats; the rest is fresh food that we both eat and freshly made sauces and condiments (see page 265). Your cleanout includes:

- Condiments
- Beverages
- Dairy
- Nuts and seeds (if stored in the refrigerator, recommended). Nuts are *not* on the Plan; seeds are.
- Vegetables
- Fruit
- Meat/protein

My refrigerator is 100 percent different now. I used to shop once a week, stocking up on all my produce and other items for the week. Now I shop every two to three days, only buying produce for specific recipes I plan to make and enough fruit for two to three days. If you can't shop this often, prep your vegetables all at once and freeze some of them in zip-top freezer bags. Keep a close eye on your fruits and veggies, and freeze them well before they go bad. The upside to this system is that we have a lot less produce that goes bad because I forget about it. Learn more about reducing food waste on page 91.

If you're used to eating packaged foods, then making the change to cooking and eating fresh foods is a big one. It's fine to start simple and find some foods that you enjoy cooking. Be easy on yourself and take your time to change this big part of your life. Over time, I encourage you to continue trying new foods, like different Plan-approved beans, grains, and greens. Ideally, you want to rotate those items in your diet, as it's not ideal to eat the exact same foods every day. In addition to nutrients, every whole food contains other compounds, antinutrients, or heavy metals that you don't want to overdose on. If you eat brown rice, kale, or canned tuna every day, you may unwittingly develop health issues if those compounds build up. For example, brown rice (even organic) naturally contains trace amounts of arsenic, kale contains oxalic acid and phytates, and canned tuna can be high in mercury. You don't need to worry about this if you make rotating food groups like grains, greens, and fish a part of your routine.

①
②
③
❹
⑤
⑥
⑦
⑧

REFRIGERATOR STAPLES

Purchased dairy products (organic and grass-fed if possible)

American cheese (purchased from the deli counter)	Cottage cheese, unsalted or reduced-sodium if available	Half-and-half	Ricotta cheese
		Heavy cream	Whole milk
Butter, unsalted	Ghee	Mascarpone	

Notes
- American cheese is not recommended for Meniere's because of the sodium content.
- If you are avoiding milk protein, replace the butter with a good quality soy-free vegan margarine.

Meat and poultry

All fresh meat, preferably local and pastured	All fresh fish and seafood, preferably wild-caught

Notes
- Make sure your fish and seafood hasn't been brined.

Vegetables

Bell peppers and hot peppers	Fennel	Root vegetables (potatoes, sweet potatoes, parsnips, turnips, rutabagas)	Salad greens
Carrots	Kale and other greens		Scallions
Celery	Leeks		

Fruits

Apples	Grapes	Nectarines	Purple plums
Blackberries	Kiwi fruit	Peaches	Strawberries
Blueberries	Mango	Pears	

Fresh spices and herbs

Basil	Garlic	Lemongrass	Shallots
Chives	Gingerroot	Mint	Thyme
Cilantro	Italian flat-leaf parsley or curly parsley	Oregano	Turmeric
Dill		Rosemary	

A *closer look at:* the quality of your protein

Ideally, those of us who eat meat should be able to buy meat produced from happy, healthy animals frolicking in the rolling fields of a lush farm. However, that's not the situation today. After reading *The Omnivore's Dilemma* and watching the movie *Food, Inc.*, my husband and I started making different choices about our meat, eventually going meat- and dairy-free for four years. Most US meat is produced on factory feedlots, with animals in poor conditions, often fed poor-quality food or food that's inappropriate for them. For instance, cattle should eat grass. That's what they're designed to eat and how they are healthiest. They get sick if they are fed corn, but because of government subsidies in the United States, corn is much cheaper than grass. So, feedlots give them corn, antibiotics to help cure them when they get sick from the corn, and hormones to grow faster. Low doses of antibiotics are routinely given to fatten up the animals more quickly. These antibiotics end up in us and affect the health of our microbiome, and they are very possibly a factor in fattening us up, too.[85]

Chickens and other animals don't fare much better. If you're concerned about your carbon footprint, smaller animals consume fewer resources. You can follow this Plan and be vegetarian, and if you're committed to being vegan, that's possible, too. Here are some tips for buying the best quality protein you can afford. Start by looking for the international 5-Step Animal Welfare Rating system; higher numbers mean better treatment of the animals. If the package doesn't show this number, assume it's a 0 (meaning, animals receive the poorest treatment).

BEEF

Look for grass-fed beef first, hormone-free second, and organic if possible. Some stores carry affordable, frozen grass-fed beef. If you have a large freezer, some families order an animal from a sustainable butchery operation and share it with neighbors, getting many cuts of beef at once and freezing them for later use. Talk to the butcher selling the meat, contact local farm-to-table restaurants, and do research on the Internet. Fattier cuts of meat and organ meats are usually cheaper. These cuts are also healthy for migraine brains (just make sure you cut back on sugar and refined grains when you begin to eat more pastured saturated fat). Meats from grass-fed, pastured animals have a lower risk of E. coli contamination and are usually higher in nutrient density, containing more antioxidants, vitamins, minerals, and a more favorable ratio of omega-6 and omega-3 fatty acids.[86] They're also lower in cholesterol and higher in beta-carotene and vitamin B12.[87]

You might be concerned about eating red meat after the 2015 WHO report came out about red meat and higher levels of colorectal cancer. However, our Plan doesn't include processed meats like bacon and sausage because they tend to be migraine triggers, and those were the ones listed as the highest risk. Use gentler cooking methods for red meats (braising, slow cooking) and marinate them in advance. Eat plenty of green vegetables. Follow those Plan guidelines and the risk of getting cancer from red meat is low.[88]

PORK

Pasture-raised pork is just as important as pastured beef. As with beef, look for pork that comes from pigs that are raised outdoors and able to eat grass, root around, and dig for insects and other foods they naturally eat. Eatwild.com is a great resource to find local, humanely raised meats all over the United States. If you live in a rural area, you may have access to meats produced with the same care, but without the labels and with lower prices. You can also find frozen ground wild boar in many supermarkets, which provides the health benefits of grass-fed beef and helps reduce the impact of feral pigs on farmland.[89]

GAME MEATS

In the United States, the Wild Idea Buffalo Company produces 100-percent grass-fed bison. Meats from grass-fed animals have five times the amount of omega-3 fatty acids over grain-fed animals, which helps restore your proper balance of omega-3 and omega-6 fatty acids. The standard American diet lacks omega-3 fatty acids, likely affecting our metabolism and possibly causing inflammation and swelling. Venison and other game meats are an excellent source of nutrients. You may be able to find frozen ground game meats—elk, bison, and venison—at some stores for around $10 per pound. When used in a plant-forward meal like stew or chili, it's still affordable.

TURKEY

Many grocery stores carry turkey year-round, and some even offer roasted turkey breast like they do rotisserie chicken. Beware, as the pre-cooked options are loaded with salt, and you don't know the quality of the turkey (you can assume it's from a factory feedlot). For example, 3 ounces of turkey breast should contain 95 milligrams of sodium, but the rotisserie turkey breast from my national grocery store contains 500 milligrams of sodium in the same serving. More options are now available for pastured turkey.

CHICKEN

Typical grocery store chickens often go on sale for $0.99 a pound, which is great if you're on a budget. Unfortunately, these birds spend their entire lives in huge warehouses under poor conditions. If you can afford it, look for birds produced in a more sustainable manner: free-range or pastured, raised without hormones or antibiotics. I have tips for saving money on groceries in Week 7 (page 83) that will help. "Cage-free" is a marketing label that often simply means the chicken was raised in a slightly better warehouse. Grocery store rotisserie chicken (unless it's pastured) is also loaded with sodium to plump it up and often flavored with MSG, yeast extract, and gluten—all potential triggers.

NONTRADITIONAL MEATS: ORGAN MEATS AND GELATIN

One of the interesting trends in recent years has been the emergence of nose-to-tail restaurants, which use all the edible parts of the animal in their dishes. This is what humans all over the world ate until the last half-century. If an animal is killed for food and the organ meat is not used, that's 22 to 24 percent of the edible meat going to waste.[90]

Many of the books I have read on the ancestral diet, and especially that of Dr. Terry Wahls, discuss the health benefits of eating organ meats, which are especially key in nutrients for brain cells. Organ meats, also called offal, are the most concentrated source of nutrients, including those lacking in people with autoimmune disease.

I have not gotten comfortable buying and cooking many organ meats yet, but I have found one brand of liverwurst that's not only made from sustainable pork, but also isn't off-the-charts high in sodium. I can only eat 1 ounce per day because of the sodium, but at least I'm getting some of those nutrients back in my diet. As it contains onion, I had to test it for a week after my four months on the diet to make sure it wasn't a trigger for me. I sometimes make my own pâté after a chef friend showed me how to cook liver properly.

I also make chicken stock from any chicken bones we have, tossing them in a zip-top bag in the freezer. When I'm ready, I buy a pound of chicken feet from the organic grocery store. While they look gross (I try not to focus on it while dealing with them), they make unbelievably rich, delicious stock that's full of collagen—excellent for migraine brains. Some stores now sell chicken backs and wing tips for making stock. (I'm told that if you have ever eaten soup in a Chinese or Thai restaurant, you have unknowingly had chicken feet, as it's a standard ingredient in most Asian soup bases.) One research team at Missouri State University has been studying the anti-inflammatory properties of chicken broth on migraine patients.[91]

①
②
③
❹
⑤
⑥
⑦
⑧

Note that some migraine trigger lists include gelatin and organ meats as triggers, likely because of the naturally high levels of glutamates they may contain. Make sure you test them for yourself.

You'll find that these meats are much cheaper than traditional cuts, so if you're adventurous and on a budget, start talking to your butcher. They are extremely knowledgeable and can help you learn to cook these meats properly. Start by buying beef heart or tongue, ask them to cut it up for you into stew meat, and add it to the slow cooker for eight hours with a bunch of vegetables.

I now order grass-fed gelatin in bulk to use in desserts and smoothies. Adding grass-fed gelatin powder to a smoothie is an easy way to begin getting these nutrients.

EGGS

Look for the Certified Humane seal on eggs, or buy from local egg producers. If you can't find that seal, "pastured" is best, followed by "free range" and "organic." "Cage-free" and "vegetarian" are fairly meaningless sales terms. Many municipalities have eased restrictions on keeping chickens; you may be able to raise them yourself if that appeals to you. Chickens are not naturally vegetarians. Pasture-raised chickens eat bugs, worms, and mice as well as vegetables, fruits, seeds, and sprouts. This varied diet adds nutrients to their eggs and meat. Purchase omega-3 eggs if you can get them, as they add this important fatty acid into the mix.

BEANS AND SEEDS

Choose organic beans and seeds whenever possible. Committed vegans will need to focus on the beans that are allowed on the Plan, supplementing with seeds, especially hemp and chia, to get enough protein. The pseudo-cereals quinoa, amaranth, and buckwheat are also high in protein; they are cooked like grains. All these foods are better for you if they are soaked for at least eight hours or overnight before cooking, as this process will eliminate or considerably reduce the amount of antinutrients (like phytates) that end up on your plate.

Once you are through the four-month period, you can test nuts one at a time to introduce more protein options back into your diet. It's not recommended to ever reintroduce soy or gluten. Be aware that soy is ubiquitous in the American diet—especially in processed and fast foods—potentially providing 10 percent of daily calories.[92]

WEEK 5
it's breakfast time!

———— ··· ————

One of the most important changes you can make, and *one of the few food-related items that all migraine experts agree upon*, is maintaining steady blood sugar levels throughout the day. The term blood sugar relates to the amount of glucose that's circulating in your blood at any given time, depending on how recently you have eaten and the types of food you ate. It's believed that peaks and crashes in blood sugar levels contribute to migraine attacks. In her book *The Migraine Brain*, Dr. Carolyn Bernstein warns that this inconsistency in blood sugar levels is something that "the migraine brain abhors."[93] In addition, eating regularly supports your adrenal glands, which are responsible for regulating stress, moods, inflammation, and hunger. After an 8- to 12-hour fast, your body needs fuel to get started. And a migraine brain needs the right fuel—that's why we're changing up breakfast this week.

① ② ③ ④ ❺ ⑥ ⑦ ⓪

WEEK 5 ASSIGNMENT: TRANSITION YOUR BREAKFASTS

———— · ————

Your Week 5 goal is to transition over to Plan foods for breakfast. If you haven't been a breakfast eater, or if you eat on the run, I'll give you some tips for how to get in the habit of starting your day with quality food, especially healthy fat and protein.

In addition to changing your breakfasts and continuing with your snacks, continue to track everything you are eating and drinking this week; track your symptoms, sodium, and steps.

BREAKFAST IDEAS

———— · ————

On-the-go breakfasts in the United States are loaded with sugar; pastries, energy bars, and blended coffee drinks are not the optimal way to start the day. High-carb meals make blood sugar levels spike and then quickly drop, which can trigger a migraine attack. Lower-carb meals that include protein and healthy fat help sustain blood sugar at a healthy level throughout the day.

DAILY TRACKING GOALS

- **Everything you eat and drink**. Do your best to eat 5 to 6 small meals (or 3 meals and 2 to 3 approved snacks) throughout the day. Have your last meal or snack three hours before bedtime if possible. Drink filtered water throughout the day.
- **Hours slept.**
- **Your symptoms.**
- **Step count**. Increase number of steps walked (via pedometer, smartphone app, or fitness device) to 7,000 per day if possible (if this feels like too much, stay at 6,000).

- **Active minutes.** Increase very active minutes to 20 per day, 2 to 3 days per week (if possible).
- **Sodium intake.** Reduce your sodium intake to 1,500 milligrams per day.
- **Caffeine intake.** Reduce your caffeine intake to half a drink (½ cup) per day, or eliminate it altogether.
- **Sugary snacks.** If you are still eating sugar at this point, reduce your intake to no more than one sugary snack *per day.*

① ② ③ ④ ❺ ⑥ ⑦ ⑧

Whole-grain gluten-free cereal, eggs, and even dinner leftovers are better bets than sugary foods for breakfast, so long as they're tweaked to follow the Plan guidelines. My husband eats eggs most days. After finding out I have a latent egg allergy (not life-threatening), I eat veggie hash for breakfast, supplemented with a protein like homemade pâté, Make Your Own Bacon (page 197), or a slice of leftover meat. Sometimes my husband adds Sunflower Seed Butter (page 195) to his plate to help him fill up. In the hot summer months when I prefer cold food, I make a green smoothie with coconut milk, coconut oil, ginger, turmeric, lightly cooked mild greens, and a small amount of fruit.

On the weekends I'll make something special like low-carb waffles with sausage patties or a Dutch baby with berries and whipped cream. We often have one slice each of Paleo bacon: uncured, low in sugar, and not too high in sodium. This type of bacon can be tested once you've completed your four months on the Plan, or you can Make Your Own Bacon. Here are some easy breakfast ideas:

- **EGG MINI-QUICHES (PAGE 202)**. Make and freeze on Sunday, heat in microwave for breakfast.

- **CREPES (PAGE 200).** Make crepes on the weekend, freeze, heat in microwave. Top with ricotta cream and berries.

- **BLUEBERRY-OAT WAFFLES (PAGE 198).** Freeze extras, use toaster to reheat. Top with Sunflower Seed Butter (page 195), berries, and butter, but skip the syrup.

- **POACHED EGGS.** Serve with spinach or kale and hot sauce.

- **STEEL-CUT OR ROLLED OATS.** Serve with berries, coconut, or whole milk; cinnamon; nutmeg; and stevia, if you like.

- **SCRAMBLED EGGS** with hot sauce.

- **VEGGIE FRITTATA (PAGE 204).** This is an excellent way to use up extra veggies from the day before.

- **MIGAS (PAGE 206).** Serve with eggs and onion-free **SALSA VERDE (PAGE 274).** This is a great way to use up corn tortillas.

- **SALMON, ASPARAGUS, AND THYME OMELET (PAGE 209).**

- **SMOOTHIES.** Make sure they include some protein from maca powder, chia seeds, sunflower seeds, flax seeds, or milk.

- **DINNER LEFTOVERS.** You'll have plenty of these once you are eating dinner on the Plan.

① ② ③ ④ **❺** ⑥ ⑦ ⑧

For more ideas and recipes, check out the Breakfast chapter on page 196.

WHY GET RID OF SUGAR?

Just like with salt, the standard American diet is sky-high in added sugar. Sugar is added to nearly every processed food in some form or other. That's because the brilliant food scientists who design those foods know that the combination of sweet/salty/fat creates a documented addictive quality to those foods. Sugar lights up the same pleasure center in the brain that heroin does; it's not your imagination that you crave it! Sugar spikes dopamine release, changes dopamine receptors, and excites reward pathways in the brain.[94] While it's not yet known how this might be related to migraine attacks, anything that causes the brain to be over active is likely not ideal for us.

Our bodies aren't designed to handle the enormous quantities of sugar found in the Western diet, and too much sugar causes glycation, the bonding of sugar molecules to proteins, fats, and amino acids. This process forms the AGEs (glycation end products) that are responsible for premature aging and implicated in Alzheimer's disease.[95] Additionally, sugar is inflammatory and causes you to gain weight.

So can I use artificial sweetener instead?

I don't recommend artificial sweeteners and here's why. Aspartame (sold as NutraSweet, Equal, and Spoonful) is a peptide (a string of amino acids) made up of phenylalanine and aspartic acid. Both are known excitotoxins, meaning they cause neurons to fire and become overexcited. Phenylalanine is a precursor to norepinephrine and may throw off the ratio of this important neurotransmitter. Aspartame includes a third component: a methyl-ester group that easily detaches and becomes methyl alcohol (wood alcohol). Methyl alcohol is poisonous if consumed, as it breaks down into formaldehyde in the liver. Not only can these substances cause panic symptoms, mood disorders, and alter seizure thresholds, but some studies also link aspartame intake to increased rates of brain cancer.[96]

And there are problems with other artificial sweeteners like saccharin. Recent studies have shown that artificial sweeteners affect the microbial balance in the digestive tract, making it possible we will absorb (and possibly store) more calories from the food we eat, shifting our weight set point higher, and triggering more hunger.[97] Research continues; there also seems to be a link between artificial sweeteners (even stevia) and higher levels of obesity and diabetes.[98] All white powder—even organic stevia—has been processed, separated from all its original plant-based nutrients, leaving only the sweetness behind.

In this Plan, I recommend using only organic stevia and in very small quantities, not every day. I use natural sugars in very small quantities in just a few recipes to achieve specific flavors. Once you get used to whole foods that aren't hiked up with added sugar, you'll find plenty of sweetness in all fruits and in vegetables like carrots, beets, sweet potatoes, and tomatoes.

If your reaction to the last sentence is, "This woman is insane!" then consider this: I would have fully agreed with you 10 years ago when I was still eating a ton of sugar—including processed foods and candy—every day. Once I got off those foods, I began to truly enjoy the sweetness naturally found in fruits and vegetables. If you are allergic or sensitive to stevia, use small amounts of coconut sugar in its place. I talk more about the sweetness level of stevia on page 298.

When you give up sugar—and foods that easily turn into sugar, such as flour, potatoes, and beer—there are lots of ways your body needs to adjust. First, you will
miss the sweets. You might have a few rough days of feeling angry, cranky, and
exhausted. And you'll need to find other foods to fill that gap.

Another invisible thing might happen internally. If you're like me and you ate a
lot of sweets, your body could have an overgrowth of yeast called Candida albicans.
Candida is naturally a part of our bodies, but given the right conditions, it can multiply if fed lots of sugar. Candida can cause headaches, itchy skin rashes, vaginal
yeast infections, fungal infections, and mouth problems. Everyone's internal biome
is different, and some people may be more prone to this overgrowth than others.
An overgrowth of Candida is believed to be the cause of leaky gut syndrome, as
the structure of the growing yeast widens the tight gap junctions inside the gut (see
page 80). This allows tiny particles of food to end up in your bloodstream, causing
any number of inflammatory problems, including in the brain.

Sugar feeds Candida, so when you pull it out of your diet, the Candida begin
to die off in large numbers, releasing mycotoxins such as alcohol and acetaldehyde.
While this die-off, known as a healing crisis or the Jarisch-Herxheimer reaction,
is a good thing for you overall, it can feel horrible while it's happening. You may
feel like you have the flu, you might develop a headache, and your joints can ache.
Symptoms usually resolve within a week.[99]

If this happens to you, know that the feelings are normal, they will go away, and
that you're doing a wonderful thing for your body.

—Ricki Heller, PhD, RHN, author of *Living Candida-Free: Conquer the Hidden
Epidemic that's Making You Sick*

① ② ③ ④ **5** ⑥ ⑦ ⑧

WEEK 6
pack a lunch!

———— ··· ————

One of my earliest memories from my preschool days is my mom making me lunch: grilled Velveeta cheese on Wonder Bread and Campbell's tomato soup. I loved those flavors and my time with Mom when the older kids weren't home. While that's not something I would eat today, I still love a good lunch. Since my husband and I both work from home now, lunch is often big salads with a protein like tuna or chicken or reheated leftovers from the night before. After lunch we take Daisy, our dog, for a short walk. For the many years I worked in an office, lunch was brought-from-home leftovers or sometimes a big salad. Eating out was a treat, both for budgetary reasons and also because back then restaurant food wasn't all that healthy. Now there are many more healthy options for eating out when you need or want to, which I'll cover in detail in Week 8 (page 93). For now, this section will focus on your midday meal.

Lunch is also the perfect time to take a break midday, set aside your work, and be present with your meal. Turn off your phone, get away from your desk, and truly have a rest, even if only for 10 or 15 minutes. Doing so will not only refresh you, but will help you digest your food better. In this section, I also discuss the benefits of mindful eating.

WEEK 6 ASSIGNMENT: TRANSITION TO PLAN-APPROVED LUNCHES

———— · ————

At this point in the Plan you've greatly cut back on your sodium, sugar, and caffeine intake. You're eating more regularly throughout the day. You're getting regular gentle movement. All your snacks and breakfasts are on the Plan. Your Week 6 goal is to transition your lunches over to the Plan, joining your breakfasts and snacks. Continue to track everything you are eating and drinking this week; track your symptoms, sodium, and steps.

LUNCH IDEAS

———— · ————

Make sandwiches open-faced to reduce carbohydrate intake. If you still feel hungry, double up the protein instead of the bread. If you have a toaster at work, toast bread right

DAILY TRACKING GOALS

- **Everything you eat and drink.** Do your best to eat 5 to 6 small meals (or 3 meals and 2 to 3 approved snacks) throughout the day. Have your last meal or snack three hours before bedtime if possible. Drink water throughout the day.

- **Hours slept.** Start going to bed at the same time each night (even weekends).

- **Your symptoms.**

- **Step count.** Increase number of steps walked (via pedometer, smartphone app, or fitness device) if possible to 8,000 per day (or stay at 7,000).

- **Active minutes.** Increase your very active minutes to 25 per day, 2 to 3 days per week (if possible, or stay at 15 to 20 minutes on those days).

- **Sodium intake.** Reduce your sodium intake to 1,200 milligrams per day if you have dizziness, vertigo, or Meniere's disease. If not, stay at around 1,500 milligrams per day for another week and see how you feel.

- **Caffeine intake.** No caffeine this week! You won't be needing it anymore.

- **Sugary snacks.** If you are still eating sugar at this point, reduce intake to one sugary snack *per week*.

① ② ③ ④ ⑤ **❻** ⑦ ⑧

before eating, then make your sandwich. Pile on the veggies: lettuce, spring mix, tomatoes, red peppers. You can also use plain homemade gluten-free waffles as bread. Below are some of my favorite lunch options, but you'll find even more ideas and the recipes in Part V (page 210).

- **ROASTED LOW-SODIUM TURKEY BREAST ROLLUPS.** My Cilantro Mayonnaise (page 268) is great on these.

- **CHICKEN OR TURKEY SALAD (PAGE 211).**

- **TUNA OR SALMON SALAD (PAGE 223).**

- **CRAB OR SHRIMP SALAD.** Eat homemade only, using unbrined seafood. Mock crab contains gluten, sugar, and salt, and usually MSG or other triggers. Note that even untreated crab and shrimp are both naturally high in sodium.

- **SUNFLOWER SEED BUTTER (PAGE 195) SANDWICH**. Thickly spread the Sunflower Seed Butter on gluten-free bread with a bit of fruit-only berry jam.

- **GRILLED BURGER**. Use grass-fed beef if available. Omit the bun, but add mayo, lettuce, and tomato, if desired.

- **LOW-SODIUM SOUP**. All ingredients should be on the approved list. You'll find several hearty soup recipes in the Lunch chapter of Part V (page 210); most can be frozen in 1-cup containers and heated up for lunch.

- **FISH TACOS (PAGE 214)** or **SLOPPY JOES (PAGE 216)**.

HOW I LEARNED TO STOP SHOVELING AND START CHEWING

In the past, eating was all about enjoyment. Make or order something delicious, then cram it into my mouth as fast as possible. I would chew each bite three times at most: whatever was the smallest possible number of chomps before I could swallow the food without choking. My fork hovered near my lips, ready to deliver another bite as fast as possible.

I would frequently be stuffed full before I realized how much I had eaten. I had little to no idea about what was happening once the food got to my stomach. I gave it no thought. If I got a stomachache, I would take Pepto-Bismol. Despite my knowledge of nutrition and food, that's the extent of my self-awareness about this critical part of my daily life.

In doing the literature review for this book, I read chapter after chapter about digestion, thousands of words on the subject. It turns out I knew little about this critical process that happens inside me five or six times a day! The more I read, the more amazed I was at the miracle that is our digestive tract.

Improving your digestion is even more important if you have migraine attacks. Digestive issues are common. Migraine patients can also have IBS, or at least digestive distress during the premonitory phase. Researchers have found that while half of migraine patients in a large study had symptoms of acid reflux or heartburn, only 22 percent of them had been formally diagnosed with gastroesophageal reflux disease (GERD).[100] Acid reflux (GERD) involves malfunctions in the ring of muscles at the base of your esophagus; either the ring relaxes and allows stomach acid to back up into the esophagus, or the ring opens too frequently.

WHAT TO EAT DURING A MIGRAINE ATTACK

This book teaches you how to eat overall. But what about when you're actually having a migraine attack? What then? Just like you probably have a little kit of meds you carry with you, having these foods in the cupboard and freezer will help nourish you during a migraine attack when you feel lousy and aren't able to cook much. They're also simple for someone else to cook for you. Focus on soft, well-cooked, bland foods, which are especially easy to digest.

- Simmer low-sodium (onion-free) chicken stock with white or Arborio rice or gluten-free noodles. If you're up to the task, grate in some carrot and cook until everything is soft. If you have shredded chicken in the freezer, add it too. You can also add jars of baby food like sweet potatoes or carrots for precooked nutrition.

- Microwave white or sweet potatoes; eat with plenty of butter, ghee, or coconut oil.

- Cook gluten-free rolled oats or steel-cut oats with coconut milk or Hemp Milk (page 255).

- Toast gluten-free waffles from the freezer; eat with butter and fruit-only jam.

- Stir cinnamon into unsweetened applesauce.

- Spread gluten-free toast with butter and sprinkle cinnamon on top.

- Brew ginger or mint tea to help with nausea.

- Heat soups from the freezer.

Stay away from strong-smelling foods like bacon and fish, even if you have tested them, as the odors might cause nausea. Don't worry about eating a "balanced" diet; just get warm, comforting food into your tummy until you feel better.

① ② ③ ④ ⑤ ❻ ⑦ ⑧

How chewing aids digestion, and other wonders of your amazing digestive tract

Think of your digestive tract as a 30-foot-long, incredibly smart, living garden hose. While it's shaped like a garden hose, it's not inert like one; it has its own brain, musculature to move food along, and the ability to churn out highly potent chemicals like hydrochloric acid to break down food. It has the same taste and smell receptors found in your mouth, in addition to sensors for fat, protein, bacteria, hormones, and plant compounds.[101] About 70 to 80 percent of your entire immune system is in your gut.[102] Anywhere from a few hundred to a few thousand species of microbes live and work there.[103] There may be as many as 100 trillion bacteria working in your gut right now.[104]

Ideally, the food stays within the hose throughout its journey, being broken down into bits of nutrients small enough to be readily absorbed by the cells in the wall of the small intestine.

When you take a bite of food, the act of chewing that food begins a complex chemical process. Your mouth begins to secrete saliva, which mixes with the food particles, helping to moisten and break them down. That critical saliva signal tells the stomach that food is coming; digestive chemicals are excreted into the stomach to make ready for the food. If you only chew a bite three times or, in the case of a smoothie, not at all, you have very few digestive enzymes ready for the food when it arrives.

Once in the stomach, the food is mixed with the enzymes and chemicals and churned around through muscle movement. It doesn't stay in the stomach long, but passes into the small intestine where it is broken down into small particles. If you chew that bite of carrot just three times as I used to, it's in chunks that may be too large to get broken down at all. Your body may not be able to pull any nutrients out of those chunks before it passes into the large intestine as part of the waste process.

The truly miraculous stuff happens in the small intestine, which has smart cells that communicate directly with your brain. The science-y term for this is the "gut-brain axis," and it's a burgeoning field of research.

The critical lining of your small intestine is only one cell thick. These cells are aligned like tiles in a floor, with a "grout" made up of a network of proteins.[105] When healthy, this alignment is called the "tight-gap junction." If you regularly eat food that your body has trouble digesting, or if there is other damage to the lining of your small intestine because of illness, food sensitivities, or celiac disease, gaps in the "grout" can become wide enough to allow larger particles of food and other toxins to pass through. You may have heard of this: leaky gut syndrome.

Leaky gut generates even more inflammation when the body reacts to those errant food particles and toxins in the bloodstream as if they are viral invaders. According to Dr. David Perlmutter, leaky gut doesn't just affect the gut, but it may also affect the blood-brain barrier. This critical barrier in brain health becomes more permeable (leaky) in response to gliadin, one of the proteins found in wheat.[106]

The small intestine is where migraine triggers like tyramine or MSG can start a chemical chain reaction that ends up affecting the brain.

The large intestine is just as important, as that's where the majority of your good gut bacteria are found. These bacteria aid digestion and sleep, help absorb nutrients, help stop viral invaders, neutralize toxins found in food, control your immune system, create neurotransmitters, and help you handle stress and inflammation.[107] That's why gut health researchers recommend eating tons of vegetables, fruit, and foods high in prebiotic fiber to feed these key microbes, while reducing your intake of sugar, starch and highly processed foods.[108]

No more shoveling

Now that I understand what is actually happening when I eat, I spend far more time chewing. I am regularly the last person finished at the table, sometimes by 10 or more minutes. If you're not used to eating quite this slowly, count 10 chews or wait until the food is pulverized and you can't effectively chew it any more. Then swallow.

If you're used to drinking lots of water or other beverages at meals, sip only enough liquid to help you swallow. Otherwise you dilute your stomach's ability to begin digesting. If you like to drink big glasses of water, have one 15 minutes before eating, so that your stomach can empty it before the food arrives. Ideally, wait two hours after a meal to drink another large glass.

When I make a smoothie, I "chew" each slurp a few times before swallowing, making sure I feel the saliva in my mouth. It seems wacky, but I have not gotten a stomachache from a green smoothie since starting this practice.

I find that if I'm in a hurry, I can eat breakfast way too fast. And when I used to eat lunch at my desk, I barely chewed at all. I'm great at remembering to chew at the dinner table. To help train myself, I have learned to put my fork down in between bites.

Adding this mindfulness practice helps me be more present at meals, appreciate the food, and recognize when I'm full, and it might also help with weight loss if that's a goal for you. Experiment with eating more mindfully this week and see what you notice.

A *closer look at*: mindful eating

One way to improve digestion, slow down, and get more benefits from your food is to practice mindful eating. When you practice mindful eating, you focus on every aspect of the meal and eating experience. Here are some tips:

- When you sit down to eat, look at your plate. Really look at it. Appreciate the bounty of each item on the plate.

- Thank all the people, animals, and plants whose energy is represented on your plate.

- Picture the food on your plate wanting what is best for you, wanting to heal you, surrounding you with love and positive energy.

- Put your fork down between bites.

- Chew each mouthful thoroughly. Chewing is incredibly important. The more you chew, the more saliva you produce, signaling your stomach to have the correct amount of gastric juices available to begin breaking down the food. The longer food stays in your mouth, the easier digestion is, making it more likely you will absorb the most nutrients from your food. Take your time, really chew everything.

- If you find that you normally eat lunch at your desk and it's impossible to eat mindfully there, try escaping from your desk at least one day a week and eating lunch somewhere quieter, even just for 10 minutes.

WEEK 7
dinner makeover

———— ••• ————

If there is one meal a day that you can share with loved ones, try and make it dinner. Having the chance to sit down, turn off screens, enjoy food slowly, and talk about your day is refreshing for body and soul. If you live alone, you can still have a Skype meal with a loved one or friend. It strengthens family bonds, improves digestion, and helps you slow down and prepare for sleep. If you're interested in learning more, check out the #SundaySupper or Slow Food movements for more information.

Our dinnertime depends on the time of year, as we have a sundown ritual at the dog park. We walk our golden retriever, Daisy, over to the local school. I sit on the grass. I leave my phone at home. She fetches the ball. My husband and I talk about our days. When sundown is early, we have dinner after our park time. During the summer months, we have dinner beforehand on our front patio, which also helps us stay connected with our neighbors. However you can make a ritual of dinner, do so. When I was single I always used my nice dishes, lit a candle, and set the table, even though I was eating alone.

After this week, you will officially be eating all of your meals on the Plan. Transitioning dinners might take a while, since this meal is often more complex and social than breakfast or lunch. If you don't get dinner totally transitioned this week, continue to experiment with it. In this section, I also give you advice for a smoother transition and tips for cooking in bulk that should help make dinners easier.

WEEK 7 ASSIGNMENT: TRANSITION TO PLAN-APPROVED DINNERS

———— • ————

Dinner is the last meal to switch over. As of this week, your food is officially trigger-free! You have an optional goal of doing some bulk cooking this week or in the weeks ahead, so you can add soups and stews to your freezer for quick lunches and dinners. Find recipes on page 224. You'll be maintaining this eating plan for the next four months. You can enjoy leftovers from any lunch or dinner for breakfast as well. Continue to track everything you are eating and drinking this week; track your symptoms, sodium, and steps.

DAILY TRACKING GOALS

- **Everything you eat and drink.** Do your best to eat 5 to 6 small meals (or 3 meals and 2 to 3 approved snacks) throughout the day. Have your last meal or snack three hours before bedtime if possible. Drink water throughout the day.
- **Hours slept.** Start getting up at the same time each morning (even weekends).
- **Your symptoms.**
- **Your steps.** Increase number of steps walked (via pedometer, smartphone app, or fitness device) to 9,000 per day, or 500 more than last week.

- **Active minutes.** Increase very active minutes to 30 per day, or stay at last week's level (2 to 3 days per week).
- **Sodium intake.** Reduce your sodium intake to 1,000 milligrams per day if you have dizziness, vertigo, or Meniere's disease. Stay at 1,000 milligrams per day for a few months to see if your symptoms improve. If not, stay at around 1,500 milligrams per day and see how you feel.
- **Sugary snacks.** This is the week to say farewell to sugar, at least for a few months.

① ② ③ ④ ⑤ ⑥ **❼** ⑧

DINNER IDEAS

Dinner is where I tend to either get more creative or eat tried-and-true favorites. I often do bulk cooking on the weekends to make dinner easier. My biggest challenge is remembering to pull out meat or fish from the freezer so it's thawed in time for dinner. While I don't do weekly menu planning, many people find it helpful. I try to have ground turkey in the freezer at all times, since I can cook a one-dish meal quickly by adding spices and pre-prepped veggies from the fridge or freezer. Pasta or rice dishes also work well. If I'm really slammed, I pick up a pastured rotisserie chicken (I can order them without salt) from a natural foods market and serve it with a salad and maybe some pressure-cooked potatoes. Below are some of my favorite dinner options, but you'll find even more ideas and the recipes on page 224.

- **STEAK AND ROASTED VEGETABLE SALAD (PAGE 244).**

- **CHICKEN CACCIATORE (PAGE 226).**

- **FISH BAKED IN PARCHMENT PACKETS (PAGE 228)**.

- Grilled burgers with side salads.

- Hearty stews or soups with gluten-free bread and grass-fed butter, like **SPICY KALE AND SPLIT PEA SOUP (PAGE 220)** or **FIREHOUSE TURKEY CHILI (PAGE 213)**.

- **PASTA WITH VODKA CHICKPEA SAUCE (PAGE 232)** or **PASTA WITH VEGETABLES (PAGE 282)**.

COOKING IN BULK

If you're unfamiliar with cooking, or if you live alone or have a small family, you might not consider cooking in bulk. This simply means making big pots of food and freezing it in individual portions. While I only cook for two people, I normally make at least six or eight portions of anything. Why cook three days in a row? In the winter I might make two large pots of soup, stew, or chili, and then freeze most of it in glass containers for eating later. When you do this regularly, you end up with a freezer full of "frozen dinners" that are high quality, migraine friendly, made to order, and ready to grab. Pack a frozen dinner in your lunch bag, let it thaw during your morning work, and it's ready to microwave for lunch. Pull out a different meal each day to thaw in the fridge so you have a steady supply of dinners that can be heated up when you get home from work. Throw a bunch of ingredients in the slow cooker and arrive home from work to a hot meal.

How and when to freeze fresh foods

When you make soup or stews for dinner, freeze the extra portions in single servings to have on hand for lunches. Your freezer can also help reduce food waste. If you realize you aren't going to eat fresh items in time, freeze them for later use. This is where doing an inventory before going to the grocery store comes in handy, so you only buy what you'll need this week. Unless noted, place cut fruits and vegetables on a baking sheet lined with parchment paper, waxed paper, or a silicone mat. Leave space between each piece and freeze until firm. Then transfer the frozen produce to a labeled zip-top freezer bag.

APPLES: Freezing is not recommended. Cut into ¼-inch dice and use in place of blueberries in Blueberry–Oat Waffles (page 198) or in gluten-free pancakes. Or sauté with butter, cinnamon, and a little coconut or maple sugar and use as a filling for Crepes (page 200). If you have one apple that's a little too soft to eat, but not moldy or spoiled, try peeling and dicing it and adding it to the Breakfast Hash recipe (page 281).

ARUGULA: Use this green in smoothies if it's not too peppery. Blend leftover arugula into a pesto sauce. Freeze the leaves in the bag they come in, closed with a clip or rubber band.

AVOCADO: Freeze cut chunks, then use in smoothies. (Avocados are not on the Plan, but hopefully you will find you can eat them once you've tested them. They're an excellent source of healthy monounsaturated fat.)

BANANAS: Freeze cut chunks, then use in smoothies. (Bananas are not on the Plan, but hopefully you will find you can eat them once you've tested them. While they are a high-sugar fruit, they add creamy texture to smoothies, become quick "ice cream" in a high-speed blender, and are an excellent source of potassium.)

BEET GREENS, KALE, OR OTHER GREENS: Completely dry the greens, roughly chop, then freeze. Add to boiling pasta water, stir-fry dishes, soup, or chili, or use them in Spicy Kale and Swiss Chard Sauté (page 243), straight from the freezer.

BELL PEPPERS: Roast bell peppers when they are starting to get wrinkly but not yet moldy. Use them in Roasted Chile Pepper Hummus (page 190). Add sliced roasted peppers to blender soup, chili, pasta sauce, or tacos. Or freeze raw pepper slices and add to stir-fry dishes.

BERRIES: Freeze whole, then use in smoothies. Halve or quarter large strawberries to make blending easier.

BROCCOLI: Freeze florets in chunks. Peel the stem, then slice and freeze it, too. Use in stir-fry dishes or soup.

CAULIFLOWER: Freeze florets and slices of the stem, but remove the core and leaves. Use in stir-fry dishes, soup, or curry.

CELERY: Wash, dry, and thinly slice. Freeze in 1-cup containers and sauté as the base for stir-fry dishes, chili, stew, or soup.

CUCUMBER: Freezing not recommended, but these juice well. Leave skin on unless very waxy or conventionally grown.

GREEN ONIONS AND LEEKS: Scrub roots well. Add root ends plus dark green leek tops to your freezer bag for making stock. If outer leaves have gone bad, pull off and compost, then cook the rest up immediately. If they are in danger of going bad or if you're going out of town, thinly slice and freeze the leeks in 1-cup containers. Then sauté as the base for most sauces, add to chili or soup, or use for making stock.

JICAMA: Freezing is not recommended, but these juice well.

LETTUCE: While I don't recommend freezing lettuce, if you have beautiful organic lettuce that would otherwise go to waste, you can freeze it in the bag and add it to green smoothies straight from the freezer.

ZUCCHINI: Freeze in chunks. Use in spaghetti sauce or stir-fry dishes.

SPEEDY COOKING TECHNIQUES FOR LEFTOVERS AND VEGETABLES

Another way to make a quick dinner is to utilize leftovers and produce. There's always something you can do with a half-full container of ricotta cheese or those vegetables you bought. If you're new to cooking, one challenge is using up all the ingredients you buy. Here are some ways to solve that:

AUTUMN SQUASH (acorn, butternut, kabocha, pumpkin, spaghetti): Wipe clean. Place in a slow cooker on low for 8 hours. Remove and let cool enough to handle. Cut in half. Discard the seeds. Scoop out cooked flesh to use in soup, or serve with a healthy fat, sea salt, and black pepper.

BEETS AND BEET GREENS: If you buy beets with the tops on, you get a second vegetable for free, but only if you handle them properly, as they spoil easily. I buy whole beets only when I have time to handle them as soon as I get home:

Greens: Slice off the tops just above the beet. Wash the tops, then spin dry like lettuce. Roll up in a clean kitchen towel, then store in a plastic bag in the fridge. Cook that night or within two to three days; try the Spicy Kale and Swiss Chard Sauté (page 243), or use them in Breakfast Hash (page 281).

① ② ③ ④ ⑤ ⑥ ❼ ⑧

Beets: Scrub the beets well, let air-dry. Store in the fridge in a plastic bag. Ideally, steam, pressure cook, or roast them within two or three days. Cooked beets can be added to salads, smoothies, or sliced on a plate and drizzled with good olive oil as a side with dinner. Freeze cooked beets in chunks for smoothies.

CHEESE: Blend cottage cheese into Quick Alfredo-Style Pasta Sauce (page 271). Small amounts of Herbed Cheese Spread (page 189), ricotta, or cottage cheese can be whisked into Quiche (page 285) or Frittata (page 280) mixtures. Sweeten leftover mascarpone with vanilla, cinnamon, and stevia, thin with whole milk or coconut milk, and serve as a dip for fruit.

CURRY PASTE AND SEED OR NUT BUTTERS: If you have a small amount of any of these items left in a jar, you have the makings of a sauce for a Rice Bowl (page 286). Just add some warm filtered water to thin it. Shake well. Add coconut milk, dark toasted sesame seed oil, minced garlic, and minced fresh ginger. Shake again. Pour over warm brown rice, chopped meat or beans, and sautéed or steamed veggies. (Note that nuts may be a migraine trigger.)

FRESH HERBS: You buy a bundle of basil, parsley, or cilantro for a recipe. But the recipe *never* uses all of it. What to do? Start by storing them properly. Trim off the bottom of the herb bundle when you buy it. Store like cut flowers in a stubby glass, and change the water daily. Or, wash, shake dry, roll up in a clean kitchen towel, and store in a plastic bag in the fridge. (It's easier to forget them if they are stored this way though.) Most herbs make lovely infused water; use organic herbs only. Or toss the herbs in a food processor, stems included, with olive oil, garlic, a touch of vinegar, and sunflower or pumpkin seeds. You now have a bright sauce for meat or fish, or to rub over a whole chicken before roasting. If it makes a lot, freeze in ice cube trays and add a cube to hot pasta, or thaw for a meat sauce. Mildly flavored herbs can go into smoothies. I added two sprigs of cilantro to a strawberry smoothie once and it was weirdly amazing. Thyme, fennel, and parsley can be tossed in a zip-top freezer bag along with leftover bones to make stock.

MUSTARD, HONEY, JAM, OR MAYONNAISE: If you have a small amount left at the bottom of a jar, you have the makings of a salad dressing, sauce, or marinade. Just add some olive oil, one teaspoon of white vinegar, a little bit of warm filtered water, and minced fresh herbs if you have them. Shake well and taste. Add ¼ teaspoon of garlic powder if desired.

OLIVE OIL: Since I buy pricey extra virgin olive oil, I want to use every drop. I turn the empty bottle upside down onto a frying pan overnight. There's usually enough for a sauté. If I have to measure olive oil for a recipe, I capture the remaining oil from the measuring cup in a cold sauté pan for my next use.

OVERCOOKED VEGETABLES: Blend into Creamy Soup (page 288).

POTATOES AND SWEET POTATOES: Wash and dry. Wrap individually in foil and place in the slow cooker on low for 8 hours. Baked potatoes for breakfast or dinner!

TORTILLA CHIPS: Crunch up and make Migas (page 206), or toast in an omelet pan and then cook with scrambled eggs.

TAKEOUT: If you have a full serving left, eat that for your breakfast or lunch. If we have enough leftovers for a full meal for both of us, I will freeze that as a future meal, especially if we have a trip coming up. I appreciate finding that in the freezer when coming home from travel. Here are some ideas to use up small amounts of leftovers that usually end up in the trash:

Burgers: Chop up, sauté for Breakfast Hash (page 281) or a Frittata (pages 204 and 280). (I will often bring half a grass-fed burger home from a restaurant to use as protein in another meal.)

Fish: Flake the fish and use in the Tuna or Salmon Salad (page 223). Or, use to make Patties (page 283) or the Salmon, Asparagus, and Thyme Omelet (page 209).

French fries or cooked potatoes: Cut into a ¼-inch dice. Sauté in a small amount of oil or rendered bacon fat to make Breakfast Hash.

Polenta: Cut into ½-inch dice. Sauté in a small amount of oil or rendered bacon fat to make Breakfast Hash.

Salsa: Use in Migas or pour over a cooked Denver Omelet (page 201).

Steak, pork chops, or chicken: Cut into ½-inch dice. Use in the base recipes for Quiche (page 285), Breakfast Hash, Chopped Salad (page 287), or a Frittata. Or stir into Creamy Soup once it's cooked.

Steamed rice: Use leftover rice as the base for a Rice Bowl (page 286). Rehydrate in a steamer or microwave, covered, with a little water in the bowl. Dried-out cooked rice is perfect for making fried rice. Use small amounts of leftover cooked rice to thicken blended veggie soup, or stir into a pot of chili or chicken soup. Warm rice with enough coconut milk to make Rice Pudding (page 262), flavoring with vanilla extract, cinnamon, and nutmeg.

Asian food: Enhance scrambled eggs or fill a Frittata with small amounts of noodle or rice dishes.

Deli foods: Toss deli salads into Chopped Salad. Rinse leftover coleslaw, drain well, and add to Breakfast Hash.

Indian food: Blend leftover curry with cooked vegetables and coconut milk for beautiful Creamy Soup.

Mexican food: Add rice and beans to a Frittata. Sauté some fresh vegetables like greens, bell peppers, and green onion, heat tortillas, and use them to fill tacos. Chop tamales and sauté (with or without chopped bacon) for Breakfast Hash.

Flavor profiles

As you're practicing your speedy cooking techniques, this chart will get you started with experimenting in the kitchen. As you get more comfortable with cooking, it will be super-helpful for the Leftovers recipes (page 279).

Cuisine	Seasoning blend	Cooking fat
Italian	Italian: oregano, Italian parsley, basil, rosemary	Extra virgin olive oil
French	Herbes de Provence: tarragon, savory, thyme, lavender, shallots	Extra virgin olive oil or butter
Mexican	Chili powder: cilantro, green onions, cumin, garlic, peppers	Grapeseed oil, mild olive oil, or grass-fed lard
Asian	Thai curry paste: mint, basil, cilantro, ginger, garlic, shallots, lemongrass	Coconut oil or sesame oil
Indian	Curry powder and garam masala: cumin, coriander, fennel, saffron	Coconut oil or ghee

For detailed information on how to choose flavors that go well together, I recommend *The Flavor Bible* by Andrew Page and Karen Dornenburg.

A closer look at: reducing food waste

Reading Kathleen Flinn's *The Kitchen Counter Cooking School* inspired me to think more deeply about leftover food and reducing food waste. When you start buying organic produce, pastured meat, and gluten-free grains, the investment adds up quickly. The last thing you want is for any of that beautiful food to spoil.

According to Flinn, we waste 40 percent of the food we produce as a country, and about 30 percent of what we bring home. This equals about 20 pounds of food per person each month.[109] If you spend $100 on groceries in a week, you are essentially *setting fire to $30 every week*. Thirty dollars is a lot of money to me!

Not only is this an issue for our budgets, but it also affects the planet. Most of that unusable food ends up in landfills, where it's estimated that it contributes 20 percent of US methane gas emissions (from rotting food in landfills).[110] Those greenhouse gases are contributing to global climate change.

If you save $30 for every hundred you spend, you could use that money (without spending any more) to buy organic produce and pastured meats. It's like magic!

Here are some tips from my own experience and from Flinn's book:

- **BUY IN SMALL QUANTITIES, ESPECIALLY PRODUCE.** While it seems like you're saving money by buying enormous amounts of items at a warehouse store, you're much less likely to eat up perishables in time. Even canned or frozen items can pile up or spoil.

- **DO AN INVENTORY OF THE FREEZER AND FRIDGE BEFORE GOING TO THE STORE.**

- **PLAN OUT YOUR RECIPES FOR TWO TO THREE DAYS, AND SHOP JUST FOR THOSE.** Search out recipes specifically to use what's in your fridge. This also keeps your items fresher and reduces the likelihood of tyramine build-up.

- **CHOOSE ONLY ONE NEW RECIPE PER WEEK THAT REQUIRES SPECIALTY INGREDIENTS.** Then figure out how to use those up before trying another recipe.

- **ONE DAY A WEEK, MAKE UP A RECIPE FROM WHAT YOU ALREADY HAVE.**
  Check your refrigerator, freezer, and pantry for ingredients. Refer to the
  Recipes That Use Leftovers section (page 279) as inspiration.

- **DON'T GO TO THE STORE UNTIL YOUR FRIDGE IS NEARLY EMPTY.**

- **IF YOU JUST CAN'T SHOP MORE OFTEN, SPEND AN HOUR ON THE WEEK-
  ENDS PREPPING AND FREEZING VEGETABLES.** This will make cooking
  much faster, too.

If you have a few random ingredients you don't know what to do with, go to
my website, RecipeRenovator.com. In the Recipe Index, type in your ingredients,
and choose Migraine Diet as the category. See if I have a recipe that will work with
what you have.

①
②
③
④
⑤
⑥
❼
⑧

WEEK 8
eating out

———— ... ————

As I found out during one anniversary dinner, eating out can be a challenge. But that doesn't mean you can't do it! This week, I'll give you some ideas for types of restaurants to try and those to avoid. I eat out all the time. I eat in airports. I attend food events. I have meals with friends. I eat at people's houses. With some meals I am more successful at being migraine-friendly than with others, but I learn each time what works better for me. This Plan isn't about you having to stay home and cook 100 percent of your meals. Who wants to do that? I don't. It's about learning what works for you, learning to plan, doing your homework, and making the best choices possible on an ongoing basis. And last, it's about enjoying being out at new places, having meals with family and friends, and trying new things without stressing out about it. It's not the end of the world if you eat a potential trigger food. If you are successful at raising your threshold by living a migraine-friendly lifestyle, you should be able to have trigger foods occasionally, enjoy them, and not suffer because of it. Savor those meals, savor time with friends, savor new experiences.

① ② ③ ④ ⑤ ⑥ ⑦ **8**

WEEK 8 ASSIGNMENT: EAT AT A RESTAURANT

———— . ————

Your Week 8 goal is to choose a restaurant or occasion to eat out, do some recon, and experiment. Go online, look at the menu, and choose something to order in advance. Experiment with asking the manager to help you with your order.

You'll continue your tracking throughout the six months of the Plan, or until you have a handle on your patterns. At this point it should be second nature, and you should be learning what foods and environmental factors trigger your headaches or migraine attacks, as well as how to take preventive measures. Once you've gone through your food testing process that begins in Month 7, you can stop tracking, unless you are tracking to prepare for a doctor's appointment.

DAILY TRACKING GOALS

- **Everything you eat and drink**. Do your best to eat 5 to 6 small meals (or 3 meals and 2 to 3 approved snacks) throughout the day. Have your last meal or snack three hours before bedtime if possible. Drink water throughout the day.

- **Hours slept**. Do your best to go to bed at the same time every night (even weekends).

- **Your symptoms**.

- **Your steps**. Increase number of steps walked (via pedometer, smartphone app, or fitness device) to 10,000 per day or a number that feels comfortable to you. Shoot for this 2 to 5 days per week. It's important to have a rest day when you need it.

- **Active minutes**. Continue very active minutes at 30 per day, 2 to 3 days per week.

- **Sodium**. Keep your sodium intake around 1,500 milligrams per day. People with Meniere's disease should try to have the level be the same each day; that seems to help reduce symptoms. You may learn that you have a sweet spot, above which you get some symptoms. Mine is between 1,200 and 1,500 milligrams.

① ② ③ ④ ⑤ ⑥ ⑦ ⑧

EATING OUT IDEAS

When it comes to eating out on the Plan, your options may seem limited, but there are usually one or two items that you can always find on a menu. One go-to option is, of course, the salad. Skip the dressing, cheese, olives, avocados, and nuts, and add grilled (no-salt-added) steak, fish, chicken, or seafood. Burgers are also a good option. See if you can order one with a lettuce wrap instead of a bun and stick with lettuce and tomato only. Note that grilled onions and mushrooms often are heavily salted (and onions are not on the Plan, because some find them to be a potent trigger). Most commercial mayos are not on the Plan, as they usually contain some form of soy or seed oils, but a primal/Paleo restaurant's mayo will be fine. Here are some of my favorite options to order at various types of restaurants:

- **MEXICAN**. Try a grilled fish taco (corn tortilla) with lettuce, cilantro, tomatoes, and cabbage only (no lime, cheese, salsa, sauce, onions, avocado). Make sure the fish is not pre-marinated; they often use lime juice. Corn tortillas are gluten-free and nearly always low in sodium.

- **SUSHI/JAPANESE**. Ask them to grill some plain fish for you, and eat it with white rice. Add a salad, if they have it, with no dressing, although sesame oil is OK.

- **ITALIAN**. Order a salad with grilled fish or meat and/or gluten-free pasta cooked without salt and finished with olive oil, garlic, parsley, and basil. If their marinara sauce is onion-free, you can ask for a small dish on the side and spoon a little on to flavor the pasta after tasting it; it's usually wicked-salty, so go easy.

- **BUFFET RESTAURANTS**. Choose from the salad bar only—lettuce, beets, tomato, chickpeas, hard-boiled eggs, carrots, celery, and cucumber (no dressing). Any meats are likely to be highly salted and possibly have MSG.

- **STEAKHOUSES**. Order grilled steak (no salt; pepper and unsalted butter or herb butter only) and a side salad (no dressing, cheese, or croutons). A good-quality steakhouse can grill vegetables with only pepper and butter or olive oil.

TIPS FOR EATING OUT

After nearly 10 years of asking for special menu items in a variety of restaurants (fast food, casual dining, fine dining, family restaurants, food trucks, and everything in between), here are my tips:

It's easier for them to **make you a special order** (a dish that's not listed on the menu) from fresh ingredients than for you to order something from the menu and request many changes to it. Restaurant kitchens are production lines. It's easy for them to mess up your order if you are ordering a salad they make 50 times a day, even if you specifically and clearly ask for five ingredient changes. Once they key in a regular menu item on their point-of-sale system, it's very easy for mistakes to get made. On the other hand, if a manager overrides the system and creates a special ticket, it's flagged for the kitchen staff.

Make sure you are working with the manager and the chef to create something special that fits your diet. Then the person making that food knows it's a special order for someone with medical dietary restrictions. Expect to pay whatever they charge; you are asking for special treatment. Here is what I say: **"Please ask the chef what he or she can** make for me that meets my special medical diet. I will be happy with whatever you bring me, and please charge me whatever is fair. I really, really appreciate it." I have found a few local places that will make things to order for me, since we eat there regularly. Any place you order from once a week wants to keep your business. Go in when they are not busy and see what you can come up with together, then drop off a typed sheet for them to use when you call in an order.

Stating that you are "on a strict diet for medical reasons" is key. Many diners have strong preferences or make special requests because they choose to be on a special diet, but you *need* this food to meet your requirements. And some people follow a gluten-free or other special diet out of preference, and then change their mind mid-meal and eat the bread in front of the server. Don't be that person; they make it harder for all of us who need servers to take our requests seriously.

Using the term "medical reasons" helps alert the staff members to make your request a priority. I have learned to start with the manager on duty and ask them to oversee my order. It may seem like you're being high maintenance, but there are fewer ways an order can get screwed up if the manager is taking ownership of your meal. The times I have relied on the busy wait staff, not wanting to "be a bother," have been the times I needed to send food back. Which is more of a bother to the restaurant: a detailed conversation or food they have to throw away? Here's what I do when I want to eat out at an unfamiliar restaurant:

- **CHECK OUT THE MENU ONLINE IN ADVANCE AND READ REVIEWS.** This often helps me determine whether I should go there at all; I can usually find one item I can have with modifications. *I nearly always arrive at a restaurant knowing what I am going to order.* Look for reviews by other diners who have mentioned how the restaurant handled special requests. Use the term "gluten-free" in your search as a starting point.

- **CALL THE RESTAURANT IN ADVANCE.** Explain why you're making a special request and ask for their help. You might get to talk to the chef, which is fun. They will thank you for calling in advance; it makes their job much easier.

- **GIVE FINE DINING RESTAURANTS ADDITIONAL ADVANCE WARNING.** If you will be eating at a fine dining restaurant, call 48 hours in advance and talk to them about your needs. Food might be prepped the day before and stocked the day before that. If they know you're coming, they are often excited at the challenge of making you something wonderful that fits your restrictions.

- **VISIT THE RESTAURANT BEFORE SOCIAL ENGAGEMENTS.** If you are embarrassed to have ordering conversations in front of family or coworkers, go to the restaurant on your own at another time. Most coworker groups have two or three favorite restaurants. Trust me, the restaurant wants your business and will try to accommodate you.

- **CHOOSE RESTAURANTS STRATEGICALLY.** Restaurants located near retirement communities are often excellent choices, as they have already reduced their sodium and are used to special requests.

- **BRING YOUR OWN SALAD DRESSING IN A LITTLE BOTTLE.** I have a small bottle of pre-made dressing that fits in my purse (inside a small zip-top bag)—just a simple mixture of high-quality olive oil, a tiny bit of white vinegar, and spices. This makes everything better, as I don't enjoy dry salad. If you don't want to bring your own dressing, olive oil and black pepper are nearly always available. Once you've tested lemons, you can squeeze lemon over a salad.

- **TRY A FOOD TRUCK.** Food trucks are even more willing to adapt for me than some restaurants. I always start by asking, "Is your meat already marinated or seasoned?" If yes, I don't try to order anything except unsalted fries or a salad. If no, then I can usually figure something out with them. And because at a food truck you are usually talking to the cook, or the cook is in earshot a step away, your order is less likely to get mucked up.

If you can't do any advance recon, you still have options. Ask the server which protein is in its natural state (unmarinated) and order it with grilled or steamed vegetables. You can assume everything is salted, especially anything made in advance. This may include grilled mushrooms (which often have onions in them), salad dressings, marinades, dips, cooked grains like rice or quinoa, and any meat or fish with a sauce.

Restaurants are in the business of selling food and making customers happy; they don't want someone getting sick as a result of their food. What restaurants gain in return are highly loyal customers. One study by the National Foundation for Celiac Awareness found that gluten-free requests accounted for more than 200 million restaurant visits in 2012.[111] Once people with celiac disease find a place they can trust, they'll go there frequently, bring friends, and book parties there. I believe this is true of all special-needs diners.

Despite the fact that food service staff members are required to take food handling and sanitation courses, I have found a shocking lack of knowledge about how to handle special diet requests. It's shocking because people can die from food allergies.[112] While restaurants are supposed to clean the table, chairs, and booths between diners, I have never witnessed that level of attention. Fine dining restaurants may change the linens between diner groups.

I took a class on managing food allergens and gluten in a commercial setting, and one of the people in the class had testified in a case in Los Angeles. A person with a seafood allergy *died* from eating French fries that were cooked in oil that had previously cooked calamari. It did not occur to that diner that French fries could be lethal, or that the oil cooking his French fries could be contaminated with enough calamari essence to kill him.

> If you or a family member has a severe food allergy, ask that the table and chairs be thoroughly cleaned before you are seated, and watch to make sure they do so.

You need to be your own advocate. This isn't about putting up a fight or being difficult, it's about your ongoing self-care. If you are concerned that your family or friends will give you a hard time about being troublesome, gently mention to them that you would rather take a few extra moments to order food that is good for you than spend three days on the couch with a migraine attack because you didn't want to "inconvenience the waiter."

THE RESTAURANT CARD

I got the idea for a restaurant card from Jessica Goldman Foung at *Sodium Girl* and have tested a few versions of it. I find it's easier to have it be a full-sized page that I can print on recycled paper, as I often don't get it back. Restaurants are usually dark, so a larger typeface is helpful for the server. You can download a full-sized sheet from my website MigraineReliefPlan.com.

Utilize this restaurant card by handing it to the manager or your server and having them suggest something that the kitchen can make. They may need to confer with the chef. (Keep extra copies with you or in your car, since you might not get the sheet back once you hand it off to a server or manager.) I'll talk in more detail about how to eat out while traveling in Month 5 (page 128). This is what I include on my card:

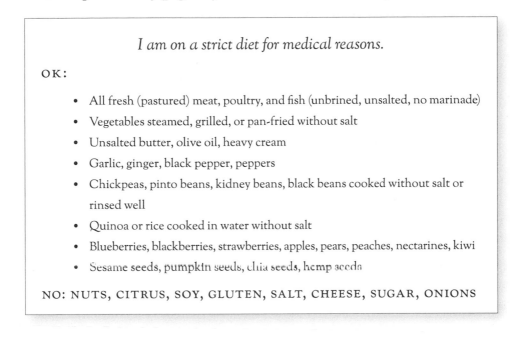

I am on a strict diet for medical reasons.

OK:

- All fresh (pastured) meat, poultry, and fish (unbrined, unsalted, no marinade)
- Vegetables steamed, grilled, or pan-fried without salt
- Unsalted butter, olive oil, heavy cream
- Garlic, ginger, black pepper, peppers
- Chickpeas, pinto beans, kidney beans, black beans cooked without salt or rinsed well
- Quinoa or rice cooked in water without salt
- Blueberries, blackberries, strawberries, apples, pears, peaches, nectarines, kiwi
- Sesame seeds, pumpkin seeds, chia seeds, hemp seeds

NO: NUTS, CITRUS, SOY, GLUTEN, SALT, CHEESE, SUGAR, ONIONS

OUR ANNIVERSARY DINNER

Our 15th wedding anniversary fell four months into my new eating plan. I was savvy enough to know that a dinner out would be tricky, but I wanted to try. We had been given a gift certificate to a trendy new Chinese restaurant, so we decided to go there. I knew it might be difficult for me to eat there, as Asian food is notoriously salty, sugary, and full of triggers like soy. That challenge competed with my desire to be able to tell our friends we had enjoyed their gift.

We sat down in the sleek dining room and began reading the extensive menu. Everything sounded delicious, and nothing seemed like it would work for me. I began having the long conversation with our waiter about options for me that were low-salt and gluten-free. He tried to be helpful, made some suggestions, and I finally settled on gluten-free vegetable tempura and ahi poke as my appetizers and a rice noodle stir-fry with oil and no seasoning.

Despite the server's help, I could feel myself beginning to get upset. Why couldn't I eat this delicious food anymore? Everything on the menu sounded amazing, and for once I just wanted to be able to order what sounded good to me, not what *might* work.

Every once in a while I get this feeling of detachment, as if I'm on the other side of thick glass looking at the people around me, feeling completely disconnected. This was one of those times. I felt the smarting of tears in the corner of my eyes. I shook them off, trying to focus on our anniversary and not the food. I reached across the table to take my husband's hand.

And then the tempura came, covered in large crystals of salt. What? How was this possible? I had had *such* a long conversation with the waiter about my salt issue.

I knew I would have to send it back; I couldn't chance it. I hesitated, two voices in my head battling it out:

I hate wasting food.

It's our anniversary!

I don't want to be a bother.

But I told him I couldn't have salt!

I finally called a waiter over and apologetically explained that I needed a new order. I was starting to blink back tears while trying to be positive and focus on being with my husband, not the challenge, again, of getting food that I can eat.

The ahi poke was delicious, but one bite was super salty. So that was another dish I couldn't have. A fresh order of tempura came back with apologies and no salt. It was crispy and tasty and I dug in. Maybe this would be OK after all. I skipped the luscious dipping sauce, likely full of soy and sugar, happy to have some fried food.

The main dishes came. Mine looked exactly like spaghetti-shaped Chinese wheat noodles. I took a tiny bite. The noodles tasted like wheat. I had my husband taste them. He couldn't tell, but I was sure. I called the waiter over again.

"Are these wheat noodles?"

"Yes, it's the lo mein."

"But I am gluten-free! I ordered rice noodles!"

"You did? I'm sorry, I didn't hear you."

This, despite a 10-minute conversation about my eating restrictions! "Do you want me to take it back?" At this point I just wanted to get out of there. We would take it home; my husband could doctor it up for lunch the next day.

I finished off the tempura and we went out for gourmet ice cream. In case you're wondering, gourmet ice cream is not on the Plan. But at that point I wanted to soothe myself with a treat. Of course the evening wasn't a total loss. We enjoyed our ice cream and our walk home. But it was the worst anniversary meal I've ever had.

I don't blame the waiter or the restaurant. But we can't eat there again, as it clearly won't work for me.

The next time someone gives us a gift card for a restaurant that I suspect will be difficult, I will just thank them warmly and pass along the card to someone who can enjoy it with no problems. We have since found better options for our special occasions.

A *closer look at:* places to avoid

When it comes to restaurants to avoid, fast food places are high on the list. They tend to use highly processed foods in addition to low-quality meats and pre-made sauces, which are problematic for people who get migraine. The same goes for cheap Mexican eateries and buffets, except those with salad bars. The language barrier can be difficult at international cuisine restaurants. If you're not sure that staff members clearly understand you, eat somewhere else, especially if you have known food allergies or sensitivities.

ASIAN RESTAURANTS

All Asian restaurants, including Chinese, Japanese, and Thai, rely heavily on soy-based sauces, fish sauce, and MSG (even if they say they don't use it), and much is pre-prepared. Many cook in peanut oil. The sodium count is very high at Asian restaurants. Your best bet at Asian restaurants is to order salad with no dressing, white rice, veggies, and meat cooked in oil only without onions (beware that there is a lot of seasoning, and usually gluten, in these woks, even if they say they're gluten-free). Check to make sure they're not cooking in peanut oil. Make sure the meat has not been marinated.

INDIAN RESTAURANTS

Indian food (Asian, but substantially different offerings) is high in sodium and almost always will have onion cooked into the sauces. However, if you have a favorite local place and can talk to the chef, you may be able to eat there or have them prepare food for you in advance if you call. Bring them your restaurant card a day early, and ask if they can accommodate you.

MIDDLE EASTERN RESTAURANTS

Middle Eastern eateries (including kebab restaurants) might be able to accommodate you if the meat they use is not pre-marinated. They use a lot of lemon in their cooking, and many of the dishes can be high in sodium. Falafel (which is made from chickpeas) might be OK if it's completely wheat-free (you need to ask them, sometimes they contain flour). Stuffed grape leaves might be OK. Ask about onion as an ingredient.

MID-PRICED AND CHAIN RESTAURANTS

Mid-priced and chain restaurants rarely make their own stocks or sauce bases. They may not even be cooking any food, but simply reheating food from a warehouse and serving it. A good rule of thumb is that if a restaurant advertises on television, the food will be high in sugar, sodium, gluten, and potential triggers, and special orders may be more difficult. For example, all the meat may be pre-marinated, frozen, and shipped to that restaurant. Bulk soup or marinade bases used in these restaurants often include triggers like MSG and yeast extract and are high in sodium. That's why I always skip anything with sauces or marinades and avoid grains unless I am sure they are cooked only with water. (White steamed rice is nearly always safe.)

① ② ③ ④ ⑤ ⑥ ⑦ ⑧

PART III
MAINTAINING THE PLAN

———— ••• ————

Over the next four months, you'll be sticking to the Plan as closely as possible. You'll keep tracking your foods, sleep, movement, and symptoms. Your tracking worksheets or apps will will show you how you are improving and if these additional lifestyle recommendations reduce your migraine frequency or severity. The next four sections guide you through this maintenance phase, giving you some additional assignments you can weave into your life each week.

MONTH 3
bodywork, meditation, and self-care

———— ••• ————

One of the key elements to this process is learning to care for ourselves. It's so easy to put yourself at the bottom of the list, skip meals, stay up too late, and forget to breathe deeply. This month, I encourage you to add yourself to your calendar. Add in five minutes of deep breathing daily; a yoga, tai chi, or Pilates class; a run or long walk—whatever makes you feel truly well, not because you think you should. Go sit on the grass in the park. Listen to the birds. Pet something.[113] Turn off your phone or leave it at home.

Part of getting a handle on migraine attacks is managing our stress. While the role stress plays in migraine isn't entirely clear, many doctors believe it is a factor. One possibility is that bodies under stress generate potent peptides and other chemicals, some of which are neurotransmitters. These may trigger the start of migraine attacks or create an environment where the brain is more excitable and reactive. Note that triggers like stress and food aren't the underlying cause of migraine, which has yet to be determined. But they are the things over which we have more control.

BODYWORK AND NON-PHARMACEUTICAL OPTIONS

———— • ————

Stress management can be achieved through movement, biofeedback, meditation, prayer, yoga, and bodywork.[114] The growing research on these techniques impacting health in substantial ways is exciting. In addition to being wonderful self-care techniques, stress management techniques greatly influence your quality of life when you practice them. Receiving bodywork such as massage is another way to honor our bodies through the healing gift of touch.

Acupuncture

This ancient Chinese healing method has thousands of years of history, practice, and (more recently) research behind it. Acupuncture can treat the symptoms of migraine,

MONTH 3

ASSIGNMENTS

- Make an appointment for bodywork.
- Buy or record a guided meditation and listen to it at least once.
- Do the priming exercise on page 114.
- Take 15 minutes to write about how you're feeling about having to give up your favorite foods. Wallow just a little, then move on.
- Talk to one friend in an open and vulnerable way about being part of your support system. Ask for one or two *specific* things they can do to help you.

headaches, nausea, and even help with vertigo attacks from Meniere's. When I was having my worst symptoms, weekly acupuncture appointments helped a great deal. I often left with acupressure beads, tiny metal balls stuck in place with sticky circles, on my ears, which continued the benefits of the session for several days. Researcher Candace Pert believed that acupuncture taps into the invisible energy communication system of our neuropeptides. Acupuncture is frequently covered by insurance with a doctor's referral and/or by a flexible spending account (FSA).

Biofeedback

Biofeedback therapy involves training sessions with equipment where you learn to reduce muscle tension in the head and neck and/or modify blood flow by focusing on raising the temperature of your fingertips. The feedback might be hearing a sound or seeing a light when you are achieving the desired state of calmness, heart rate variability, or watching a digital thermometer on your finger. In most cases, biofeedback is combined with relaxation training. Because it trains the nervous system to be calmer, it's shown to reduce headache frequency and severity by 45 to 60 percent, which is as good as some medications without the side effects. Once you've learned the techniques, you can practice them at home without the equipment.[115] Biofeedback may be covered by insurance with a doctor's referral and/or by an FSA. You can purchase a fingertip thermometer online for about $22 and teach yourself, or you can order biofeedback supplies from headachecare.com.

Chiropractic

A skilled chiropractor can realign bones in your neck and spine that may be triggering or contributing to headaches. Ideally, find a chiropractor who incorporates massage techniques before their adjustments. Chiropractic may be covered by insurance and/or an FSA, although it sometimes requires a doctor's referral. You might ask your doctor or dentist about an NTI mouth splint (which is prescription only) if you think teeth grinding might be related to your migraine.

Deep tissue massage

Deep tissue massage assists with relaxation as well as headaches generated by muscle tension in the neck and shoulders. I can only afford a massage every few months. I finally bought an electric massager from Canada called Thumper, which uses a patented percussive technology. Using this when I wake up and before bed has greatly reduced my body aches and tension. It costs less than two massages; for me, it was well worth it. Massages may be covered by insurance and/or by an FSA if recommended by your doctor.

Electrical stimulation devices

Researchers have been studying whether stimulation of the vagus nerve (which starts deep inside the brain and connects to all major organs and the gut) can help with migraine. Researchers have been focused on medical devices, either implanted within the brain or using electrodes on the skin that send a signal to the vagus nerve, which calms the nervous system down. Stimulating the vagus nerve releases the neurotransmitter acetylcholine, which has a calming effect on the body.[116] These devices are most effective for chronic migraine, as they need to be used daily.[117]

You can experiment with one type of nerve stimulation without equipment. The following techniques all have a positive effect on the vagus nerve:

1. Breathe in so deeply that the breath expands your belly.

2. Press gently on both eyelids with your eyes closed.

3. Massage the carotid body on your neck for a few minutes.

The carotid body is a nerve bundle located on the carotid artery, just under your jawbone. Find the pulse in your neck, and then place a finger above it in the hollow under your jawbone. Massage there for a few minutes while you take deep belly breaths as in Step 1.

MEDITATION

I have heard prayer described as talking to God and meditation as listening to God. Whatever your view of religion, meditation is not a religious practice, but a way to calm your mind and body for a few minutes. If the idea of meditating doesn't feel comfortable to you, you can achieve some of the same results by combining the deep belly breaths described above with your prayer practice.

Meditation lowers blood pressure, reduces stress hormones, increases positive peptide production, and deeply relaxes muscles. It calms busy minds, helping us be more present in our lives.[118] It also helps improve sleep. Willpower researcher Dr. Kelly McGonigal also reports another huge benefit to meditation: It rewires your brain, increasing self-control skills and the size of your pre-frontal cortex. You'll see these results in just eight weeks of daily meditation practice, and possibly with just five minutes a day.[119] In addition, remember that our brains are constantly changing and adapting. By focusing on positive thoughts, we can literally rewire new neural pathways. A 2011 Harvard study found significant changes in brain structure after just eight weeks of meditation practice, compared to a control group.[120]

Types of meditation

There are a number of meditation methods. The most familiar to you might be guided visualization, which often includes full-body relaxation techniques as part of the instruction, and mindfulness-based stress reduction (MBSR). MBSR is the most widely studied to date.

Guided visualization specific to migraine attacks might include instructions to visualize holding a ball of white light in your hands, which redirects blood flow away from the brain and may provide relief during a migraine attack. MBSR is a technique taught by trained professionals over a several-week course. It can reduce both pain and the emotional reaction to pain.

A 2015 study at Wake Forest showed that MBSR reduced pain by activating regions involved in the self-control of pain while deactivating the thalamus, the gateway that determines if sensory information is allowed to reach the brain's higher processing centers.[121]

I have been impressed with the eight-week guided visualization program in *You Are Not Your Pain* by Vidyamala Burch and Danny Penman. The eight recorded tracks are soothing, and the program is well tested. Burch and Penman, both chronic pain sufferers themselves, have helped many people through their program. They espouse paying "kindly attention" to our lives as they truly are, without harsh judgment and with loving intention.

I have found that my daily morning practice using guided meditations of just 10 minutes has transformed me in ways noticeable to myself and to others. I don't worry about things the way I used to. I take life's rapids more in stride. I bounce back more quickly. People tell me I seem calmer, more peaceful, and nicer to be around.

Meditation resources

The least expensive way to learn meditation is to buy or download a guided visualization. Listen to one per day. Guided visualizations are powerful tools that tap into our subconscious. Use them in a quiet place, either in a comfortable seated position or lying down with your eyes closed. Do not use them while driving. Here's a list of some of my favorites:

- *Meditation for Optimum Health: How to Use Mindfulness and Breathing to Heal* by Andrew Weil and Jon Kabat-Zinn (the Lovingkindness meditation is my favorite)
- *Meditations to Relieve Stress* by Belleruth Saperstek
- *Yoga Nidra* by Bhava Ram and Laura Plumb
- DawnBuse.com, Dr. Dawn Buse's website
- *The Soul of Healing Meditations* and *Chakra Balancing: Body, Mind, & Soul* by Deepak Chopra
- *The Inner Practices of Yoga—Self-Healing* by Michele Hebert
- Kaiser Permanente offers a number of free podcasts you can download, including ones for headaches, sleep, and relaxation
- HeadSpace app, which is available for Apple and Android
- My online program MigraineReliefPlan.com includes a number of guided meditations

Guided meditation—by you, for you

You can also record your own guided meditation.[122] Here's one I've written to get you started; use the voice-recording app on your smart phone. You can record this as is, or change the wording to perfectly suit you. If you like, play instrumental music or ocean sounds in the background while recording for your personal use:

Sit or lie down in a comfortable position. Make sure you are warm and feel safe and relaxed.

Close your eyes. Take a calm, rich, deep breath, [pause] then let it out, relaxing completely.

Imagine your toes relaxing completely. Continue to take easy, deep breaths, imagining that your toes, and then your feet, are being covered in gentle golden light.

Imagine the light moving up your calves, relaxing them.

All is well with your world. You are surrounded by people who love you, people who wish the best for you.

Even people you have never met in person are surrounding you with healing golden light.

The light moves up your thighs, relaxing them completely. It moves up into your hips, buttocks, and lower back. As you breathe deeply into your belly, the golden light meets your breath.

You are willing to release anything in your consciousness or body that might unknowingly contribute to your headaches or migraine.

You lovingly forgive and release all of the past. You choose to fill your world with joy. You love and approve of yourself.

As you continue to breathe, the light travels up your lower back, both arms, your stomach, into your chest and shoulders. You see the light like a candle flame right behind your breastbone. It's the beautiful light of your soul.

You trust the process of life. Everything you need is always taken care of. You are safe.

The light continues up your neck, relaxing every single muscle in your neck. It covers your face, and you release your tongue, cheeks, the tiny muscles around your eyes, and your forehead.

The light quiets and calms your neurons and heals inflammation in your brain.

The light covers your head, and hovers in a beautiful golden ball right above the top of your head. You are completely relaxed.

Any pain you are feeling dissolves and melts away.

You recognize your self-worth. Life is easy and joyful.

You love and appreciate and take care of yourself.

You relax into the flow of life, letting life provide all that you need easily and comfortably.

You move forward with confidence and joy, knowing that all is well in your future.

Take three more complete, deep breaths, letting each one flow out softly.

Picture the light above you floating up, into the heavens, taking any pain, tension, or headaches with it.

You are free.

When you are ready, slowly open your eyes.

MINDFULNESS IN MOVEMENT

If sitting quietly and meditating doesn't float your boat, there is another way to reap the benefits of meditation. Learning mindfulness practice—that is, fully focusing your attention on the activities of your everyday life—helps you be completely present, not reliving the past or worrying about the future. If you'd like to learn more, reading *Peace Is Every Step* by Thich Nhat Hanh is an excellent starting point.

Mindful walking

You can do a walking mindfulness meditation by being fully present and noticing every single thing you can on your walk: the sounds of nature or the city, the colors of plants and flowers, the smells, the way your body feels as you walk. Take this one step further and try walking a labyrinth, a repetitive path traced on the ground that has been used in mindfulness meditation practices dating back 4,000 years; research "labyrinth walk" to find out if there is one in your city or town and to learn more.

Mindful Cooking

To practice mindful cooking, don't multitask. Turn off all media and just focus on the food. Look at the colors of the vegetables and fruits as you wash them. Utilize the repetitive nature of chopping or slicing; feel the rhythm, focus on your hands as they move. (This has the added benefit of lessening the likelihood you will cut yourself.) After you finish cooking, try mindful eating, described on page 82. You may also want to try a mindful meal in silence, which is common practice at meditation retreats.

SELF-CARE: HARNESSING THE POWER OF OUR THOUGHTS

Neuroscientists have learned that our brains are wired for a negativity bias, developed over time to help humans survive. We see threats everywhere—in as little as a tenth of a second—but take many times longer to register pleasant things. Negative experiences also generate far more intense brain activity than pleasant ones do.[123]

When you add long-term chronic pain to that inherent bias, it's a double whammy. Feeling lousy for a long time shifts your self-perception; it molds your identity. When I was sick in 2003 with what they thought was chronic fatigue syndrome, it became very difficult to remember what it felt like to be well. I couldn't remember what it was like to have energy. Even in my dreams I was exhausted, unable to move, or feeling like I was moving through Jell-O. One sign that I was recovering started in my dreams, when I found myself running easily with energy. My subconscious mind had not forgotten what feeling well was like, and I clung to that hope until my physical body recovered.

My chiropractor assured me that my body wanted and had the innate power to heal. Just hearing that made me cry. But it's true. Our cells regenerate quickly; the average age of the cells in our body may only be seven years, with many regenerating in days or weeks. Even genetic tendencies are not set in stone; we can alter them. How we respond to our environment and life events determines which genes get switched on.[124]

Words matter

You may have noticed that I have chosen not to use the term *migraineur* in this book, nor do I call myself one. It's a commonly used term in both the medical literature and support groups. It's easier and more elegant when writing. But I'm deliberately avoiding the term.

The first few times I saw it my reaction was first, "That's French," followed by, "That's odd." It took me a while to put my finger on why it felt odd to me. One day I realized I wouldn't find it helpful to describe myself as a "fusioneur," even though I have had a spinal fusion surgery. If I call myself (or think of myself) as a migraineur, it's hard to think of myself as a person who never gets migraine attacks, or one who might never have them in the future. This is not a critique of anyone who does use the term, just an observation about what's helpful for me.

I have found it helpful to pay attention to language and my inner dialogue. I don't want any health-related label to unwittingly become part of my identity. I believe that words and inner dialogue are incredibly powerful.

After reading Ellen Langer's book *Counterclockwise*, I am even more convinced that words, which frame our thoughts, have an actual physical effect on our bodies. I'm not suggesting that using the term *migraineur* causes migraine attacks or makes migraine attacks worse, only that it seems useful for me to be aware of my inner dialogue and frame it in the most helpful way possible. Langer and other researchers have extensively looked at the nocebo effect, which is when being told you are ill impacts your health negatively.

Priming

Try a little experiment. Read the following list of words, then close your eyes and think about how the list makes you feel:

Patient, doctor, diagnosis, chronic, illness, debilitating, neurological, prescription

Now, try this list:

Health learner, consultant, plan, supplement, healthy, vibrant, energetic, powerful, strong

How does the second list feel compared to the first?

Choose a word from the second list that resonates with you and add it to your personal identity. Begin describing yourself using this term on a regular basis. You might tell a friend that you feel powerful and strong today. You might tell your mother that you've been doing research as a health learner and it's making you feel more energetic.

Each week, take a few minutes to write out what you're doing right and how you're improving. Seattle nutritionist Jennifer Adler recommends this approach to her clients. You'll begin to see how much you are doing to feel well, and that alone may help you feel better emotionally. I can tell how I'm feeling overall by whether a certain street in my regular walking loop feels like a long way to walk that day, or when I seem to get there without a second thought. And I note on a calendar above my desk when I have to take my migraine medications. Just seeing how seldom those notations now appear is encouraging.

Focusing on what's working, and how you can do more of that, is what authors Chip and Dan Heath call the "bright spots" in their book *Switch*. Even when my health is not where I want it to be, having these types of positive mental images helps me to feel better emotionally, and sometimes that leads to physical improvement, too.

The need to grieve (but not wallow)

When you find out you have to change your diet, it's a loss. It's a loss of lifestyle, of ease, of being like everyone else. It's a loss of being able to (easily) go out to lunch with your office mates, to go out to dinner, to eat out anywhere without having to pepper the server with questions and special-order something off the menu. It's the pain-in-the-ass of reading labels on every grocery trip for an entire month.

It's tiring having to talk about what I can and cannot eat over and over again. I prefer to have an interesting conversation involving other people. I don't like being the center of attention unless I'm on stage. I don't want to be the difficult one, the odd person out. I'm already redheaded, left-handed, born on the Gemini–Cancer cusp, and untannable. I don't need another weirdness stuck to me. Instead, I like to focus on all the positive words and actions I am using to feel as well as possible.

I now look back on the days when I was *only* gluten-free with longing and nostalgia. How easy that was!

All of these aspects need to be grieved. But that's not the same as feeling sorry for yourself. When I got very sick in 2003, I made up a rule. If I was feeling crappy, I would set a timer for 10 minutes and feel super sorry for myself, crying if needed. And then, the timer would go off and that was that. Move on.

It's the same now. There are times where this feels just too hard and I nearly cry in a restaurant. But most of the time, I arrange my life to make it work as well as possible. And I try to focus on the many positives. The diet works. I'm feeling better. I may not go deaf. My friends and family love me. I can eat a whole bunch of foods again, as they're not a trigger for me!

Building your support team

One of the most gratifying things about working on this Plan has been meeting people online who also struggle with Meniere's and migraine. The support communities online are pretty amazing, and I continue to appreciate aspects of our virtual world that allow me to connect with people all over the world who share in this experience. This was especially true when I found recipe testers from all over the United States and three other countries. A sixteen-year-old named Gabbie wrote me a note when she sent in her final recipe testing sheets:

"Thank you so much for allowing me to work with you on this project. It really made me feel, through my year of isolation and slow progress, that I was doing something important."

This experience can feel lonely. Being in pain is lonely. Eating differently is lonely. Having weird or invisible symptoms that people don't understand is lonely. And it's especially difficult because overall I look just fine. I look like I should be able to be spontaneous and go out to lunch, or for a walk at lunchtime on a bright-hot sunny day, or to jump in the car for a road trip. But I can't always do that. It might make me sick.

So what happens when I start feeling this way? I start saying no, a little here and a little there. I tell the work gang to go ahead to lunch without me. I skip the party. I stay home, slowly isolating myself to make life easier. And that's not OK.

If that also sounds like you, I would encourage you to create allies for yourself, build yourself a little pit crew, one team member at a time. Have heart-to-heart talks with these folks, expressing in a deep way how hard it can be for you, how much you could use their support in these very specific ways, until you have a few people in your corner.

Migraine doctors Dawn Buse and Romie Mushtaq encourage their patients to remain hopeful, connected, and to stay engaged with their lives and work as much as possible. They caution against catastrophizing (fearing the worst) because it shifts the focus onto negative fears. And they encourage you to seek out people who can "hold hope for you."[125]

One change I've enjoyed is to make walking dates instead of lunch dates. I shift the focus from food to conversation, and as a bonus we get some movement in. Think of activities that would allow you to see friends in a way that also supports your health. It can be focused on a specific activity you both enjoy, instead of on food.

MONTH 4
detoxing body, home, and work

———— ··· ————

Last month, I suggested you add some self-care techniques to your routine. This month, we're going one step further, looking at potential toxins or triggers in your life that may be contributing to your migraine attacks and headaches. We'll look at whether you should consider a supervised cleanse, talk briefly about migraine medications, and cover skin care routines and beauty products. Then we'll expand out from you to the items in your home and your workplace.

INSIDE: DETOXING YOUR BODY

———— · ————

In medical terminology, this Plan is an elimination diet. You eliminate all known migraine triggers from what you're eating, then gradually test them to see what you can safely add back. Because we also gradually eliminate sugar, excess sodium, and processed foods, this Plan has aspects of a detoxification diet as well. A practitioner you work with may recommend a stricter detoxification diet or cleanse, depending on your health status and symptoms. Or if you have a sense that you need a stricter diet than this Plan offers, find a functional medicine practitioner in your area, discuss the Plan with them, show them the list of foods you can eat in this book, and do a supervised cleanse if they recommend it and can monitor you. I don't recommend fasting (skipping a day of meals) or juice fasting (eating only juiced fruits and vegetables for a day or longer) if you get migraine attacks; these methods can lead to more attacks because of the blood sugar spikes and drops that are common. But you may find a supervised detoxification plan helpful if you have other health conditions in addition to migraine. Just be certain any supplements your practitioner recommends are free of all triggers until you are clear what yours might be.

You may find that you need to rebalance your gut bacteria to help with your symptoms. I would encourage you to read *Brain Maker* by Dr. David Perlmutter to get more

ASSIGNMENTS

- Try dry brushing one morning to see how it makes your body feel.
- Go barefoot on the grass or at the beach.
- Choose one room in your home and do a little audit. Is there one simple change you could make that would make that room healthier for you?
- Choose one aspect of your work environment and see if you can make a change to reduce your headaches.

information on this topic and specific recommendations, including using a probiotic enema, which he describes.

What about medications?

While we're talking about removing toxic elements from your body, you might wonder about medications. I take prescription medications at times (about twice a month now, at the first sign of an attack), although my goal is to use them as little as possible by following the Plan. There was a lot of discussion at the 2016 American Headache Society meeting about the issues with medication overuse headache (MOH, previously referred to as rebound headaches, page 5). Note that this term isn't an indicator of patients misusing medications outside of how they are prescribed; it refers to the problem that occurs when medication use unfortunately begins to cause additional headaches.

One thing to remember is that all doctors want to help you feel better as quickly as possible. If they have limited appointment times with you, the most effective course of action is to prescribe something they know will work quickly. They may not have time to consult with you on alternative methods. Promote yourself to the head of your medical team, become your own health advocate, and think of your doctors as valued consultants.

All medications have side effects. You and your doctor need to weigh the benefits of taking the medication versus weaning yourself off of it. Triptans, the most effective migraine meds, are effective in reducing pain for 70 to 80 percent of people, and cut short migraine altogether in about half.[129] They work best when taken as soon as you're

HOW IS MEDICATION OVERUSE DEFINED?

Medication overuse is defined as the regular use of one or more of the following medications **for a period of more than 3 months**:

Regular use (per month)	Type of drug
15 days	• Non-steroidal anti-inflammatories (NSAIDs) (aspirin, ibuprofen, and naproxen sodium)*
10 days	• Triptans (such as Imitrex or sumatriptan) • Ergot alkaloids (such as dihydroergotamine and Migranal)
5 days	• opioids (such as codeine and oxycodone) • combination analgesics (Excedrin Migraine)[126] • butalbital compounds (Fioricet and Fiorinal)[127]

Note that headache specialists no longer recommend either opioids or butalbital compounds for migraine patients. According to Dr. Stewart Tepper, headache worsens with the medication overuse, and these medications can cause MOH even if they are used for something other than headache. Combining days still results in MOH. For example, five days of triptans plus five days of Excedrin (on the same or different days within the month) would equal 10 days of acute treatment and likely lead to MOH, in Dr. Tepper's experience.

* Doses of NSAIDs are listed on the bottle, e.g., one dose of ibuprofen is a single 200mg tablet. Acetaminophen, known as Tylenol, is not known to cause MOH and could be taken according to package directions if needed. [128]

aware of the migraine coming on. This is an easier task for people with aura or clear premonitory symptoms.

Preventives don't carry the risk of medication overuse headache, but they come with their own set of side effects. Preventives are prescribed for people whose migraine attacks are considered chronic (more than 15 days a month) and are only effective for 50 percent of people 50 percent of the time.[130] One study found that regular exercise was just as effective as the most-prescribed preventive.[131]

Current guidelines suggest triptans are safe up to twice per week, which is why most insurance policies will cover nine doses per month. Note that taking other medications along with that number of triptans can put you into MOH territory.

If you are taking any of the medications listed in the box on page 119 over the guidelines or you are not seeing good results from my Plan after six months, it's possible you could be getting MOHs from the medication itself. You may have to go through a painful short-term period to get off that medication; this should be done only under your doctor's supervision.

To explore weaning yourself off your medications with your doctor, make a plan with her to help you with the transition and any acute symptoms you might experience over the first two to three weeks.

Chronic migraine is defined as more than 15 headache days per month, although this is not a hard and fast rule. If you have chronic headaches, MOH may be playing a part and it may take you longer to see results with this Plan. If at any time you notice your attacks are becoming more frequent or intense, be sure to see your doctor right away. You don't want to move from periodic to chronic migraine, as it is more difficult to treat.

For women who are pregnant or planning to become pregnant, be aware that many migraine medications and some migraine supplements (such as feverfew and large doses of riboflavin) will not be safe during pregnancy and breastfeeding. Be sure to have your migraine doctor and your OB/GYN confer about this. For a more detailed approach to migraine and pregnancy, check out the Resources (page 304) in the back.

OUTSIDE: TAKING CARE OF YOUR SKIN AND HAIR

We tend to think of our skin either as inert or as something to be "dealt with": fighting acne or wrinkles, getting a tan, or avoiding the sun. But it's so much more than a blank canvas. It's our largest organ, a complex and beautiful protective covering that works in tandem with the rest of our body. Covered with about five million hairs, made up of trillions of cells, our skin is an active, changing part of our bodies throughout our lives. It converts sunlight to vitamin D, creates and excretes chemicals, regulates temperature, and bends and flexes thousands of times in our lifetime. Your skin cells are constantly rebuilding, and the top layer of your skin renews itself completely every two weeks.[132]

Healthy, nurtured skin supports our overall health and immune system. As the largest organ in the body, it absorbs almost everything it comes into contact with. Chemicals or nutrients on your skin can make their way into your bloodstream and, possibly, your brain. What you put on your skin matters. A rule of thumb at the Optimum Health Institute in Lemon Grove, California, is to avoid putting anything on your skin that you can't eat or drink. Think about it. You wouldn't drink makeup remover or body wash, yet we use items like those on our beautiful bodies nearly every day. Let's look at a few ingredients in a typical skin lotion.

Do you know what each of these ingredients is and whether you could eat them? I didn't; I had to look them up:

HAND LOTION INGREDIENTS

DIMETHICONE: Lubricant; defoaming agent; main ingredient in Silly Putty.

ALOE BARBADENSIS LEAF JUICE: The juice from aloe plants.

ASCORBIC ACID: Powdered form of vitamin C.

ASCORBYL PALMITATE: Fat-soluble vitamin C; from palm kernel oil.

CETYL ALCOHOL: Fatty alcohol; thickening agent; sensitizing for eczema.

CHOLECALCIFEROL: Form of vitamin D3; from wool.

CITRIC ACID: Weak acid; from citrus fruit; natural preservative.

CITRUS AURANTIUM DULCIS PEEL OIL: Valencia orange peel oil.

DIAZOLIDINYL UREA: Antimicrobial; byproduct of formaldehyde and allantoin + sodium hydroxide + heat. Neutralized using hydrochloric acid, then evaporated.

GLYCERYL STEARATE SE: Emulsifying agent; used as a food additive.

HYDROXYTYROSOL: Plant-based chemical from olive leaves and olive oil.

METHYLPARABEN: Antifungal agent; produced from fruits or chemically; may have an estrogenic effect.

PROPYLENE GLYCOL: Attracts and holds water molecules; hydrating to skin; from fossil fuels.

That's a list I'm not too excited about eating *or* putting on my skin anymore. So what to use instead? I have found an organic lotion that, while I wouldn't enjoy eating it, would be edible. And I usually mix it about half and half with coconut oil to moisturize my face at night.

I have simplified my beauty routine, using as few products as possible and making sure each one has natural ingredients, ones that I understand. You don't have to throw everything in your bathroom away, just start investigating better choices so that when something runs out you can buy a replacement that's simpler and healthier for you. As you're doing this, be aware that many products contain fragrance, which may itself be a migraine trigger. In her book, *Eating Clean*, Amie Valpone has excellent resources on specific brands, as well as tips for detoxing your home and office.[133]

Beauty products

I've gone through phases where I wore far more makeup than I do now. Makeup is another area to read labels and find companies making simpler, organic products. I have switched over to mineral makeup by a company that is completely gluten-free and doesn't test their products on animals. Daily, I generally wear only homemade sunscreen, under-eye cover stick, and a mineral lipstick that doubles as blush. I have also recently found a natural deodorant that works for me called Schmidt's. For occasions where I need to dress up, I have a cream mineral foundation, a simple eye shadow color, eyeliner (the cake kind), and natural mascara. If you get excited about making your own beauty products, Amy at ABlossomingLife.com has recipes for homemade mascara, foundation, blush, and bronzer. Nutritionist Jennifer Adler details her natural deodorant-free beauty routine in *Passionate Nutrition*.[134]

Dry brushing

I have adopted dry brushing, a technique used in Ayurvedic medicine and also at many wellness centers like the Optimum Health Institute. Dry brushing is an excellent way to begin the day before a shower or bath. Using long strokes, always directed towards your heart, it exfoliates dead skin cells and stimulates the skin, blood flow, and the lymphatic system. The lymphatic system moves toxins around and out of your body. You want your lymphatic system to be revved up, not sluggish and sticky.

Using a natural bristle brush, or a rough-textured washcloth mitt, begin with the sole of one foot, brushing along it 10 or so times with some force. Then brush up your calf about 10 times, moving around to get each side. You should feel zinginess, not pain. Then do your thigh. You always want to be moving in the direction of your heart. Now switch to the other foot, calf, and thigh. Now brush each arm, starting with your hands. Then your torso, front and back, moving towards the heart as much as possible. You'll feel awake and energized afterwards. While I don't get around to this every single day, I always feel better if I do, especially on a headache or migraine day.

I often find I don't need to shower daily; I just wash the parts that need it after dry brushing. This saves water, especially important in the drought-stricken West. If the idea of skipping a shower repulses you, feel free to hop in there after you dry brush.

Scents

It's well known that strong smells can trigger migraine attacks. For me it's certain perfumes, especially patchouli- and musk-based perfumes. I switched to unscented everything a few years ago and have found that the switch reduced my headaches, too. The downside is that I can't use any regular perfumes; they all smell far too strong and fake. I can use essential oils like lavender, and I often just add a few drops to my organic body lotion dispenser.

Hair care products

A few years back, I read a blog about skipping commercial shampoo, and it intrigued me. The motivation for the blogger was to save money and also to see if natural, homemade shampoo did as good a job as store-bought shampoo that is full of chemicals. I tried it (search "baking soda shampoo") and found my hair looked amazing after the short adjustment period. I spend virtually nothing on shampoo and conditioner and only need to wash my long hair every three or four days, so the styling products I do use (from Aveda) last seemingly forever. I simply spritz my hair with water and run my fingers through it, scrunching as needed. It also helps that I no longer fight my hair's natural texture and now have it cut to work with my wavy curls. If you get excited about making your own hair products, search "flaxseed hair gel" on the web for more DIY recipes.

Connecting with the earth

Other ways to support your overall health and immune system include getting out in nature, getting in touch with the earth, and petting an animal. I try to spend 30 minutes each day outdoors with our dog. I sit on the grass at the park. If it's warm enough, I put my bare hands and feet on the grass. There's something deeply healing about connecting to the earth. Some health advocates believe that physically connecting to the earth's magnetic field and free electrons has a positive effect on the electrical currents in our bodies, and some early research shows it has a positive effect on our blood, sleep, chronic pain, stress hormone levels, and blood-borne micronutrients.[135] That may be part of why we get such innate pleasure and comfort from walking barefoot on the beach or grass.

In his book *The Urban Monk*, Pedram Shojai talks at length about the importance of our feet connecting with soil, sand, gravel, and seawater. I was fascinated to read that our "flattening" of the earth's topography through paving and sidewalks might have negative effects on our balance system, brain, and spine, starting with our biomechanically sophisticated feet. Shojai recommends being barefoot anywhere that's safe, gradually adapting to barefoot shoes, and walking or hiking on uneven surfaces as a way to re-ground ourselves.[136]

I am not advocating buying any of the Earthing products for sale; be a smart consumer and read the reviews. Regular, physical contact with the earth on your skin is free.

DETOXING YOUR HOME

We all like to think of our homes as safe havens, but modern life has changed that in some ways. This section is not intended to make you paranoid. Just read through it and pick one thing to address at a time, using your intuition to guide you. I have done most of these items over the course of two years, certainly not overnight. For more ideas on detoxing your home, check out *The Wahls Protocol*.

> **PLASTIC**. Plastic is an amazing substance, and it's hard to imagine our world without it. It was invented around 1900, but it wasn't until after World War II that advances in technology brought us the myriad of plastics we take for granted today: plastic bags, food storage containers, carpet foam, and shower curtains. Most plastics off-gas, meaning that they release chemicals in the form of gas for weeks or months after manufacture. Off-gassing is responsible for "new car smell." No one knows the health risks of this. So, to be safe, I have reduced the plastics in our house.
>
> *Kitchen.* I always store hot foods in glass containers. The issues are greatest when storing hot foods or oil-based foods in plastic; the heat and oil leaches chemicals from the plastic into the food.[137] I transfer large pots of soup into smaller containers to quick-chill in the fridge before freezing. I have bought a few clamp-top glass jars of various sizes, and I also reuse glass jars as much as possible. I do

use zip-top bags for their convenience, but not with hot or oily food. I always use waxed or parchment paper to cover food in the microwave, never plastic film. When possible, I choose foods sold in glass jars. When we switched back to organic grass-fed butter from margarine, we greatly reduced our consumption of plastic tubs. Many healthy-living advocates forgo microwaves altogether; we still use ours fairly frequently for the convenience. In her book, *The Paleo Approach*, Paleo and autoimmune author Sarah Ballantyne cites repeated scientific documentation that microwaved food is perfectly safe, and explains that microwaving preserves the vitamins and minerals better than other cooking methods and reduces the production of carcinogens when cooking meat.[138]

Bathroom. Since glass isn't safe in bathrooms, I use plastic containers for my homemade shampoo and conditioner, refilling them as needed. I refill my plastic container of organic body wash at the co-op. This reduces my consumption of plastic overall. Non-toxic ("PVC-free") shower curtains that don't off-gas are now widely available. I tried using just the fabric shower curtain for a while, but it got moldy pretty quickly, which may be worse for our health than plastic.

Living room. Carpet foam is a huge off-gasser. I plan on using an old rug under newer rugs as padding, instead of buying new foam next time. When renovating or repainting, look for "low-VOC" (volatile organic compound) materials and check out eco-friendly options, especially relating to odors and off-gassing.

CLEANING AND HOME SCENTS. Keeping your home clean and reducing allergens may also help with your headaches. My hometown of San Diego, being a coastal desert, is very high in airborne particulates, meaning that our house gets filthy no matter how often we clean. In addition, our golden retriever, Daisy, does her part by shedding everywhere, every day, and tracking dirt in on her paws. We use a HEPA-filter vacuum and change the bag frequently, plus a cloth dusting system. We clean with Simple Green and use Murphy Oil Soap for the hardwood floors. These items are nontoxic and low odor, which helps with headaches. I try to limit my spraying of anything, after reading that spray cleaners can increase the incidence of asthma and lung problems (possibly because the act of spraying aerosolizes tiny particles).[139] I use white vinegar and water as a simple cleaner as well. I have not had any luck finding a natural dish soap that actually works in cutting grease, so that's one area where I still use a conventional product, especially now that we have dishes with saturated fat on them. I wear gloves while washing dishes to help protect my hands, as we don't have a dishwasher. Bleach is one odor that can trigger migraine attacks, so be aware of this and ask housemates to go easy and use lots of ventilation.[140] You may be triggered by any artificial scents, such as candles, plug-ins, or air fresheners. I avoid them.

LAUNDRY. Switch over to unscented, Earth-friendly products and ditch the scented dryer sheets and fabric softener. Not only will you remove potential scent triggers, but both types of products also contain chemicals known to be toxic with long-term exposure. [141]

LIGHTING. I have chosen warm compact fluorescent bulbs, which don't seem to bother me. You could also try warm-spectrum LED bulbs, which are even more energy efficient. (Cool LED bulbs give me an instant headache.) I have to be careful about having the light on with the ceiling fan, as sometimes the strobe effect can trigger a headache. It's important for me to avoid working in over-bright or dim conditions. Paying attention to your home lighting might reduce your headaches and migraine attacks, so take a look at your light bulb choice when you can. You can also purchase migraine glasses to wear both indoors and out, which reduce and filter the light that triggers migraine attacks.[142] About 90 percent of migraine patients are light sensitive during a headache, while 60 percent say a type of light can trigger a migraine. One-third to one-half are chronically light sensitive, especially to artificial indoor light.[143] Learning this made me feel less crazy, as light has always been a big issue for me.

I had my car windows tinted, because riding in the car on bright days was a big trigger. It has helped tremendously. Some people with migraine, including high-profile athletes, have had success wearing tinted contact lenses to reduce the light to their eyes.

DETOXING YOUR OFFICE

You might think that even if there are headache-inducing issues in your office, there's nothing you can do about them. However, your employer is required to provide you with a safe workplace that's ergonomically sound. If you have a known medical condition, it's perfectly fine to ask for some accommodation to reduce your sick time. Some employers will be great about this; others will not. It's worth investigating to see if there are aspects of your physical workspace that could be changed to make your life better. Your employer wants you to be well and productive, so proactive requests framed in those terms should be honored.

ERGONOMICS. If you sit at a desk and use a computer, it's worth checking the ergonomics of your chair, desk, and monitor to make certain your head and neck are in alignment while working. Similarly, if you have a job with any kind of repetitive motion, ask your HR department if they can do an ergonomic audit to make sure everything is optimal for you.

CLEANERS AND PERFUMES. If you think the cleaning supplies being used in your workplace might contribute to your headaches or trigger migraine attacks, ask to talk to the manager of the cleaning staff to see if you can research other options that are cost-effective. If you have a coworker who wears strong perfume that gives you a headache, have a little heart-to-heart with them about it. I had to do this at my last job; the perfume wearer was a lovely woman who is still a friend. She wore a heavy, lingering musky scent so strong that it remained in the office after she had left. I finally spoke with her privately and told her it gave me a headache. She had no idea; she had been wearing it for so long she didn't smell it anymore. She was happy to switch it up and wear less.

LIGHTING. Buzzy, fluorescent fixtures get me every time. If your office has these, that's the first thing I would ask about. See if you can talk to the building supervisor, explain the problem, and work out a solution, even if it's only over your desk and not the entire space. This is where migraine glasses would be especially helpful if nothing can be changed about the lighting fixtures. Dr. Bradley Katz, an expert in light sensitivity in migraine patients, cautions against wearing standard dark sunglasses indoors, as they will make your eyes even more light-sensitive.[144] Ironically, doctors' offices almost uniformly have terrible lighting for migraine.

SICK BUILDING SYNDROME. One issue with some older, hyper-efficient office buildings is that the ventilation systems are closed, so air is recirculated over and over. People throughout the building pass viruses back and forth, and any indoor contaminants from off-gassing are recirculated as well. These buildings, sometimes called "sick buildings," are prone to developing mold in the HVAC systems.[145] Now that this problem has been identified, buildings are being built with windows that open for fresh air. If you suspect you're working in a sick building, talk to HR to see what can be done. Sometimes a few windows can be replaced with ones that can be opened. It's in your employers' interests to work with you, as reducing absences saves them money in the long run.

MONTH 5
planning to fail

————— ••• —————

While it may be unconventional for a wellness book, this section will help you gain a better understanding of your decisions to eat off the Plan. It's inevitable that you will, so the best option is to be prepared, expect that it will happen, and think through why it might happen. I'll give you tips for a variety of social situations to think through in advance, as well as some suggestions for building a support system for yourself.

WHY SHOULD YOU PLAN TO FAIL?

————— • —————

Wait a minute now . . . this book is all about positive reinforcement. This is a bulletproof, well-thought-out, eight-week plan that will change my life forever. This is the magic bullet! It's effortless!! It's foolproof!!! It's a miracle!!!!

Except it's not.

Real life isn't like that. You *will* go off the diet, fall off the wagon, cheat, or however you describe it. We all do. I do. Frequently. That's life. It's human nature. It's choices.

It's running low on willpower because you're tired of having to work so damn hard to be well, when everyone around you can blithely eat whatever they want and feel fine. (Everyone around you may not *actually* feel fine, but you're not them, so you don't know.) From the outside it looks like everyone in the world can eat whatever they want with no consequences. Except us. It's hard and it's tiring.

So we go off the diet, fall off the wagon, cheat. Or as I prefer to say: *I made an unhelpful choice.*

The words you choose are important here. Because this is an ongoing lifestyle. It will likely need to be your new reality for the rest of your life if you want to feel well long term. (Once you've completed your trigger testing, you'll find that the diet isn't restrictive, especially once you're used to it.) And I've learned that forgiving yourself is an important part of the process, too.

Because "diets" are temporary. If you're "on a diet," in your mind there is an end point, a finish line when you achieve your goal, and then you can go back to your real life.

ASSIGNMENTS

- Pick an upcoming work or social lunch and do some restaurant recon in advance.
- Imagine going to visit relatives for the next big holiday coming up. What is one thing you could do to make that visit work better for you?
- If you have a vacation coming up, start researching hotels or places to stay that will accommodate your eating plan.
- Imagine you just spectacularly went off the Plan, i.e. failed. What is your inner monologue? How can you shift it to be more supportive and helpful? How can you forgive yourself? How can you be as loving and understanding toward yourself as you would be to a friend?

They're a detour. You go off diets—and back on them—over and over. That's why I call this book a Plan.

Writing this book helped gel thoughts I've had about the word *dieting* for many years. We, especially women, tend to use modifiers like *good* and *bad* in relation to food. You have probably heard someone say, "Oh, I was *so bad* last night. I ate two desserts!" We use other loaded terms, too. *Staying on the wagon* implies an above-ground balancing act, when clearly the ground and gravity will never stop calling. *Cheating* runs the gamut from passing the answers in fourth grade to being caught in a tawdry motel room. *Being bad* sounds like a kindergartener being scolded.

I have worked to change how I think about food altogether, and instead, frame the daily food decisions I make as helpful or unhelpful choices. I try to forgive myself, let those unhelpful choices go, and move forward.

Unhelpful choices are made one at a time. They're not irrevocable. Making an unhelpful choice doesn't mean I am weak, a terrible person, or bad. It was simply an unhelpful choice that I—an adult—made. It may have tasted really good. It may have been a really fun party. When there are consequences, I own up to them.

Instead of pretending—as every weight loss show and diet book does—that *this* time it's going to stick, let's assume it won't. At least not forever. And learning to shift your mindset, from a fixed mindset to a growth mindset, is key.

According to researcher Carol Dweck in her book *Mindset*, people with a fixed mindset believe that they are who they are; they can't really change. They don't like to try new things because they are afraid they will fail or be bad at them. They believe that working hard shows you are vulnerable. They label themselves as: stupid, bad at math, fat, lazy.

People with a growth mindset believe that they can change and learn with hard work. They know they will fail at new endeavors, but they try them anyway. They see setbacks as motivating, informative, and providing a new opportunity to learn. They expect that they will change and grow over time. And the great news is that the growth mindset can be taught.[146]

Here are some key phrases to learn the growth mindset:

- Everything is hard before it is easy.

- I should never give up just because I don't get it the first time.

- My brain is like a muscle; it can be trained to learn amazing new things.

- I can learn how to do this if I work hard at it.

Think about the military. When they design a battle plan, they don't make just one plan. They prepare for three or four contingencies:

- The best-case scenario: We take the hill.

- Plan B: We hold the field.

- Plan C: We fall back to the stream.

- Plan D: When all hell breaks loose, we regroup behind the ridge.

Your best-case scenario is that you stay on this Plan forever. You are never tempted. You never make an unscheduled restaurant stop. You're completely in control of everything you eat at all times. You never get tired of cooking for yourself. You never entertain or eat with friends. You never travel.

It's not realistic, is it?

ABOUT WILLPOWER

Researchers have found in study after study that willpower is a finite resource. If we use it up on one task or area, we have less to apply to another area.[147] It's also physically draining to keep it up constantly. That's why I made this Plan a gradual shift, so you could integrate the changes into your lifestyle over two months, making it more likely that you will succeed. Do be aware that if you're in a series of situations where you are tempted to eat off the Plan, you have a finite amount of willpower to resist those temptations. To quote authors Chip and Dan Heath: "What looks like laziness is simply exhaustion." Let's see how this plays out in real life situations.

The single temptation

You're shopping for something other than food. For some reason, some very tempting food falls into your path. You're at the checkout counter of the garden store with a cart full of petunias, minding your own business, and you spy a display of handcrafted French caramels with gray sea salt. You weren't expecting to have to use willpower at the garden store, so your defenses are down. If you've been doing great with the Plan and are feeling well, will two caramels hurt?

If I've been on a few weeks' run of no sugar, the caramels won't call to me as strongly as they would if I recently had some or recently turned down sugary treats. Willpower is finite each day; my experience is that it also gets used up over time. If I'm devoting a lot of willpower to staying on the Plan, those caramels will really be calling to me. And I might give in.

Dallas and Melissa Hartwig, creators of the popular Whole30 Program, advocate an all-or-nothing approach for their 30-day experiment: no sugar, dairy, grains, legumes, or alcohol. The Hartwigs explain that classifying food as a gray area, such as "I only eat natural sugar" is tiring for our brains, because it keeps the decision making front and center.[148] Literally, the frontal cortex needs to be constantly engaged, assessing each and every possible choice. I am definitely an all or nothing person. So it helps me to say that I don't eat any food that contains any kind of sugar. Then the caramels aren't a decision I have to make, they are just a "no."

That's great in theory, but I don't always hold to it. So if I choose to buy the caramels, I try to really, truly savor them. I eat them slowly. I don't wolf them in the car while I'm driving, because then I don't remember them. Waiting until I get home provides the bonus side effect of keeping my pants and car upholstery free from chocolate stains. Not that I have ever dropped bits of chocolate on my lap in the car and had to use upholstery cleaner to remove the stains. Nope. Not me.

If I eat the caramels slowly and mindfully, I register that I had them, they were delicious, and I enjoyed them fully. I may get a small headache from the chocolate. The salt shouldn't be too much of a hit, but I'll need to read the package to make sure. I am present in the moment. The caramels are delectable.

For me, the bigger issue seems to be that having a little sugar tends to make me want more. And more. And more. So that single temptation often turns into a week or two of unhelpful choices. There is quite a bit of evidence that sugar lights up the same pleasure center of the brain, with the same intensity, as cocaine and heroin do, so sugar's powerful influence is not in my imagination.

The Hartwigs provide some helpful questions to consider when you're looking at a tempting food: Do I have a specific desire for this particular food, or am I just emotional, hungry, or craving? Is the food special, significant, or delicious? (Meaning, homemade for you by your Mom versus a peanut butter cup.) How much is it going to mess me up?[149]

The party

You've been invited to a party. You go, and suddenly there is a maze of unhelpful choices, plus a few helpful ones.

There are a couple of ways this can go for me. If the hosts are good friends, they already know I have eating restrictions and ask me what I can eat. I always tell them I will be bringing food. (I don't have any friends who cook sit-down dinner parties; everyone in my world does some sort of potluck.)

I bring enough food to eat and share that blends with what the host is serving: chili or tapas or Irish. I bring enough so that I can fill up completely, like a hearty salad or main dish and a dessert.

If it's a food event or a catered party where I cannot bring food, I eat first. And I mean, I eat. I have a healthy serving of protein plus healthy fat, so that I am not hungry at all when I get there.

If that sounds awful to you, then your party strategy might look different than mine. That's OK.

You could decide that you are absolutely going to fail here, and fail big time. Consider a couple of things when developing your failure plan: How sick will it make you, and how much time will you have to recover before you need to be functional? If you plan to fail, you could take a preventive medication, eat super clean the day before and up until the party, and hope for the best. If it's a Friday party, you will have the weekend to recover, provided you don't have other obligations like family or work.

> I have had to train myself out of the expectation that "parties are for eating." For me to be successful overall with this Plan, parties must be for socializing, with a tiny bit of nibbling and mostly drinking of sparkling water or something similar. You can train yourself to think this way, too.

WHAT IF YOU HAVE FOOD ALLERGIES OR SENSITIVITIES?

If you have any food sensitivities, you shouldn't "plan to fail." If you are allergic to particular foods or have celiac disease, you shouldn't knowingly eat those foods. Instead, what would be more helpful for you is to recognize where in your eating habits you can be less strict when needed, and where you absolutely can't risk it.

If you have any serious reactions to particular foods, come up with an accidental failure strategy. If you accidentally ingest this ingredient (usually due to failure in labeling or the restaurant server's faulty information), what do you need to have with you to address that? An EpiPen? A supplement to help you digest it? Benadryl? A list of approved treatments on your MD's stationery for the ER? Also note that if you have life-threatening food allergies, a medical ID bracelet would be a smart investment.

If you have food allergies or sensitivities and are traveling overseas, write out a note describing what they are (keep it brief) that you can give to servers; use a translation program to translate it for you. If possible, ask a native speaker to check the translation for you. Just in case you need to purchase items in a pharmacy to deal with your allergies, write that out and translate it as well. I've tried buying Noxzema for a wicked sunburn, contact lens solution, and estrogen patches in different countries overseas, and it isn't easy to communicate!

If you do have an accidental exposure, here's what I recommend. Utilize your deep breathing techniques and meditation to keep your anxiety in check so you don't make any symptoms worse. Use my list of What to Eat During a Migraine Attack (page 79) for the first day or two and then use my 3-Day Get-Back-on-Track Plan (page 140) to fully recover. See your doctor as needed.

Another thing to consider: How often do you go out to events like these? It's only once or twice a month for me, so it's more manageable. If your work or social life revolves around events, you'll need to take that into account.

You get to think this through and *make the decision you want.* You're a grown up, that's what grownups do. Before a party, you might want to pre-stock the fridge with clean recovery foods to make your weekend easier.

One summer I was invited to a cupcake tasting for food bloggers. They assured me there would be gluten-free options, so I decided to go. I knew I would be eating sugar and chocolate, so I took ibuprofen before I went.

My willpower failed mid-event, and I ended up tasting *all* the cupcakes, not just the gluten-free ones. I ate too much sugar, chocolate, dairy, eggs, and sodium in addition to gluten. I drank lots of water the rest of the day, took more ibuprofen, and ate a clean dinner. I had a pretty bad headache, ringing in my ears, and a little bit of dizziness afterward. The next morning my hands and joints were stiff and achy.

While I didn't end up getting a migraine attack, this event, a week before my birthday, set off a cascade of unhelpful choices that lasted for two weeks. I finally got myself back on track, but it took a lot of effort. In retrospect, not going would have been a better choice, but it didn't kill me.

Would I do it again? Probably not. It just wasn't worth it overall, although it was delicious at the time.

The let's-get-takeout

You are bone tired after a horrible workday. Cooking is the last thing you want to do.

Do you get tired of cooking? Me too. Really *tired*. And I love to cook. I might not spend as much time cooking as a professional chef, but between cooking our meals, recipe development, and cooking and shooting photos for my websites, some days it feels pretty close. So getting takeout is a treat as well as a break for me. But because I'm more likely to do it when I'm tired and not planning, I find that it's an area that tends to lead to unhelpful choices. Read my tips for eating out (page 95) and spend a little time thinking about your takeout tendencies so you can be better prepared.

The holiday weekend

You're heading home from work for a holiday weekend. It's time to relax, and relaxing means fun food and drinks.

Three-day weekends, and holidays in general, are difficult because food is woven into memories, family expectations, and media images about these holidays. Whether you celebrate Christmas, Hanukkah, Kwanzaa, or Diwali, it's likely that you binge on sugar in the winter months, because everyone in the United States does. This "holiday season" goes from Halloween through Valentine's Day, with a brief break for resolutions and cleanses in early January. I find that I start craving peanut butter cups in mid-October, which apparently are my "Halloween treat." I start craving peppermint bark by Thanksgiving. Just being aware of these pre-programmed mental tapes helps me decide what choices to make.

Holidays are all about planning. Take a long hard look at your calendar. If there is one party after another, or the holiday weekend is just before a super-stressful workweek, think about how you can plan in more helpful choices than unhelpful ones. Can you pre-select restaurants and dishes that will allow you to enjoy them while staying on the Plan? Can you make yourself some treats that will truly satisfy you while not being too far off the Plan, like gluten-free cookies without nuts or chocolate? Can you pre-stock the fridge and freezer with great options to balance out the unhelpful choices?

CREATING A TRAVEL KIT

Thinking strategically about migraine relief means lots of planning. Current research has shown that during a migraine attack, people are not able to think clearly. So creating rescue plans and travel kits is something you need to do when you are feeling well.[150] One way I've been able to improve my migraine while traveling is by spending more time planning before I go. In addition to the meds that I keep in my purse at all times, my travel kit also includes ibuprofen and naproxen sodium tablets, sumatriptan, and Cambia. If I'm staying overnight somewhere, I pack all my other medications as well. Be sure to pack enough for a stay two days longer than you planned. I recently got stuck in Denver for two extra days and ran out of a daily medication.

Also in my travel kit: soft ear plugs (for the airplane and hotel room), white noise app on my phone, phone charger, blackout eye mask (essential for sleeping on the plane and in the hotel), and foods that work for me, like pop-top canned salmon and sardines. I have two tennis balls in a tube sock that I use for self-massage on tight muscles, and two inflatable travel pillows to allow me to sleep comfortably on long flights.

The family visit

You're heading home to visit family members. What could possibly go wrong?

At family gatherings, you will not be at your best, because everyone automatically reverts to their inner 12-year-old when they visit with their family. Unless you've done a lot of therapy. In that case, rock on. You won't have trouble being assertive.

My family has gotten used to what they describe as my "weird diet" over the years, and yes, there is a lot of discussion about it, far more than I would like. I have found that not staying at the hosting house helps—just being mobile and having a place with a kitchenette allows me to make better choices. Some of my family is very supportive and will cook specifically for me; others not so much.

But it's up to me, the 50-something-year-old me—not the 12-year-old me—to stay the course as much as possible, so I can feel well and enjoy the visit. Enlisting an ally (a sibling, partner, or cousin) in advance is very helpful, as is actually planning out what you want to eat and what will work for you. While I always did that for vacations, for some reason family visits were just blank slates between flight arrival and departure. I did no planning. Not only was this frustrating for me, but it led to lots of unhelpful choices.

Keep in mind that families can be a great source of stress. In addition to planning your food, come up with suitable exit strategies and a stress management plan (make time to meditate, walk, or simply spend time on your own).

If you're traveling to visit family, do the research on restaurants and places to stay exactly as you would for a vacation (page 137). If you "always" do a certain thing, that is when you are likely to fail. And only you can decide if it's worth it or not. Think back to your last few trips there. Did you always get a migraine or headache? Did you miss out on activities because of it? Thinking this through might help you decide that it's worth it to rock the boat and change the dynamic. Maybe you decide that eating properly is worth it, as is staying in a hotel or bed-and-breakfast and renting a car instead of being picked up. (You might not have these options because of budget, and that's OK, too.) Maybe changing those dynamics also shifts your migraine pattern. Experiment and see. Having agency in the situation helps me feel stronger.

Maybe you decide to get more engaged in helping to cook, planning what will be served, and making sure you'll have plenty to eat. You can still eat family recipes if they are reasonably close to the Plan. Maybe you just carve out a portion before adding the salt and sugar, for example.

A therapist I saw a long time ago said something that always stuck with me: "A family is like a boat. Everyone's in the boat. You can't stand up or jump out without it affecting everyone else. But that doesn't mean you can't stand up or jump out. The boat will still float and regain its equilibrium, and once it settles down, so will everyone left in the boat."

The vacation

You're finally getting a week away.

Travel gets easier once you have an idea of what types of restaurants are most likely to work. Do your research before you go, so you know how much food you'll need to pack, what you can buy there, and where you can eat out. If it's possible to stay at a place with a kitchen (rental or hotel with a kitchenette), that is your best option, as eating out meal after meal will tax both your willpower and your sodium intake, in addition to exposing you to your triggers. Eggs and fresh fruit for breakfast are available nearly everywhere in the United States. Undressed salad and unmarinated grilled protein are your safest bets for lunch and dinner. Focus on the non-food activities as much as possible, and really put your intention there instead of on the food.

For my first trip after my diagnosis, we chose Portland, Oregon. We stayed with highly accommodating friends, cooked a lot at their home, and had some pretty successful meals out. Was it the carefree visit to Portland I had enjoyed in the past? No. Did we go to all my favorite restaurants? No. But it was a great trip, and I found an amazing new Paleo food truck that I would never have tried otherwise. Check out Amie Valpone's book *Eating Clean* for more helpful tips on living a full and happy life while on a restricted diet.[151]

The overseas trip

You love to travel, and going overseas, for work or pleasure, is part of your life. Is it possible to do it while staying on the Plan?

Yes and no. With planning and research, you can learn what kinds of foods you will likely find in that country. If it's possible to rent a place with a kitchen, then my general travel strategy will work here, too. Stick to fresh fruits and vegetables, eggs, steamed rice, potatoes, and grilled meats and fish. Have your diet list and special request card translated into that country's language.

Keep it simple.

Don't ask if they can make you a gluten-free croissant in Paris. If you research typical foods and customs before you travel, it will go a long way. Bring your meds, anything you need to help reduce symptoms, and as many safe snacks as you can pack. Drink a ton of water. Order a salt-free and gluten-free meal from the airline. You need to call ahead; United, Lufthansa, and Virgin Australia have all accommodated me on recent trips. Eat about half of what is provided, plus your healthy foods. I brought hard-boiled eggs in a zip-top bag and asked for ice to keep them cold, which I changed out midway through an overseas flight. I also packed Paleo jerky (reasonably low-sodium), one serving of home-made granola, and two pieces of fruit. Check agricultural restrictions before packing; most countries don't allow fruit to enter but will allow unopened packaged foods. I had additional sealed packages of Paleo jerky, Paleo wraps, and energy bars free of triggers that I was able to bring through customs.

Search for food blogs from that country to see in detail what the cuisine is like. You can use Google Translate if the blogs are not in English. You can also email the bloggers directly with questions; most of us are thrilled to help readers.

Contact hotels in advance to find out how they can help you, and if possible, pick ones where they seem interested in working with you. It's much more common for ho-tels (rather than bed-and-breakfasts or hostels) to have travelers with allergies and other life-threatening conditions, so contact them in advance and stay at the places that seem willing to help you. The more advance notice you can give them, the better. If you are renting an apartment, be aware that the cookware has almost certainly been used to pre-pare foods containing gluten. Clean all pans, cutting boards, and utensils thoroughly be-fore using them if you're gluten-intolerant, have celiac disease, or have a life-threatening allergy. Colanders are nearly impossible to clean.

Ultimately, you're spending a lot of money to see another country, and you don't want to miss out by feeling sick.

PLAN YOUR BINGES

It seems counter-intuitive, but when you have to be as disciplined as we are to feel well, you need to have some release valves built in. Willpower researcher Dr. Kelly McGonigal makes it clear that constant willpower is too much of a burden to maintain long-term and encourages people to "give up the pursuit of willpower perfection." A regular deep relaxation practice is helpful to release this tension.[152]

A friend of mine, who follows a very strict anti-cancer diet, told me that she plans quarterly three-day binges on each solstice and equinox. For those three days, she eats whatever she wants. And then she returns to her vegan diet.

I have 15 days each year where I *know* I will want to eat off the Plan: New Year's Day (we host a brunch), Valentine's Day, three days in March, my birthday and anniversary in June, the Fourth of July, three days in September, Halloween, Thanksgiving, Christmas, and the day after Christmas.

Just knowing that I have those days to look forward to helps me stay on track. Ricki Heller has a chapter in *Living Candida-Free* that is full of strategies for success. The anti-Candida diet is also quite strict; Heller deals with cravings by making small batches of treats that still align with her plan.[153] Gretchen Rubin suggests creating a list of treats (not food-related): small pleasures or indulgences that align with our desired goals. My list includes buying new kitchen tea towels, visiting a hardware or crafts store just to wander, and having tea with a friend with no time limit.

Rubin also points out that some people are wired as Abstainers and some as Moderators. The names are a little confusing. Moderators are able to be moderate. Abstainers are all-or-nothing people, finding it exhausting to keep track of any gray area.[154] Not sure which you are? Moderators can eat one square of chocolate a day. Abstainers have to finish the entire bar. I'm an Abstainer for sure. I used to have a roommate who would buy packages of Vienna Fingers cookies. She could *eat one cookie*, and then not touch the package for a week or more. They would often go stale. That package of cookies called to me constantly. Stale cookies are not a concept I understand.

> Rubin suggests thinking of time away from a habit as a pause (rather than a fail), and setting a specific day on your calendar to pick the habit back up.

Ironically, I had a complete-and-totally-off-the-rails binge while I was writing this book. I had been dealing with a lot of change in my diet, a lot of change in my life, some negative health news I wasn't expecting (on top of the migraine attacks and Meniere's), and some still-recent deaths in our family circle.

I was trucking along, experimenting on myself, developing recipes, thinking I was handling it. And then something *terrible* happened to someone I loved very much. I was devastated. I fell apart. I was crying all the time. I had trouble concentrating. I was feeling depressed.

I started buying peanut butter cups. Every day. And then more sugar. And then more food truck choices that weren't helpful, like egg rolls in sugary dipping sauce. Until one day when someone offered me Oreos, I ate them, too. Oreos! I hadn't had Oreos in 10 years. They're junk food. They're full of gluten and sugar and GMOs. There is absolutely nothing about Oreos that aligns with my health goals. And that's when I knew I was in trouble. It was too much to do alone.

I called a friend, had a long talk, and set up accountability for my food choices, emailing her every day for a week until I felt like I was making progress. I found a professional grief counselor. I talked to a nutritionist. I reconnected with local friends. And finally, I accepted that I needed to be gentle and compassionate with myself.

I share this not so you will feel sorry for me, but because s#*t happens. Sometimes the eating plan takes a backseat. If this happens to you, don't beat yourself up. Be as kind to yourself as you would be to a friend. Get the help you need to start feeling better emotionally, and then you can retool.

And when you're ready, follow this three-day plan to reset yourself. If you've gotten hooked on sugar again, know that it takes three days for the cravings to subside. Make it to day four and you'll feel less crazy.

MY 3-DAY BACK-ON-TRACK PLAN

Since making unhelpful choices is inevitable, I've found it helpful to have a plan at the ready to get back on track, complete with shopping lists and meal plans. Do your best to give yourself a 12-hour fast between dinner and breakfast. This allows your body time to rest, digest properly, and detox. Since I usually eat at 8 a.m., I try not to eat any food or snacks after 8 p.m. If you need something sweet in the afternoon on any of these days, have the Vanilla Ricotta Cream (page 263) as your afternoon snack and chicken broth or liverwurst for your evening snack.

Shopping list

2–3 (4-ounce) cans albacore tuna fish, no salt added, wild-caught if possible

Low-sodium mayonnaise (or homemade olive oil mayonnaise)

½ dozen cage-free eggs

1 (15-ounce) tub whole milk ricotta cheese

Unsalted grass-fed butter, such as Kerrygold

1 bunch kale

1 bag mixed salad greens

1 bunch beet greens or Swiss chard

1 bunch flat-leaf Italian or curly parsley

3–4 mint leaves (optional)

12 sprigs fresh thyme or ¼ teaspoon dried thyme (optional)

1 bunch green onions

1 bunch asparagus

1–2 red or golden beets

4–6 carrots

2–3 bell peppers

1 jalapeño

1 bunch broccoli

1–2 cucumbers

2 pints organic strawberries or 2 bags no-sugar-added frozen strawberries

3 grass-fed burgers, fresh or frozen

Reduced-sodium liverwurst or pâté (optional)

6–8 ounces frozen wild-caught Pacific salmon fillet

1 chicken breast

Notes

- This list is for one 5'6" woman; double or triple the amounts if needed.
- If possible, buy organic products.
- Omit the ricotta if you don't eat dairy and replace the butter with ghee if you don't eat lactose

Check to make sure you have in your kitchen

Low-sodium, onion-free chicken or beef broth

Hemp seeds (optional)

Chia seeds (optional)

Flax seeds

Pumpkin seeds

Sesame seeds

Sunflower seeds

Organic stevia packets

Garlic

Best-quality pure vanilla extract

2–3 (14-ounce) cans regular (full-fat) coconut milk

Hemp Milk (optional, page 255)

Dark toasted sesame oil

Hot sesame oil (optional)

Extra virgin coconut oil

Old Bay seasoning

Extra virgin olive oil

Maca powder (optional)

Notes

- The chia seeds and hemp milk are for Vanilla Chia Pudding (find the recipe on RecipeRenovator.com) and Beet–Strawberry Smoothie (page 187).

What you need to make or purchase in advance

Vanilla Ricotta Cream (page 263), Coconut Whipped Cream (page 254), or Vanilla Chia Pudding

Chopped Salad (page 287), enough for three servings

Chicken stock (optional)

Olive oil mayonnaise (optional)

Notes

- If you don't want to purchase chicken stock, use the Golden Bone Broth recipe from meljoulwan.com minus the vinegar and onions.
- Find the olive oil mayonnaise recipe on RecipeRenovator.com.
- If you are pressed for time, feel free to prep all the vegetables and fruit the night before, so you can just add them to the plate, pan, or blender.

3-DAY BACK-ON-TRACK PLAN

MEAL	DAY 1	DAY 2	DAY 3
Breakfast	1–2 eggs cooked in coconut oil and either 1 ounce liverwurst *or* 1 cup hot chicken broth with 1 pinch curry powder	1–2 eggs cooked in coconut oil and either 1 ounce liverwurst *or* 1 cup hot chicken broth with 1 pinch curry powder	1 Salmon, Asparagus, and Thyme Omelet (page 209) with either 1 ounce liverwurst *or* 1 cup hot chicken broth or bone broth with 1 pinch curry powder
Mid-morning snack	Beet–Strawberry Smoothie (refrigerate half for tomorrow)	Beet–Strawberry Smoothie	Vegetable smoothie *or* green juice (blend or juice all the remaining veggies, leaving enough for your dinner stir-fry)
Lunch	Tuna Salad (page 223) with 1 serving Chopped Salad	1 grass-fed burger topped with mayonnaise and 1 serving Chopped Salad	1 serving Tuna Salad with the rest of the Chopped Salad
Mid-afternoon snack	Chicken broth *or* liverwurst (whatever you did not have in the morning)	Chicken broth *or* liverwurst (whichever you did not have in the morning)	Chicken broth *or* liverwurst (whichever you did not have in the morning)
Dinner	2 grilled grass-fed burgers and Spicy Kale and Swiss Chard Sauté (page 243)	1 grilled salmon fillet (save ¼ for tomorrow morning) with grilled asparagus topped with unsalted butter and spices (save ¼ for tomorrow morning, chopped up)	1 chicken breast cut up into pieces, stir-fried in coconut and dark sesame oil with the last of the veggies and sprinkled with sesame seeds
Dessert or Snack	1 cup sliced strawberries with ½ cup Vanilla Ricotta Cream, Coconut Whipped Cream, or Vanilla Chia Pudding	1 cup sliced strawberries with ½ cup Vanilla Ricotta Cream, Coconut Whipped Cream, or Vanilla Chia Pudding	1 cup sliced strawberries with ½ cup Vanilla Ricotta Cream, Coconut Whipped Cream, or Vanilla Chia Pudding

MONTH 6
sleep and movement

——— ⋯ ———

This month we're going to be taking a deeper dive into two critical components of a migraine-friendly lifestyle: getting enough sleep on a regular schedule and including gentle exercise in your daily routine. All migraine experts agree that these two factors are key to managing migraine attacks, as well as maintaining good overall health and wellness. If you followed the Plan guidelines, you should be on a fairly consistent sleep pattern by now and getting some regular, gentle movement. You may already be seeing improvements in your health, weight, and migraine pattern. Now we'll go deeper into the science, which has helped motivate me to protect my sleep and make time for movement.

SLEEP

——— · ———

I used to have terrible insomnia. I would have trouble falling asleep, avoid going to bed, and often have to get up, watch TV, and then try again. I even went to a sleep clinic and had electrodes stuck to my body. For a hyper-vigilant insomniac, trying to fall asleep in a sleep clinic is like having a Doberman watching you eat a steak when you're afraid of dogs. They had to drug me to fall asleep.

Most, if not all, migraine experts suggest regulating sleep, as a regular sleep pattern is known to help reduce migraine and headaches. Some fascinating ongoing research out of Germany may in the future be able to link circadian rhythms (or other biorhythms) to migraine attacks.[155]

Americans are chronically under-rested. Too little sleep over time can put you at a higher risk for heart disease, heart attack, high blood pressure, and stroke. Lack of sleep also affects sex drive, depression, memory, and weight gain, and it can also impair your judgment, leading to accidents or other risky behavior.[156] Too-short nights of sleep affect the expression of 117 different genes, stimulating the immune system response and turning on genes that increase inflammation.[157]

In addition, it's important to allow your gut to do its work, unencumbered by food. Gut-health expert Dr. Gerry Mullin recommends having your last meal three to four

ASSIGNMENTS

- Take a look at your bedroom and see how you can make it a sleep haven. Ideally this means no TV or phone, room-darkening curtains, and restful images.
- Try listening to white noise or a guided sleep meditation for a few nights to see if it helps you.
- Think about what you really love to do that's active rather than what you

think you "should" do.
- Make a date with yourself to do that activity one time this week. If you love it, then put it into your calendar for next week, too. If you don't love it, then pick something else to try next week. Focus on lots of little movements rather than "getting exercise" or "working out."

hours before bed. This allows what he calls the "cleansing wave" of gut contractions to clear your stomach and small intestine, critical to preventing small intestinal bacterial overgrowth (SIBO). The later you eat, the less effective these waves will be at cleaning out the small bowel while you sleep.[158]

I finally improved my sleep situation by taking an online insomnia course that taught me the basics of good sleep hygiene. I dealt with some issues from my past. I started practicing yoga and meditation. I changed my diet. And I finally sleep well.

I hope what I learned will help you, too.

Establish regular bedtime and wake time
We aren't following the rhythms of nature any longer, so our bodies aren't being supported to sleep naturally. We have artificial light disrupting our circadian rhythms, blue light from screens suppressing release of the sleep hormone melatonin,[159] and irregular schedules.

It's not realistic for me to tell you to go to bed at sunset and get up at sunrise. I don't. But I do try to head to bed by 10 p.m. at the latest. I read for 30 to 45 minutes from a book or magazine, not my tablet, and then turn out the light. If you use a tablet to read, turn down the brightness as much as you can so it doesn't affect your body's natural release of melatonin. There are also apps that automatically adjust your phone or tablet's screen hue after sunset.

I try my best to do this every night. I try not to stay up later on weekends. If you currently have an irregular schedule, think about a median point where you could reasonably go to bed seven days a week and start there. It might be later than you want some nights, but it's better at first to have less sleep and be more regular than have a consistently irregular schedule. Slowly shift your bedtime forward until you are getting seven to eight hours of sleep, if at all possible, but no more than nine. I average 8.25 hours.

In her *Body Book*, Cameron Diaz talks about the importance of creating a bedtime ritual and sticking to it every night, no matter where she is in the world. Some elements of a sleep ritual might include closing out the world, setting your alarm, preparing your bed, brushing your teeth, and washing your face.[160]

My gentle alarm goes off at 6:15 every morning—every morning—and if that doesn't work, my dog, Daisy, sticks her nose in my armpit shortly thereafter. Whether I feel like it or not, I get up. (If I'm in a migraine/headache period, I cut myself some slack and take another 30 minutes, or I plan on a nap later if needed.) This allows me to start my day with 30 minutes of walking, 10 minutes of yoga, and 10 minutes of meditation; I eat around 8:30 a.m., roughly 12 hours after my last meal.

Utilize guided meditations to relax muscle tension and promote sleep

One thing I learned following the insomnia program was that insomniacs tend to hold a lot of tension in their bodies. That was certainly true of me in the past. I was *wound up*. Unsurprisingly, it's difficult to fall asleep when your whole body is full of tension. If a hard-core Type A person like me can change, anyone can. One inexpensive tool is an acupressure mat to help induce the relaxation response.[161]

Using guided meditations (see page 110) that teach you how to relax each muscle group systematically works wonders to release this tension. During the insomnia program, I would take a short break every afternoon to listen to a 15-minute guided meditation. Sometimes I would fall asleep and have a brief nap. Within a few weeks, I noticed great improvement in my ability to fall asleep at night.

I have used a few guided meditations over the years that are specifically designed to help me fall asleep, plus a white noise machine every night. When I started exploring guided meditation, I had a portable CD player next to the bed. If you need your phone to access your meditations, that's a smartphone exception. Just make sure you use the phone solely for that. You'll find that, over time, hearing the white noise or even the beginning of the meditation will start to make you sleepy, as you'll become conditioned to have a sleep response.

While I'll never be a world-champion napper, I'm happy to get 7.5 to 8.25 hours of sleep consistently every night.

Make the bedroom a sleep haven

The consensus among sleep experts is that the bedroom should be reserved for two things: sleep and sex. This is difficult for a lot of people because our digital lives have crept into the bedroom. Many people sleep with their smartphone next to or even *in* their bed, and many people watch TV in bed. Neither of those behaviors is ideal for proper sleep. The light from TVs and computer screens is particularly unrestful, as the blue

---

TAKE A NEWS OR SOCIAL MEDIA FAST

I have found that going on a news fast helps me be more calm and peaceful. How does this work? For a set period—like a day or week—don't listen to, read, or watch any news. If you're a news junkie, or feeling informed is really important to you, this might sound very difficult. You might feel like I'm suggesting that you don't care, and you may argue that educated people need to stay informed and that it's impossible to avoid news. I originally had all those reactions as well. What you may find is that:

- Truly important events come through.

- You will feel better not absorbing all the noxious filler, panic, and fear mongering that infuse most newscasts.

- You will have more time and compassion to focus on things that matter to you and that you can actually do something about.

I spend my time meditating instead, which I hope helps me be a better person and serve the world in the way I'm meant to do so. Ingesting the news does not support that in me.

Consider trying a social media fast for a day, for the weekend, or at least after a set time in the day. I'll be honest: This has not been easy for me. I'm experimenting with no phone or computer between 8 p.m. and 8 a.m., and none at all on Sundays. Dallas Hartwig, cofounder of the Whole30 Program, now has a free four-week program called More Social Less Media if you'd like to explore this concept further.[163]

---

spectrum of light depresses our natural release of melatonin. In addition to removing screens, install warm light bulbs in the bedroom to encourage sleep. You can order light bulbs from lowbluelight.com to use in the evening.

Even if I fast-forward through the commercials, processing TV's many images for hours at a time is stimulating for my brain. Often the content is upsetting. If you watch the news before bed, your mind is filled with horrible things happening around the world, things you have no control over but are now aware of. That's not a great recipe for sleep.

Make sure your mattress, bedding, and pillows are all comforting. I have found a fluffy down pillow works best for my tender head, and my husband and I have a dual-control electric blanket, so the temperature is good for us both. Many health advocates will tell you to avoid electric fields in the bedroom. Our room is so small and cold in the winter that I literally cannot fall asleep without the blanket prewarming the bed. I don't sleep with it on, but my husband really likes it.

I don't bring my phone or tablet into the bedroom, as its presence tends to call to me even when it's off. This is called hypervigilance, and it's becoming a real problem, especially for younger people. One recent study found that 63 percent of people ages 18 to 29 sleep with their phone *in* bed.[162] It's not yet clear if that's causing health or mental problems.

I use a white noise machine as well. If you want to try this, there are many white noise apps available. That's an exception I would make for the phone, using it to play a white noise app. That's what I do when I travel. The last thing I recommended is room-darkening curtains. I recently added room-darkening and sound-dampening curtains and wished I had ordered them years ago.

Avoid stimulants

Caffeine, chocolate, decongestants containing pseudoephedrine, regular and decaffeinated tea, and even spicy foods have kept me up at night. Some people find alcohol to be a stimulant as well. A regular cup of coffee in the morning will keep me up until 2 or 3 a.m., as will chocolate after 2 p.m. I have always had to be careful, even before I started getting migraine attacks. Removing these things from your regular routine, as we do on this Plan, should help with your sleep.

Eat early, rather than later

Our bodies use a lot of energy to digest food. Not only can that be an issue with sleep, but it also means your body isn't able to use energy for other key tasks while you sleep, like rebuilding muscle tissue and healing. While I don't recommend daytime fasting for people prone to migraine attacks, one way you can get the benefit of fasting is to have 12 hours between dinner and breakfast. If you try this and regularly wake up with a migraine, that 12-hour fast might not work for your body. In that case, eat a small protein snack right before bed and see if that helps.

Take a magnesium supplement 30 to 60 minutes before bed

I had no idea that magnesium might help me sleep; it's a supplement that was recommended by my acupuncturist and every migraine book I read. Taking it before bed seems to turn on my sleep clock, and I often conk out as soon as I turn out the light, which is bliss. (Dr. Wahls has specific recommendations for additional sleep supplements in her book *The Wahls Protocol*.[164]) Magnesium helps our bodies store fat properly and absorb nutrients. Inadequate magnesium is linked to systemic inflammation. Magnesium-rich foods on the Plan include pumpkin seeds, sesame seeds, spinach, black beans, and quinoa.[165] I now take a migraine-specific supplement that contains the proper amount of magnesium in addition to feverfew and riboflavin. Magnesium alone is safe to take during pregnancy. Soaking in a warm bath of baking soda, Epsom salts (magnesium sulfate), and lavender essential oil (if it doesn't bother you) can help you absorb more magnesium through your skin and may help with a migraine attack. See Appendix B (page 300) for a complete list of recommended supplements.

Get your hormones balanced

One thing that will wreak havoc on your sleep if you're female is hot flashes as you head into menopause (the cessation of your periods). Perimenopause can last 10 years while your body slowly moves out of its reproductive phase, with wildly fluctuating hormone levels that can make migraine worse or better. My perimenopause symptoms started around age 42 and went undiagnosed. If I had found a doctor who recognized what was happening then, I might have gotten a lot more sleep. I have chosen to use bio-identical hormone replacement therapy to even out my estrogen level and address my hot flashes and other symptoms. It's not right for everyone, but I have read enough about it to feel the small risks for me are worth it for the quality of life it provides.[166]

Make a list

I have always had a busy, busy brain. It's better now, but one thing that has helped me with sleep is using to-do lists in a specific way. I read *Getting Things Done* by David Allen a while back, and use his "next actions" list every day, plus his "someday-maybe" list for long-term ideas.[167] Having all my ideas captured somewhere allows me to let go of them. If I find that I'm lying awake, it's usually because I have come up with still more ideas of things I want to do or think I *should* do. In that case, I get up, go into the other room, and write them all down. Only then do I go back to bed where I fall asleep, knowing they are taken care of for the moment.

MOVEMENT

We all know we're "supposed to exercise." In fact, exercise has become such a loaded word that I use it in this book as sparingly as possible. Instead, think of any and all types of movement you can add to your life: parking farther away, taking the stairs instead of the elevator, standing during a phone call. Whether we are working out to lose weight, look better, or to meet a goal like running a 5K or a triathlon, we know that movement is good for us. And it is—it's good for our hearts, lungs, and organs. Movement sends positive signals to your body to increase your level of human growth hormone, which tells your body to stay vigorous and vibrant. It bathes your brain in happy chemicals and blood flow that helps prevent the plaque deposits that cause Alzheimer's. It helps expend excess stress; it may help us meet like-minded people.[168] For people with autoimmune disorders, regular low to moderate movement helps regulate essential hormones.[169] What exercise *isn't* good for is weight loss.

Why exercise doesn't help you lose weight

Like everyone else, I believed what I was taught: that you have to burn more calories than you eat in order to lose weight. This is referred to as "calories in, calories out." You will see this concept being taught today in nearly every health magazine, article, and book, excepting the ancestral/Paleo literature. It's logical.

And it's wrong.

Science writer Gary Taubes spent five years researching and writing his book *Good Calories, Bad Calories* to better understand the obesity epidemic, the public health recommendations about diet (and whether they are helping or hurting), and the quality of the research that has been done on obesity and metabolism in the last 150 years. The book has 450 footnotes and hundreds of books and articles in the bibliography. Unlike many popular diet books, Taubes's project is not based on a particular point of view.

Reading Taubes's book has convinced me that "calories in, calories out" is a dangerous myth.[170] Your body is extraordinarily complex, able to regulate your metabolism based on your food intake and energy output. Taubes makes the case convincingly that our bodies are so complex that weight loss is not simply a mechanical process. If "calories in, calories out" were true, eating just 20 extra calories a day would guarantee that you would gain 50 pounds over 20 years. Everyone would be overweight. Instead, here is the latest research about weight gain:

1. The most problematic food group in weight gain is starchy carbohydrates like sugar, flour, and beer, which screw up our insulin response. Weight loss can be achieved by removing or greatly reducing these foods in our diets and replacing them with low-carbohydrate vegetables and healthy fats. Eating fat calories does not make us gain weight. Eating starchy carbohydrate calories does. Research has shown time and again that *eating carbohydrates stokes feelings of hunger*, while eating fat does not. Because I think calorie counts are overly emphasized, we have not included them in the nutritional analysis in this book.

2. Where you put on weight tends to be genetic.

3. Not all calories have the same effect on the body; their effect can be radically different. Usable calories (what's listed on the package) are not the same thing as metabolized energy (what your body actually does with the calories).[171] In addition, everyone is different in how they metabolize fat, carbohydrate, and protein. So some people are able to eat a lot of carbohydrates (think of those rail-thin vegans you know) while others cannot.

4. Having an imbalance in our gut biome (the good bugs and bad bugs in our small and large intestines) can greatly affect whether we are overweight. If we have too many Firmicutes bacteria—which are more efficient at extracting energy from food—we are more likely to be overweight.[172]

Dr. Mark Hyman and other high-profile health professionals now recommend a high-fat, lower-carb diet for long-term health and weight loss (specifically, good fats like coconut, olive, and avocado oils, and ideally eating them as whole foods rather than as oils).[173] Reading Taubes's research profoundly impacted my thinking on what constitutes a healthy diet, especially for migraine management. While it may not be an easy or effortless approach, eliminating sugars and refined flours may be the cure we've been seeking for the diseases of civilization, including obesity, diabetes, heart disease, Alzheimer's, and cancer.[174]

During my six months of symptom tracking I learned that I could eat up to 500 more calories per day than my tracker said I burned and not gain weight, so long as my carbohydrate intake was low and I moved my body regularly. That convinced me more than any book I read. If you don't believe this either, because it goes against everything you know to be true, then do the experiment on yourself. I had to unlearn 30 years of nutrition reading and training before coming to this position.

By all means, move daily for the many health benefits, especially to improve your migraine. If weight loss is your goal, you'll need to shift away from starchy carbs or your efforts will be frustrated. You may also need to rebalance your gut microbiome by working with a functional medicine doctor. If everything else doesn't work, you may need to reduce your portion sizes.

The main thing is to be patient. Long-term weight loss is best achieved through a gradual process: a pound a week for a month, then maintaining that loss for another month. Then repeat. These alternating rest periods allow your metabolism to reset. Rapid weight loss featured on shows like *The Biggest Loser* has been found to permanently alter peoples' metabolisms.

> This Plan isn't written as a low-carb diet. You can decide how to eat within the Plan in a way that feels best for you, whether that's low-carb, Paleo, Mediterranean, pescatarian, vegetarian, or vegan.

Nearly all the winners of that show have regained all the weight they lost, and more.[175] While it looks like those contestants just work out all day and lose miraculous amounts of weight, that's a poor strategy because:

- Our bodies adjust to our higher energy output.
- We have to exercise *a lot* to burn enough calories to make a difference.
- We tend to eat more when we exercise because we're hungry and need fuel.

The problem with belly fat

I used to think of extra fat on my body as simply annoying or ugly. I had no idea that those excess fat cells act as an active hormonal organ, excreting inflammatory hormones called cytokines every day. Cytokines trigger inflammatory pathways.[176] Belly fat is the most active and problematic of all the fat cells. The more belly fat cells you have, the more inflammatory hormones are excreted. And the more inflammation in your brain and body, the more likely you are to have a migraine attack. Working towards slimming down should provide benefits in terms of your pain experience, not just your appearance and overall health. Any weight you lose, even five pounds, is helpful if you are overweight. You can focus your energy on weight loss after you've been on the Plan for a while and are starting to feel better.

How to get more movement into your day

For me, getting regular exercise has always been a challenge, especially when I thought of it as "working out." I have followed the pattern throughout my life of feeling pretty good, exercising regularly, then getting hurt or sick, "quitting" exercise, feeling poorly for a while and terrible about myself, and then starting the cycle all over again.

Some people's bodies are built for heavy-duty exercise. Mine is not. Instead of beating myself up about this, I have found some strategies, outlined below, that work for me, which started with focusing on movement rather than on working out. Note that for some people, intense activity can trigger migraine attacks. Even a brisk walk on a hot-bright day, especially if I have not eaten or drank enough water, is certain to trigger a migraine attack for me.

Stop thinking about "getting in shape"

I'm in my mid-fifties, so at some point, I had to come to the realization that uber-fitness was not going to happen for me. I try very hard to simply be in my body and love it where it is right now, today. I'm able to walk to the park, I'm able to do a little yoga, I'm able to travel, and my clothes fit. I focus on moving more throughout the day. Those are all great things. I wasted so many years feeling inadequate about my fitness. I try hard not to continue those thoughts today.

Find something you love to do

I have a friend who has transformed her body through classes at a studio that combine ballet, Pilates, and yoga. She looks amazing, healthy, and strong. I have done the studio's DVDs and class a few times. It's really hard. It makes me super sore. I don't love it the way she does. I want to, but I don't. I feel like I *should*, but I don't.

What does it for *me* is yoga. Not hot yoga, not even regular yoga. (Note: Hot yoga can trigger migraine attacks.) Mellow, mostly floor, yoga. There is something about the combination of the spiritual side of the practice and the physical that resonates deep inside me. I use a ton of props (pillows, folded blankets, and blocks) to hold the poses properly, as I am not that limber and my lower back still gets tender since my fusion. I am not pretzel woman.

That might not happen for you with yoga, and that's OK. I have a friend who confessed to me that she thinks she *should* love yoga, but she hates it. She loves spin class. Maybe for you it's dancing in your underwear, having sex with your partner, going kayaking, hiking a trail, or walking your dog. Whatever it is, find it and do it. Even a little each day or a few times each week.

Recognize that all movement is good

One thing I loved about Mark Sisson's book *The Primal Blueprint* was his suggestion to play more, and quit doing what he calls "chronic cardio." Instead, he advocates lots of easy walking, play, and then a little sprinting or heavy, intense activity in short bursts once or twice a week only.[177] This more closely replicates the hunter–gatherer lifestyle for which our bodies are designed. It was the first book whose exercise recommendations ever felt realistic for me. Specifically, he says that you can get healthy and fit with this bare minimum of intentional movement:

- 2 hours of walking around per week
- 1 (10- to 15-minute) strength workout per week
- 1 (30-minute) strength workout per week
- 1 (15- to 20- minute) sprint session every 7 to 10 days

Wearing a fitness tracker has helped me see how much I am moving and encouraged me to gently set goals to move more. I can tell where I'm at in terms of a goal and whether a slightly longer walk will help me get there. I try not to focus too closely on step goals, as it doesn't feel helpful for me. I focus on the fun of seeing how the steps add up. I don't have my fitness account connected to friends', as I find it stressful to compare myself to others. If adding that friend component makes it fun for you, go for it!

Dr. Dale Bond offers these simple tips for reducing sedentary (too-much-sitting) behavior: Put your remote next to the TV, walk or stand during commercials or while fast forwarding, stand while talking or texting, take every piece of recycling to the bin individually, carry every grocery bag from the car separately, and drink more water to create bathroom breaks.[178]

Give yourself permission to have off or rest days

I used to think I needed to work out every day, and if I didn't I was some kind of failure. Reading Sisson's information about the dangers of chronic cardio—and the need for rest days for our bodies to rebuild—allowed me to enjoy those days without guilt, especially if I was dealing with a headache or migraine attack. As you gradually work towards regular movement, plan in rest days to allow your body to recover.

Create a movement routine that truly fits into your life long term

I have had periods in my life where I exercised very regularly, and in every case it was because it was part of my lifestyle at that time. I biked to work almost every day for years in Chicago (despite the Chicago weather and having that pesky broken vertebra masquerading as sciatica). It was a given. I would pack my lunch and clothes the night before, and have my riding gear laid out. There was no thinking or willpower involved.

I find that putting out my yoga outfit the night before greatly increases my chances of putting it on and doing yoga in the morning. I often go straight from bed to my mat, with only a brief bathroom stop on the way. I don't check email or look at my phone until I am finished. Once you've found a movement routine that works for you, build the habits into your life in a way that helps make them stick.

Acknowledge that some fitness goals aren't in the cards

Although there have been brief periods in my past where I was in pretty good shape, I am not a competitive athlete. I will never be that. I am never going to run a marathon, compete in a ballroom dance, try out for *American Ninja Warrior*, or do CrossFit. I can *guarantee* you that I will never post a selfie wearing a bikini. I will never own a bikini again. So why, in the back of my head, do I still feel I fall short in this area? It's something I continue to work on but mostly have come to terms with. I'm not saying those aren't great goals for other people or, if that's what really excites and motivates you, that you shouldn't set that goal. I have simply come to realize it's not helpful for me. Think about what expectations you have for yourself, where you feel you are falling short, whether that's true, and whether those expectations bring you joy. And then, perhaps, allow those expectations to fall away.

PART IV
CREATING A
LONG-TERM
LIFESTYLE

———— ••• ————

You've spent the past four months maintaining the Plan—congratulations! This part of the book includes two sections to help you continue on your healing path through Month 7 and beyond. The first will lead you through the process of testing trigger foods to see if they actually are a problem for you, giving you several ways of approaching this process. The second will cover some additional specialty diet information that may be useful to you for optimal health long term. The goal of this part of the book is to help you customize the Plan to suit your body and your needs.

MONTH 7 AND ON
trigger testing and adjusting your diet

———— ••• ————

At this point, you are now ready to begin adding foods back. If you're like me, you already have your food-testing list ready to go, and you know exactly in which order you want to test possible trigger foods. You can download a worksheet from MigraineReliefPlan.com to help you form your own list.

Or perhaps you had it all planned out and then you saw that Whole Foods had this bacon that's reduced sodium, sustainable, and uncured, and you threw the list out for that week and decided you really missed bacon and you were going to test it your first week. Not that I did that. Oh, wait, I did. Because: bacon.

The beauty is, *you* decide what order you test things and how long the process lasts. You may be doing this testing over a few months, as there are a lot of foods. You may get tired of it, skip a week, or just take your chances. But know that you can always come back to this section and start again if you need to. If you stopped tracking your symptoms and your intake because you were having success on the Plan, you will need to print out some new tracking sheets and keep close attention during this process.

I also cover some additional diet tweaks you might want to explore if you're not seeing the results you want. The beauty of the Plan is that it's designed to be a structure to help you find your individual sweet spot, learn what brings you below your migraine threshold, and to be as healthful as possible even though you still get migraine attacks.

HOW TO TEST TRIGGER FOODS

———— • ————

In *Heal Your Headache*, Dr. David Buchholz describes his recommendations for reintroducing foods by testing them **one at a time for an entire week**. If a few days of eating the food causes headaches or migraine attacks, then you can end the test there and try another food the next week. Remember that the window for food triggers is estimated to be 4 to 96 hours. He says most of his patients just cheat here and there, learning what

ASSIGNMENTS

- Make your list of foods you want to test.
- Restart tracking if you have stopped for a while.
- Follow the trigger testing guidelines and experiment.

- If you aren't seeing great improvement in your migraine pattern, consider going lower-carb over a few weeks.

works and what doesn't without structuring their reintroductions. He cautions to never add caffeine or soy back in, as in his experience they are too potent of triggers. He says most of his patients find it easier to remain on the baseline plan, as they feel so much better, and then they add in trigger foods from time to time.[179] Since triggers are cumulative, meaning they add up over time, I try to live on the Plan as much as possible as a day-to-day rule so that I can add in triggers without reaching my migraine threshold.

Below are my recommendations, which blend Buchholz's experience with patients (he does not get migraine attacks) and my personal experience with trigger testing. The cumulative nature of triggers means that this process will never be black and white, but this approach helped me truly understand which foods bother me and which are now OK. I still don't overdo trigger foods, but it's nice to have more options, especially when eating out.

1. **MAKE A LIST OF THE FOODS YOU MISS THE MOST, THEN PRIORITIZE THEM.** I recommend testing onions and fermented foods as early as possible, as they are important sources of prebiotics (feeding your good gut bacteria) and probiotics (adding healthful bacteria to your gut). If onions don't bother you, then adding them opens up more prepared foods, like organic chicken broth, that will make cooking easier.

2. **CHOOSE YOUR NUMBER ONE FOOD TO TEST THE FIRST WEEK.** This is the beginning of Month 7, unless you decided you couldn't wait and are doing it sooner.

3. **HAVE AT LEAST ONE SERVING OF THAT FOOD PER DAY FOR SEVEN DAYS.** You can have the food at any time of day, unless you're testing chocolate. I recommend testing chocolate no later than 2 p.m. if you are at all sensitive to the stimulants in it.

4. **NOTE ANY CHANGE IN SYMPTOMS IN YOUR TRACKING PROGRAM.**

5. **IF IT'S CLEAR THAT THE FOOD TRIGGERS A MIGRAINE ATTACK, DON'T KEEP EATING IT**. I recommend finishing out the week on the baseline Plan to allow your body to recover.

6. **TEST THE FOOD EACH DAY**. This is important, as you need to allow for other variables that might also be affecting you. (Ideally, you are having few symptoms at this point, so it will be easy to tell.)

7. **IF THE WEATHER PATTERNS DURING A WEEK OF TESTING WILL AFFECT YOU, DON'T TEST THAT WEEK**. For me, the hot, dry winds called Santa Anas that come with high barometric pressure, high temperature, low humidity, and bright skies *always* trigger a migraine attack no matter how well I eat, so if we had that weather, I did not test during that week, and sometimes waited a week afterwards to get back to normal. For you, it might be thunderstorms. Flying also negatively affects many people with migraines, so I would skip testing if you're traveling somewhere

8. **ONCE YOU HAVE FINISHED TESTING A FOOD, REMOVE IT FROM YOUR DIET (AS MUCH AS POSSIBLE) AND START TESTING THE NEXT FOOD**. Unless you had a bad reaction and need time to recover, you can move straight into testing the next food.

9. **REMEMBER THAT TRIGGER TESTING IS NOT ABSOLUTE**. It's best to keep yourself at the Plan baseline while testing one food per week, as most experts believe there is a cumulative effect of triggers.

10. **TEST SEAWEED EARLY**. Because seaweed (often a trigger) is an incredibly rich source of nutrients and is recommended by most nutritionists, test adding seaweed powder (½ teaspoon per day) early on to see if you can incorporate it into your diet. While seaweed does contain glutamates (which is why it's likely a migraine trigger), it removes heavy metals from our bodies and provides a rich array of minerals.[180]

11. **TEST EACH OF THESE FOODS SEPARATELY, IF POSSIBLE**:

   - *Onions.* Cooked red onions should be tested separately from cooked white, yellow, and brown onions, which can be tested as one group. Additionally, you might want to test raw red onions and raw white/yellow/brown onions separately from their cooked counterparts. A chef's tip is to soak raw onions in ice water, then drain well before adding to a dish. This helps mellow the flavor.

- *Fermented foods.* Real sauerkraut and pickles (in the refrigerated section), kefir, live yogurt, kombucha, kimchi, and miso or tempeh should all be tested individually.

- *Citrus and other fruit.* Lemons, limes, oranges, and grapefruit should all be tested separately. Pineapple and bananas should also be tested on their own.

- *Vinegars.* Ideally, each type of vinegar is a separate test: apple cider vinegar, white balsamic vinegar, white wine vinegar, rice wine vinegar, etc. However, if one light/clear vinegar doesn't seem to bother you, then the rest of this group should also be OK in small amounts. Once you have tested it, I recommend using unpasteurized apple cider vinegar for its many documented health benefits. If you wish to try dark vinegars (balsamic, sherry, red wine), note that they are much more likely to be triggers, and try them at the very end of your testing period.

- *Cheeses.* Each type of cheese (e.g., Swiss, cheddar, brie, mozzarella, Parmesan) is a separate week.

- *Nuts.* Each type of nut (e.g., cashews, pistachios, pecans, etc.) is a separate week. I don't recommend adding peanuts back into your diet, as they tend to be highly allergenic.

- *Chocolate.* Ideally, test chocolate without sugar (unsweetened cocoa powder or cacao nibs) instead of chocolate bars, so you can see the effect of chocolate itself, not chocolate plus sugar.

The reason you can't simply test citrus fruits interchangeably is that they contain different compounds. You might not be sensitive to anything but grapefruit, or you might react to everything but grapefruit. If you test them interchangeably, you won't know which foods specifically cause a problem for you. It would be a shame for you to avoid all citrus, which is delicious and loaded with nutrients, if only oranges trigger you.

Migraine symptoms can show up as long as 96 hours after eating a food, so be aware of this if you use a shorter process.

My results

Here is the order in which I tested food, along with my results. It shouldn't surprise you to learn that I was pretty anal about tracking everything. I found the process fascinating, liberating, and tedious all at once. But for me it was worth the time and trouble, because now I truly know my own patterns.

Food	Notes	Results
Heritage uncured bacon	I tried the Whole Foods 365 brand in small quantities due to sodium	OK
Avocados	I was missing them, and they are such a great source of healthy fats and nutrients	OK
Chocolate	Do I need to explain?	Not OK. Sad face.
Lemon	I was missing acidity; it's such a staple in my cooking	OK? I might need to test again, as I did have some headache issues that week
Apple cider vinegar	For more options with salad dressing	OK
White/yellow onion	Such a basic for cooking, plus an important prebiotic food	OK
Low-sodium Swiss cheese	I was really missing that cheesy component	Borderline OK. It gives me a headache within 15 minutes, but doesn't seem to trigger a full migraine attack. Have since learned I have a dairy allergy, so I can't eat this for other reasons
Bananas	For the potassium, and for smoothies	OK
Almonds	Missing my nuts and easy protein	OK
Pineapple	Because we would be traveling overseas and I expected it might be very common on the trip	OK

A *closer look at:* food allergies and migraine

A recent study of 500 clients seeing a migraine physician found that 36 percent of participants tested positive for a highly allergic response to eggs, 32 percent had a similar highly allergic response to dairy, and 23 percent to grains.[181] Another study in Turkey of 30 clients found that food allergies seem to play a role in migraine, possibly by adding inflammation to the body. In this small study, top allergens included milk, guar gum, flours (including gluten-free flours), coffee, aloe vera, egg whites, malt, vanilla, crayfish, peanuts, sunflower seeds, and sweet peppers. Each client's allergy profile was different. The clients halved their migraine attacks when they avoided their specific allergic foods.

If you are still having migraine attacks after following the Plan for six months, I recommend having allergy testing done to see if you have specific allergies, then eliminating those foods from your diet entirely.[182] I had delayed food allergy testing done via blood test through a functional medicine physician; that's how I learned I have a latent allergy to dairy and eggs, and I don't eat them any longer. According to nutritionist Ayla Withee, the best test to use is mediator release testing (MRT) offered by Oxford Labs; the process that complements this test is called LEAP (Lifestyle Eating and Performance). While you can order the test yourself to learn if you have allergies, Withee recommends working with a certified LEAP therapist to translate the results into a personalized diet plan that is designed to reset your immune system. It can be tricky to identify food sensitivities, and some interpretation of the lab results by a trained professional is needed.[183]

other specialty diets to consider

———— ···· ————

At this point, you may be feeling absolutely fabulous. In that case, just continue with what you are already doing and be well.

If not, I wanted to share some additional information that may be helpful to you, and explain how I have incorporated some of these recommendations into my daily life. You'll find checklists for all the options summarized in Appendix A (page 299). While it is comforting to try to figure out "the best diet," everyone is different. What works for me might not work for you, or might not be the best way for you to eat forever.

I was struck by something I heard from lifestyle medicine expert Dr. David Katz. He said that if you got a whole bunch of diet experts together for a meal, their plates would look remarkably similar: loaded with greens, some bright organic vegetables, maybe a little fruit, and some healthy protein and fat.[184] Some might have wild-caught fish or pastured meat on the plate. Some might have avocado for fat but no oil. But all those plates would be far more similar to each other than any random trays in a mall food court. Keep that in mind as you read this section.

ANCESTRAL DIETS

———— · ————

The Migraine Miracle by Dr. Josh Turknett was my first introduction to the ancestral diet, where I learned that it specifically helps with migraine and Meniere's by reducing carbohydrates, eliminating sugar, and increasing healthy fats. I erroneously thought that Paleo diets were just another fad, with no research behind them.

Before reading Turknett's book, I firmly believed that the following described a "healthy diet": low-fat foods; lots of fruits, veggies, and whole grains; lean meats in moderation; low-fat dairy products; or perhaps a vegetarian or vegan version of the same. Instead, after reading Turknett's book, I was fascinated to read in Gary Taubes's *Good Calories, Bad Calories* that this notion of "healthy diet" became gospel *without any rigorous scientific evidence to back it up.* A gluten-free and vegan version of this "healthy diet" is exactly how I was eating when I was diagnosed. It happened to be a diet full of migraine triggers.

Ancestral, primal, and Paleo diets are closely related; some of the terms are used interchangeably. In this section, I discuss several versions of these diets. The Weston A. Price Foundation has been promoting a version of the ancestral diet, which includes functional foods like sauerkraut and yogurt, for many years. The Wahls Protocol by Dr. Terry Wahls is a version of the ancestral diet focused on reversing multiple sclerosis symptoms. Dr. Sarah Ballantyne's Autoimmune Protocol (AIP) is a strict Paleo diet specifically designed to heal autoimmune conditions. A new iteration is the Viking diet, which is recommended for people in Norway, as it includes grains and other foods native to Norway, such as rye (rye is not gluten-free).[185] All of these diets approximate what humans ate for two million years, up until the invention of agriculture 10,000 years ago. The shared belief is that agriculture shifted human diets to include beans, grains, dairy, and eventually sugar, which were not found in nature in large quantities before then.

Proponents of these diets believe that humans are not at optimal health when beans, grains, dairy, and sugar are a regular part of our diets. For instance, hunter–gatherers might have found a small patch of wheat growing wild and eaten the grains when they were ripe, or most likely after sprouting or fermenting them. But they would not have had wheat again for a year, and certainly not multiple times per day. Similarly, they might have found a hive of honey, eaten it right away, and then not had honey for six months. The idea is that our bodies evolved to be sustained on fatty meat, organs, and animal fat (not lean protein, which was left behind for other animals); small amounts of fruits (mostly lower-sugar wild berries); and nuts and seeds. The bulk of the diet was anything else that was edible in the landscape (green vegetables and roots).

Taubes, who has studied the medical literature extensively to learn more about obesity and the diseases of Western civilization (e.g., heart disease, diabetes, and cancer), believes the evidence is strong for eliminating or greatly reducing our intake of sugar, refined flour (bread, cereals, pasta), liquid carbohydrates (beers, fruit juices, and sodas), and starches like potatoes, rice, and corn. He is not a proponent of any one of these diets in particular.

Each diet has its supporters, many of whom are highly passionate. It's difficult to find and separate each one into a tidy category. Instead, I've created an overview by food groups—relating each specifically to migraine—and given you my recommendations.

Meat and poultry

All the ancestral diets encourage regular consumption of meat, but *not grocery store meat from factory farms*. Most specify using the whole animal and eating the organ meats, fat, and skin. Dr. Wahls talks at length about the important nutrients found in organ meats that likely help heal our cells' mitochondria, which seem to be broken in people with autoimmune illnesses like multiple sclerosis.[186] Most diets encourage buying high-quality meat from pastured animals and avoiding meat from factory-farmed animals. The Weston A. Price Foundation recommends eating pastured meat on a regular basis, and occasionally raw meat like steak tartare.[187]

Many recommend making "bone broth," vegetables and animal bones simmered with water, spices, and apple cider vinegar to help draw out the collagen and gelatin. Bone broth is a rich source of collagen and gelatin as well as other nutrients, which may help repair skin, bones, and brain cells.

My recommendations: Unless you are a vegan or vegetarian, eat fresh meat and poultry of the best quality you can afford. Try to incorporate organ meats into your diet whenever possible. If the idea is repellent, do so gradually with more familiar options, such as a high-quality liverwurst or pâté. Make your own salt-free stock from bones or buy low-sodium organic chicken broth (check the label for trigger ingredients; most store-bought stocks contain onions). Purchase grass-fed gelatin and add one tablespoon per day to smoothies, or make gelatin desserts. Note that some migraine diet lists include gelatin and organ meats as possible migraine triggers, so test these foods as you would any other.

Utilize your freezer to stock up on good-quality meat when it goes on sale. Eat it right away or freeze it while it's still fresh. Try to avoid meat sold in Tetra Paks, which may have been treated with a sodium solution to maintain freshness. Ask whether it was packed at the store, as that is likely safe.

Cook meats to recommended safe temperatures. My public health degree included a course in epidemiology: the study of human disease transmission. To me, raw meat and fish aren't worth the risk of parasites or other serious illnesses. If you wish to eat steak tartare or sushi, choose it only if you are positive it comes from a high-quality source and has been handled properly.

Fish and seafood

All the diets encourage a regular consumption of fish and seafood. A few talk about eating the whole animal, including the head and bones of fish. Some talk about fish and seafood quality and avoiding farmed fish. Fish and seafood are also each on the list of the eight most common food allergens.

My recommendations: Most wild-caught fish is fine if you are not allergic. If you're able to buy and prepare whole fish, make stock from the head and bones. Use Seafood Watch or other reputable seafood information to help you make the best purchases both for your health and for the health of the ocean—unsustainable fishing practices are bad for us and the ocean. For example, a recent study found that only 10 percent of the shrimp eaten in the United States was US farmed or wild-caught. The other 90 percent came from shrimp farms in Asia and South America, which have much lower environmental and farming standards. They might be contaminated with antibiotics (banned in the United States) or antibiotic-resistant bacteria. Even US–produced shrimp has issues: Nearly all is treated with sodium bisulfite, sodium tripolyphosphate (which quadruples the sodium content), and/or Everfresh (4-hexyl-resorcinol, a xenoestrogen that may increase breast cancer risk if ingested at high levels).[188] Vary the types of fish you eat to reduce the possibility of contamination and heavy metals from a particular type of fish or location. Dr. Mark Hyman does not recommend eating tuna or swordfish, due to their high mercury levels. Our neighbors give us wild-caught yellowfin tuna, and we also eat salt-free albacore. I try to vary the types of fish we eat each week. Choose seafood carefully because of the sodium content. Avoid sushi unless you are absolutely certain of the origin and quality of the fish. (Sushi nearly always includes soy sauce and sugar.) Canned fish may be high in tyramine or contain MSG; read the label to be sure it contains only fish and water as ingredients. For more information, see page 51.

Dairy products

Dairy is one area where these diets diverge. Some allow full-fat dairy products; others are opposed. One allows full-fat dairy but only if it is raw. Some omit it altogether and give lengthy explanations why. The autoimmune protocol diets described by Dr. Wahls and Sarah Ballantyne exclude all dairy. Dairy is one of the top eight food allergens.

My recommendations: If you are not lactose-intolerant, consuming whole-milk, organic, grass-fed dairy products is fine. There are so few dairy products that are allowed on the Plan; sometimes it's helpful to have that protein. Before I found out about my dairy allergy, I occasionally ate whole-milk ricotta cheese, heavy cream, half-and-half, and one kind of Swiss cheese that's low in sodium and that I tested for myself. Milk and cheese from goats and sheep may be more digestible for you, so test them if you like. Fresh (soft) cheeses are less likely to be triggers than aged, harder cheeses because they will not have high levels of tyramine. Note that milk tested high as a food allergen with migraine sufferers in at least two studies, so this may be a problem for you. It's an area you might come back to down to the road, once you are comfortable eating on the Plan and feel you might be able to incorporate another big change.

Eggs

All the diets except the Wahls Protocol and the AIP allow eggs. Ballantyne suggests eliminating eggs until your autoimmune symptoms are markedly improved, then trying just egg yolks. Most plans specify pastured or local eggs from healthy chickens, not factory farms. Eggs are on the top eight food allergens list.

My recommendations: If you are not allergic to the protein in eggs, then enjoy them. I buy eggs for my husband that are certified humane and free-range. Sometimes we get local eggs from friends. If you need to reduce sodium, toss the egg whites and use more yolks. Most of the fat is in the yolks; most of the sodium is in the whites. Egg labeling is not consistent. Look for the "certified humane" label if you can find it. The next best is organic and free-range. The term *cage-free* sounds good but doesn't guarantee the chickens are humanely treated, as chickens can be labeled as cage-free and still be housed in giant warehouses, never seeing daylight for their entire lives. Chickens are omnivores, so "all vegetarian feed," a common phrase on packaging, is not the optimal diet for them.

Grains

Most of these diets are gluten-free. Some allow grains in small amounts. Some allow grains only if they have been pre-sprouted to help with digestibility. The Viking diet allows whole-grain rye, which contains gluten. The diets described by Dr. Wahls and Sarah Ballantyne exclude all grains, in part because it's believed to be necessary to heal leaky gut syndrome. Wheat is one of the top eight food allergens.

My recommendations: Eat gluten-free whole grains in small quantities. When I started on the Plan myself, I did not restrict grains, as it was difficult enough to make all the other changes. Once I got the hang of the Plan, I cut back on grains, starting by making my portions smaller. Next, I tried not to have more than three servings per day of beans and grains total. Many days I am free of both. I find it too difficult and limiting to be completely grain-free with all the other restrictions. I focus on the pseudo-cereals, which are botanically seeds and not related to the grass family: quinoa, teff, amaranth, buckwheat, and millet. I do have sprouted brown rice on occasion but in small servings. One final note: Reducing starchy carbs also acts like a diuretic, which may be helpful for people with Meniere's disease. Recent research by Consumer Reports suggests limiting rice consumption on a weekly basis, as it naturally contains organic arsenic in small quantities.[189] As with all foods, rotate your grains to limit this potential problem. Down the road, if you are having any digestive issues, you may want to try going grain-free.

TWO DAYS ON, ONE DAY OFF

If giving up beans and grains feels like too much for you, then try a version of Mark Sisson's 80/20 rule. He encourages readers to follow the diet 80 percent of the time in order to be successful long term. I suggest eating bean- and grain-free for two days, then have one to three servings on the third day. Continue this as needed. You can plan these days to give you more choices when eating out. This will reduce your carbohydrate intake overall and help you stay on the Plan long term.

Beans (Legumes)

Most of these diets do not allow beans; the Weston A. Price Foundation includes them if they are properly prepared (soaked and sprouted). The belief is that beans are difficult to digest and contain proteins called toxic lectins (prolamines and agglutinins) that are thought to damage the gut barrier and cross into the bloodstream. The Wahls Protocol and AIP exclude all beans. Soybeans are one of the top eight food allergens.

My recommendations: If you like beans, eat the ones allowed on the Plan as needed. I have found that I now get very bloated when I eat beans and grains, even though my entire diet used to depend on them. I have reduced my servings to no more than three per day (total) of beans and grains; I still avoid soy altogether. I choose organic beans whenever possible. Canned beans are fine if they are low-sodium or no-salt-added. If you are a dedicated vegan, you'll need to continue to eat all the allowable beans for protein. You'll likely want to test each of the beans at the top of your list once you get to the trigger-testing phase.

Nuts

While it's easy to imagine our hunter–gatherer ancestors feasting on nuts, all of these diets differ in their recommendations. Most allow them, some only with pre-soaking to improve digestibility. Many ban peanuts, which are actually a legume, not a tree nut. One recommends focusing on macadamia nuts, as they have the best types of fats. The AIP excludes all nuts. Once you are feeling well, Ballantyne describes a phased approach to reintroducing nuts. Nuts (tree nuts and peanuts) are on the top eight food allergens list.

My recommendations: Since nuts are a known migraine trigger, they are not allowed on the Plan until you test them. I recommend testing them one at a time. Ideally, eat them after soaking for at least four hours in filtered water to improve their digestibility. If you have tested a type of nut and it doesn't trigger migraine attacks, then enjoy them as a rich, nutrient-dense source of fat, protein, and fiber. I would not go back to peanuts, which are a legume, can contain mold, and seem to be the most problematic in terms of allergenic reactions. After peanuts, cashews and pistachios may cause the most problems because they are related to poison ivy.[190]

Seeds

Most of these diets allow seeds, such as chia, sunflower, pumpkin, and sesame. Some recommend pre-soaking seeds for 4 to 24 hours. Nature provides nuts and seeds with a protective coating that has two benefits. First, it allows the seeds to pass undigested through animals or birds, spreading the seeds in their droppings as they move around, helping the plant propagate. Second, it allows for optimal conditions for sprouting, as it requires a good soaking from rain to remove the protective coating.[191] The compounds in this protective coating make it difficult for our bodies to digest them, hence the need for soaking. The AIP excludes all seeds, including seed-based spices. Once you are feeling well, you may want to seek out Ballantyne's process to reintroduce seeds. Although it's quite complex, you may find it helpful.

My recommendations: If you have time, pre-soak larger seeds. I usually use tiny seeds like chia, flax, and teff in such small amounts that I don't bother soaking them; their tiny size makes them almost impossible to strain. Seeds are packed with protein, important if you wish to eat vegan or vegetarian on this Plan. Dr. Buchholz includes seeds in his approach, so I gratefully include them as a protein source in my Plan, too.

Vegetables

Most of these diets allow vegetables, with a few exceptions. White potatoes are hotly debated. Some ban nightshades (white potatoes, tomatoes, tomatillos, peppers, and eggplant) because they may be inflammatory. Some reduce the intake of sweet root vegetables like sweet potatoes, beets, and carrots because of the natural sugar content. Some allow sweet potatoes as a special treat. Some encourage eating starchy vegetables with a healthy saturated fat. Some plans encourage juicing; one does not allow it but says that smoothies are fine if made in a high-speed blender. The AIP excludes all nightshades because they contain toxic lectins.

Dr. Wahls strongly recommends eating vegetables in equal ratios: deeply colored vegetables (up to three cups per day, depending on your body size), greens (lettuce and all hearty greens, up to three cups per day), and sulfur-rich vegetables (up to three cups per day of onions, kale, asparagus, artichokes, mushrooms, rutabagas, cabbage, Brussels sprouts, and turnips).[192] You can eat fewer than nine cups per day on her plan, but she recommends keeping the ratio even for optimal nutrition: 1:1:1, 2:2:2, or 3:3:3. If it works better for you to think in weight instead of cups, you can eat one pound of vegetables and fruit per day, mostly vegetables (not blended or juiced).[193]

My recommendations: Eat as many vegetables as you can that are allowed on the Plan. Once it's second nature and you are easily incorporating vegetables every day, try Dr. Wahls's ratio, as it will give you optimal nutrient balance. Experiment with more bitter vegetables, like those from an Asian market, as they are higher in phytonutrients. When eaten, bitter vegetables help your body release hormones that trigger satiety (feeling full). Wild-foraged foods, like dandelion greens from safe fields or chemical-free yards, have much higher levels of phytonutrients than even organically grown crops. For instance, dandelion greens beat spinach seven times over in phytonutrients.[194] In *The Dorito Effect*, author Mark Schatzker makes a passionate case for expanding our taste horizons and experimenting with unfamiliar vegetables, because our palate is a growing, living thing. He recommends trying something 10 times before deciding you don't like it.[195]

If you are wavering between any kind of vegetable and a sugary snack or processed food, and the vegetable wins, then I think that's awesome. Juicing or blending vegetables into smoothies is fine by me if it means you'll eat them. To avoid spiking your blood sugar, try not to overload juices with sweet vegetables (carrots and beets) and fruits. If possible, throw everything in a high-speed blender so you get all the fiber, too. If buying a cold-pressed juice, check the carb count and shoot for under 15 grams of carbs per serving. See page 80 for tips on improving your digestion if you have smoothies.

I have no trouble eating plenty of brightly colored veggies and greens; I am often short on my sulfur-rich veggies. But I try.

Fruits

Some of the diets limit fruit or types of fruit to lower-sugar fruits like berries. One plan recommends eating fruit with healthy fat like coconut oil or organic, grass-fed heavy cream. Our Paleolithic ancestors didn't have access to fruit every day or year-round, so it's believed that our bodies aren't built to handle that much sugar. Most Paleo or ancestral plans encourage only limited fruit consumption, up to one serving per day.

My recommendations: Since we are quitting sugar on this Plan, and many fruits are off limits because of triggers, do whatever you need to do here. You may find, as I did, that your sugar cravings are so greatly reduced that you don't need much fruit unless you're in binge mode. I usually eat just one serving of fruit per day, and I try to focus on berries. Berries are recommended on the MIND diet, which is focused on brain health and reducing dementia and Alzheimer's. Blueberries are the fruit that seems to offer the most protective brain effects, with strawberries a close second.[196] When stone fruits are in season in the summer, I also enjoy those as an occasional local treat.

Keep in mind that today's fruits have been hybridized to contain far more sugar than they used to, so try not to go overboard on sweeter options like peaches, pears, or tropical fruit. As you enter fruits into your tracking program, you'll learn how many carbs different foods provide, and you'll see how quickly your carb count jumps up when including fruit. Going through that process has helped me make the most helpful choices.

It makes sense to eat fruit combined with some kind of saturated fat to lower the blood sugar surge. Try ricotta cream, coconut cream, coconut milk, heavy or whipped cream, or a cheese that works for you.

Fermented foods

Most of the diets recommend eating fermented foods like sauerkraut, yogurt, kombucha, miso, raw vinegar, and kefir—anything with live cultures, as they are natural sources of probiotics. This would include pickles only if they have been fermented (most traditional store-bought pickles are not fermented). This category doesn't include cured meats, cheeses, or foods like chocolate or coffee that may include a fermentation process in their manufacture but don't include probiotics. Most don't encourage alcoholic beverages.

My recommendations: Fermented foods are not allowed on the Plan because they are high in tyramine, may contain glutamates, and can be high in sodium. You'll need to test these one by one, as they are all possible triggers. I was eating tons of home-fermented foods before I was diagnosed, which may have been the reason I had headaches every day. They do seem to be strong triggers for me. It's difficult to find ones that don't include high sodium levels. Use your best judgment. Kombucha and kefir are fermented with sugar. Soy sauce, fish sauce, and Bragg's liquid aminos are fermented and sky-high in sodium. Fermented foods that add umami flavor are also high in natural glutamates, another trigger. I take a probiotic capsule daily, with 50 billion organisms, to try to provide some of these benefits without the triggers. I sometimes use coconut aminos (which I had to test before adding to my diet) in very small amounts for adding soy-free Asian flavor to certain recipes.

Fats

Most of these diets encourage a shift away from the plant-based oils recently introduced to the human diet (soybean, canola, corn, grapeseed, cottonseed), back to oils that have been eaten by humans for far longer (extra virgin olive oil, coconut oil, and animal fats from healthy pastured animals).

Most recommend the liberal use of saturated fats, which are solid and stable at room temperature, such as ghee, tallow, lard, rendered bacon fat, and coconut oil. Cold-pressed extra virgin olive oil and avocados or avocado oil, which provide mainly monounsaturated fats, are acceptable additions. Some do not recommend cooking with anything but saturated fats, as they have a higher smoke point and won't add carcinogens as easily as plant oils with a lower smoke point.

My recommendations: I have switched from cooking with grapeseed oil to cooking with extra virgin olive oil, coconut oil, ghee, or high-quality rendered bacon fat. The bacon fat is either from Make Your Own Bacon (page 197) or one I have tested: pastured, uncured, low in sugar, and reduced in sodium. I now use my expensive extra virgin olive oil on salads or drizzled on vegetables after cooking to get the most benefit from it. Olive oil contains a potent anti-inflammatory called oleocanthal. It's what gives good olive oil that peppery bite that makes you cough. (The more coughing, the better it is for you. And the more you get used to it, the more your body perceives a health benefit and acquires the taste.[197])

While some sources contend that heating olive oil destroys the polyphenols that make it so good for us, others claim it is fine at the temperatures and times common in home cooking. It was difficult to get used to, after years and years of low-fat living, but now I enjoy the taste of higher fat meals and feel much better.

Processed foods, sugar, and artificial sweeteners

Most of the diets ban processed foods like bread, pastries, frozen dinners, and chips (basically, all the foods found in the aisles, not the perimeter, of the grocery store); a few allow the use of sweeteners like xylitol or stevia. The AIP excludes even stevia.

My recommendations: Do your best to avoid everything in this category. Make treats as needed from allowed ingredients to help you stay on the Plan. Be sure to read labels, as many processed foods are now using artificial sweeteners to increase the sweetness factor. Use only stevia as a sweetener on a semi-regular basis, and try not to use it daily.[198] Small amounts of coconut sugar, raw honey, molasses, and maple syrup are probably OK from time to time, and some of the recipes in this book use them in very small amounts to achieve particular flavor profiles. Do not use any artificial sweeteners; many health experts believe they create long-term negative effects on the body, and a recent study showed that they may contribute to diabetes.[199]

Chocolate

Some diets don't recommend it. Some allow small quantities of high-quality, low-sugar dark chocolate or raw cacao nibs or cocoa powder as a special treat.

My recommendations: Chocolate is a potent trigger and one that does bother me. Some early results from a new migraine tracking app called Curelator suggest that chocolate can be a protective factor for some people with migraine.[200] It may be on the top of your list to test. If it works for you, use it in low-sugar forms (super dark chocolate bars), cacao nibs, or cocoa powder, sweetened with stevia. Be aware that it's a stimulant and may also affect your sleep. Carob powder is a chocolate alternative that's on the Plan. Make Carob Squares (page 251) or Creamy Not-ella Carob Butter (page 188) and see if they fulfill your craving. Be aware that carob chips contain soy lecithin and milk powder.

THE KETOGENIC DIET AND MIGRAINE

The goal of a ketogenic diet is to switch your body from burning sugar for fuel (glucose) to burning fat for fuel (ketones). It's believed that this type of diet most closely matches what our ancestors ate, as they had infrequent access to starchy carbohydrates, fruit was rare and lower in sugar, and their primary sources of calories were wild animals (or seafood) and edible green plants, tubers, nuts, and seeds. Since reducing carbohydrates may have positive benefits for migraine brains, and many of the proponents of ketogenic diets fall into the ancestral diet camp, I wanted to share what I've learned.

The ketogenic diet defined

Ketogenic diets contain **fewer than 50 grams of net carbohydrate per day** (total carbs minus fiber). After a few days at this level of carbohydrate intake, the body will likely achieve **ketosis** when it switches from burning glucose to primarily burning fat in the form of ketones. Ketones are a special type of fat that's created by the liver, and they are small enough to cross the blood-brain barrier. In contrast, when we eat a diet high in carbohydrates (like the standard American diet), our bodies run on sugar all the time, which means our brain is running on glucose. The fatty acid particles that are created by this high-carb diet and end up in our bloodstream are too large to cross the blood-brain barrier, so our brains can't burn them for fuel. Brains running on glucose are thought to be more reactive (and therefore likely to trigger) as well as more sensitive to highs and lows of blood sugar.

Ketogenic diets should not be confused with high-protein diets; the recommended protein intake for ketogenic diets is calculated per pound of lean muscle mass. To do a rough calculation for yourself, figure 1 gram of protein per half pound of your ideal body weight: a 140-pound person would eat around 70 grams of protein per day.[201] In percentages, ketogenic diets are 10 to 20 percent carbs, 20 to 30 percent protein, and 50 to 70 percent fat.[202] Fat replaces the calories from carbohydrates—generally saturated fat from pastured animals, coconut oil, or a special kind of coconut oil called MCT (medium-chain triglycerides) oil.

Pro-Paleo authors like Mark Sisson, Dr. Mark Hyman, and Dr. David Perlmutter advocate following lower-carb diets, so I wanted to clarify the differences between what they recommend and a true ketogenic diet. Dr. Terry Wahls' Paleo Plus diet (the strictest version of her Wahl's Protocol) is an MCT ketogenic diet.[203] (She utilizes MCT oil to achieve ketosis with a somewhat higher carb intake, thus allowing for optimal nutrient density.) The diets described in Dr. David Perlmutter's *Grain Brain* and Dr. Mark Hyman's *Eat Fat, Get Thin* are low carb but not quite as strict as ketogenic diets. For example, for optimal brain health Dr. Perlmutter recommends 60 to 80 *total* carbs per day with added coconut oil to facilitate ketone production.

What are the benefits?

Ketogenic diets are used primarily for **weight loss** and have been used successfully to treat epilepsy and multiple sclerosis. They are being explored as a treatment for other degenerative brain diseases such as Alzheimer's, Parkinson's, dementia, and ALS, as well as stroke, autism, and migraine.[204] These explorations to date have been small, short clinical trials.

Reducing carbohydrates **suppresses appetite**. Ketogenic diets have no calorie restrictions, but people report eating far less than they used to once they have transitioned onto the diet. (This has been my experience, plus feelings of satiety that last for hours.)

Ketogenic diets are believed to help migraine because the low levels of carbohydrates force the liver to convert existing fuel from body fat into ketones (a normal process that happens any time we fast, such as the 12 hours overnight between dinner and breakfast). Ketones are particles small enough to cross the blood-brain barrier. It's believed that brains running on ketones may be slower to react to triggers and may therefore have a reduced migraine response.[205] Ketones may also prevent cellular injury.[206] Dr. Perlmutter recommends gradually cutting back on carbs over a few weeks (as we do in this Plan) to allow your body to adjust and become keto-adapted. He calls it "a super-cool thing for migraine patients to pursue over a period of a few weeks."

What are the risks?

You have to be very disciplined and intentional when adopting a ketogenic diet, as you must pack a ton of nutrients into the few carbohydrates you do eat. I would not recommend a long-term ketogenic diet (under 50 grams of carbs per day) without the ongoing supervision of a nutritionist or functional medicine doctor, as they need to monitor you closely to make sure your body is responding well, you're getting enough nutrients, and none of your lab tests are indicating imbalances.

The research on ketogenic diets is still underway, and some results are conflicting. Sarah Ballantyne, author of *The Paleo Approach*, notes that studies of ketogenic diets in autoimmune disease are very limited and that long-term use of a ketogenic diet could potentially have other negative effects, such as raised cortisol levels and non-alcoholic fatty liver disease.[207] In contrast, one study suggests that being on a ketogenic diet has no long-term side effects.[208] Another study found that a ketogenic diet raises good high-density lipoprotein (HDL) levels, lowers serum triglyceride levels, and lowers blood sugar, all of which should lower heart disease risk.[209] Dr. Mark Hyman covers the ketogenic research extensively in *Eat Fat, Get Thin*; he has seen reversal of fatty liver disease in patients on ketogenic diets.

In *The Primal Blueprint*, Mark Sisson recommends doing a ketogenic diet for two days to two weeks (under 50 grams of net carbs a day), and then easing back into the 50 to 150 grams per day range. Sisson recommends 50 to 100 grams of carbohydrates as the weight loss "sweet spot" and 100 to 150 for "effortless" weight maintenance. Dr. Wahls herself maintains an MCT ketogenic diet (Wahls Paleo Plus), because she has seen the best results for slowing her multiple sclerosis symptoms.

If you want to try this approach

Start with your tracking sheets to see where your net carbs are currently. Cut back a little each day until you are under 150 net grams per day. Priorities are to remove sugar, grains, and beans first, then higher-carb fruits and vegetables.

If after two weeks that doesn't help with your migraine attacks, try getting carbs under 100 net grams per day for a couple of weeks. Experiment with living in the 60- to 80-gram range for a while to see how you feel.

You're looking for *net carbs*, which is total carbs minus fiber. It's difficult but not impossible to follow these guidelines. Finally, remember that carbohydrates aren't evil, they're simply one type of food energy, providing four calories per gram. Protein provides four calories per gram, alcohol provides eight calories per gram, and fat provides nine calories per gram. Vegetables, fruits, grains, nuts, seeds, and any type of sugar all provide carbohydrates. Appendix C (page 302) has all of these recommendations in one place for easy reference.

PART V

MIGRAINE-FRIENDLY RECIPES AND MEAL PLAN

———— ••• ————

In this section you'll get into the kitchen to explore some of my favorite dishes that work within the Plan: tasty, hearty, and healthy, starting with a 14-day meal plan. I have eclectic tastes, so I draw inspiration from world cuisines as well as some tried-and-true American recipes. My assumption is that most readers are eating a standard American diet when they start, including processed foods, restaurant foods, and fast foods. It's my experience with my recipe testers that most people aren't comfortable cooking, so we have chosen the simplest recipes for this book. It's important to keep a couple of things in mind:

- All recipe instructions assume that produce has been washed and items such as garlic cloves and shallots have been peeled. Recipes calling for root vegetables like carrots and potatoes should be scrubbed but not peeled unless otherwise specified. All recipes using green onions use the white and green portions together unless otherwise indicated. All recipes use large, free-range eggs and large garlic cloves. All recipes calling for coconut milk use full-fat canned coconut milk unless otherwise specified.

- Some recipes call for stevia in its sugar equivalencies. Most stevia packets are the equivalent of 2 teaspoons sugar, but it varies by brand and whether they include fillers. Five drops of liquid stevia usually equals 1 teaspoon of sugar.

- Because triggers are so different from person to person, you may still have to tweak the Plan's recipes as you go. For instance, if you know you are sensitive to stevia, you will need to make an adjustment to any recipe containing stevia in the Desserts section.

Some of the ingredients may not be familiar to you, so please refer to my Glossary (page 296) to get you up to speed. If a spice is unfamiliar to you, I encourage you to be bold and try it.

These recipes have all been tested multiple times: three times in my home kitchen and critiqued by friends and family, and then by at least three volunteer recipe testers in their kitchens. My recipe testers came from four countries, and many are migraine sufferers. More than 30 people helped test recipes, making the book so much better. Most recipes include:

- **NUTRITIONAL INFORMATION.** Do note that I chose not to include calorie counts in the recipes because focusing on calories is not the most helpful way to look at food, reinforcing the myth of "calories in, calories out" (see page 149). I did have the recipes analyzed for people who need to track macronutrients like carbohydrates or fat, or specifics like sodium, potassium, or saturated fat. Remember that saturated fat is good for us if it comes from healthy sources like pastured animals or coconuts, as long as you have lowered your intake of starchy and sugary carbs. Notice that often in my recipes the potassium count is 8 to 10 times the amount of sodium, which is the appropriate balance when you eat whole foods and don't add much salt.

- **BUDGET-FRIENDLY INDICATORS.** Recipes are listed as Very or Moderate, meaning that ingredients are either readily available and less expensive (Very) or a bit more expensive or available online (Moderate).

- **TIME INDICATORS**. Prep Time includes time organizing ingredients, preparing raw ingredients (peeling, chopping, slicing), and/or stirring before cooking. Cook Time includes all active cooking time on the stove or in the oven. Passive Time includes any additional time that ingredients need to soak, marinate, or cool.

- **DIETARY ICONS**. I've created icons for each recipe to guide readers who follow special diets or have food sensitivities. A recipe includes that icon if it can be made to fit that diet: Vegan/Vegetarian (no animal products or meat included), Dairy-Free (no dairy products or an alternate to dairy given), Egg-Free (no eggs), and Grain-Free (no grains). All recipes are gluten-free, free of processed sugar, free of added salt, and anti-inflammatory.

🌿	**Vegan/Vegetarian**
🧀	**Dairy-Free**
⊘	**Egg-Free**
🌾	**Grain-Free**

If you're looking for more recipes, any South Beach Diet Phase 1 recipe should work, so long as it doesn't include migraine triggers or Splenda. Substitute stevia packets for Splenda if their recipe calls for it, or skip it.

Paleo blogs also offer a good starting point for more recipes, as they are grain-free/gluten-free and focus on veggies, pastured animals, and healthy fats. Just avoid triggers in their recipes and cut back or eliminate sodium, which they generally don't address.

I look forward to hearing your thoughts about the recipes on my website, MigraineReliefPlan.com.

food list summary

———— ••• ————

Food	Plan-Approved	Exclusions
Grains	gluten-free grains	*wheat berries, couscous, rye, barley, spelt, triticale, einkorn, farro, garfava flour, white, wheat, or all-purpose flour*
Vegetables	all, except for exclusions	*broad beans, fava beans, Italian beans, lentils, lima beans, navy beans, onions, pea pods, sauerkraut, snow peas*
Fruit	all, except for exclusions	*avocados, bananas, citrus or citrus zest, dates, figs, pineapple, papayas, passion fruit, raspberries, raisins, red plums*
Sweeteners	stevia	*sugar (all forms), artificial sweeteners*
Proteins (fresh and freshly cooked; grass-fed, pastured, free-range, and salt/additive-free where applicable)	beans (except exclusions), beef, eggs, fish, pork, poultry, seeds (sunflower, flax, chia, sesame, hemp), shellfish, tuna/salmon/sardines (if canned, no salt or other additives)	*dried or smoked fish, smoked or preserved meats (like sausage), favas, limas, navy beans, lentils, nuts, soy products, seitan*
Dairy	American cheese (good-quality from the deli—not recommended for Meniere's), cottage cheese, chèvre (fresh goat cheese), cream, cream cheese, mascarpone, milk, ricotta	*hard, aged cheeses, processed cheeses, yogurt, kefir*
Fats and Oils (organic, grass-fed, extra virgin, and unsalted where applicable)	butter, coconut oil, ghee, lard or rendered bacon fat, olive oil, sesame oil (regular and toasted), sunflower seed oil (in small amounts), tallow (beef fat from grass-fed cows)	*trans fats; corn, cottonseed, canola, rapeseed, soybean, peanut, nut oils*
Herbs and Spices	all, except exclusions	*blends containing MSG, salt, seaweed, yeast, "flavorings," or onion powder*
Drinks	coconut water, filtered or spring water, herbal teas (except exclusions), infused water, milk, seed milks, sparkling water (except exclusions), and white wine and vodka (small amounts; may be triggers)	*nut milks, boxed milks that include carrageenan or gums, soy milk, red wine, hard liquors, beer, soda (regular or diet), caffeinated tea, teas containing citrus, coffee (decaf coffee is OK but might still be a trigger); do not use wine in cooking for the first six months, then test it for yourself*

14-day meal plan

————— ••• —————

Use this meal plan to fit these recipes into your busy life, once you've completed the first eight weeks (Month 3). Start on a Saturday or Sunday and do some cooking for the week.

I don't indicate serving sizes here; eat mindfully until you feel not quite full. Skip the snacks if you aren't hungry between meals. Listen to your body. The goals of this meal plan are: (1) Never be hungry. (2) Time your evening meal or snack to fall 12 hours before breakfast and 3 hours before bed, to allow your gut to clear and digest your food. (3) Eat enough healthy fat so that your blood sugar levels are sustained throughout the day.

Eating enough fat reduces your cravings for sugar and other starchy carbs. Nutritionist Jennifer Adler believes that sugar cravings are directly related to a shortage of protein. She recommends eating protein at breakfast, lunch, and a 3 p.m. snack. Shoot for protein in grams equal to half your body weight: a 150-pound person needs 75 grams per day.[210] Whole30 founders Dallas and Melissa Hartwig recommend one to two "palm-sized" servings of protein per meal.[211]

This Plan makes leftovers, which are incorporated into the meals the next day. All items are stored in the refrigerator unless otherwise noted. Choose beverages from the Plan-approved drinks list on page 180. Smoothies are considered meals or snacks.

To Make or Purchase in Advance

Pork Sausage Patties (page 208, freeze most of them)

Egg Mini-Quiches (page 202, enjoy one or two hot from the oven the day you make them, freeze the rest)

Salsa Verde (page 274)

Spice Rub from Seared Pork Chops recipe (page 240)

Brown rice

Sunflower Seed Butter (page 195)

Salad dressing of your choice (page 265)

Tuna or Salmon Salad (page 223)

Vanilla Ricotta Cream (page 263)

Coconut Whipped Cream (page 254)

Olive oil mayonnaise

Reduced sodium or salt-free Old Bay or seafood seasoning

Organic, low-sodium ketchup

Organic, onion-free chicken stock

THE 14-DAY MEAL PLAN: WEEK 1

MEAL	DAY 1	DAY 2	DAY 3
Breakfast	Scrambled eggs with low-sodium ketchup or Salsa Verde and Pork Sausage Patties	Egg Mini-Quiches (place foil-wrapped baking potatoes in the slow cooker on Low if you want them ready when you get home from work)	Potato–Green Onion Frittata (page 280)
Mid-morning snack	Cold-pressed green juice or Beet–Strawberry Smoothie (page 187)	Carrot slices with Sunflower Seed Butter	Pumpkin seeds
Lunch	Tuna or Salmon Salad	Chicken Salad on greens with dressing	Tuna Salad with large green salad and dressing
Mid-afternoon snack	Carrot slices with Sunflower Seed Butter	Pumpkin seeds	Salt-free or low-sodium tortilla chips with Salsa Verde
Dinner	Sautéed greens and grilled chicken breast with steamed broccoli	Baked potato with chopped steamed broccoli, ricotta or mascarpone, and butter	Spice-Rubbed Seared Pork Chops with Sweet Potatoes and Pear–Cranberry Sauce (page 240) and steamed broccoli with butter or olive oil
Early evening snack	Berries with Vanilla Ricotta Cream or Coconut Whipped Cream	Berries with Vanilla Ricotta Cream or Coconut Whipped Cream	Berries with Vanilla Ricotta Cream or Coconut Whipped Cream
Prep for future meals	Make Chicken Salad (page 211) from leftover grilled chicken; chop leftover steamed broccoli	Dice leftover baked potato; thinly slice two green onions; season pork chops with Spice Rub	Slice leftover Spice-Rubbed Seared Pork Chops; prep fruit for smoothie and salad; hard boil eggs

THE 14-DAY MEAL PLAN: WEEK 1

DAY 4	DAY 5	DAY 6	DAY 7
Peach–Mango Power Smoothie (page 194)	Egg Mini-Quiches (from freezer)	Eggs your way with Pork Sausage Patties	Blueberry–Oat Waffles with berries and butter; freeze leftover waffles
Hard-boiled egg	Sunflower Seed Butter on rice cakes	Pumpkin seeds	Herbed Cheese Spread with cherry tomatoes or veggie sticks
Salad with peaches or grapes and sliced Spice-Rubbed Seared Pork Chop	Egg salad with green salad or as an open-faced sandwich on toasted gluten-free bread	Salmon–Potato Cakes	Burger (beef, turkey, or bean) with olive oil mayonnaise and/or low-sodium ketchup and green salad with dressing
Carrots with Sunflower Seed Butter	Pumpkin seeds	Mascarpone and fruit on rice cakes	Fruit salad
Burger (beef, turkey, or bean) with olive oil mayonnaise and/or low-sodium ketchup and green salad	Salmon–Potato Cakes (page 237) and green salad with dressing	Steak and Roasted Vegetable Salad	Meatloaf (page 230), steamed broccoli, and Spicy Kale and Swiss Chard Sauté (page 243)
Berries with Vanilla Ricotta Cream or Coconut Whipped Cream	Fruit	Herbed Cheese Spread on veggie sticks	Sunflower seeds
Make egg salad by mixing mashed hard-boiled eggs with mayo	Prep ingredients for Steak and Roasted Vegetable Salad (page 244); make Herbed Cheese Spread (page 189); cut up veggie sticks	Make fruit salad; veggie sticks; Blueberry–Oat Waffle batter (page 198); Granola (page 205); salad dressing (page 265); Chile Pepper Sauce (page 267)	Make Berry Cobbler (page 248) and Chunky Tomato Sauce (recipe-renovator.com); thaw frozen fish (2 meals); pack leftover Meatloaf, tomato sauce, zucchini ribbons

THE 14-DAY MEAL PLAN: WEEK 2

MEAL	DAY 8	DAY 9	DAY 10
Breakfast	Broccoli–Ricotta Frittata (page 280)	Leftover toasted Blueberry–Oat Waffles topped with berries and butter	Migas
Mid-morning snack	Chicken stock with pinch of curry powder	Chicken stock with pinch of curry powder	Granola with coconut milk or Hemp Milk
Lunch	Meatloaf with zucchini ribbons and Chunky Tomato Sauce	Meatloaf with zucchini ribbons or meatloaf sandwich on gluten-free bread	Firehouse Turkey Chili
Mid-afternoon snack	Herbed Cheese Spread on rice cakes	Granola with coconut milk or Hemp Milk	Herbed Cheese Spread with veggie sticks
Dinner	Fish Baked in Parchment Packets (page 228) with Smoky Mustard Sauce (page 273) and green salad with dressing	Fish Tacos (page 214) with Chile Pepper Sauce	Scallop Corn Chowder (page 238)
Early evening snack	Berry Cobbler	Berry Cobbler	Berry Cobbler
Prep for future meals	Make Firehouse Turkey Chili (page 213, freeze individually) and Herbed Cheese Spread (page 189); pack leftover Meatloaf, tomato sauce, and zucchini ribbons	Chop leftover fish taco veggies for Migas (page 206); cut veggie sticks; thaw frozen scallops; pack a serving of frozen Firehouse Turkey Chili	Pack leftover Scallop Corn Chowder; pack one serving of frozen Firehouse Turkey Chili

THE 14-DAY MEAL PLAN: WEEK 2

DAY 11	DAY 12	DAY 13	DAY 14
Egg Mini-Quiches (from freezer)	Granola with coconut milk or Hemp Milk	Poached eggs with kale and Chile Pepper Sauce	Salmon, Asparagus, and Thyme Omelet (page 209) with Smoky Mustard Sauce
Pumpkin seeds	Beet–Strawberry Smoothie (page 187)	Chicken stock with pinch of curry powder	Granola with berries and coconut milk
Scallop Corn Chowder	Tuna Salad with greens	Chicken Cacciatore with pasta, green salad, and dressing	Firehouse Turkey Chili
Beet–Strawberry Smoothie (reserve one serving for tomorrow)	Chicken stock with pinch of curry powder	Carrots with Sunflower Seed Butter	Pumpkin seeds
Firehouse Turkey Chili with mascarpone and brown rice	Chicken Cacciatore and gluten-free pasta	Grilled salmon and asparagus	Beef, turkey, or bean burger with olive oil mayonnaise and/or low-sodium ketchup and green salad
Berry Cobbler	Fruit or sunflower seeds	Granola with berries and coconut milk or Hemp Milk	Leftover protein or veggies (if needed)
Make Chicken Cacciatore (page 226) and Tuna Salad (page 223)	Marinate salmon; slice carrots; pack Chicken Cacciatore and pasta	Chop leftover grilled salmon and asparagus; pack one serving of frozen Firehouse Turkey Chili	

snacks

———— ••• ————

Snacks are fun. They're also small and non-threatening, so they're an easy starting point for making changes to our life in an area that's as fraught with drama as food. I focus on just a few key snacks to get you started: two tasty smoothies (which can double as breakfast), two sunflower seed–based spreads, and two savory dips. Finally, you'll find an easy cracker to make, in case you can't find any crackers locally that fit the Plan.

Beet–Strawberry Smoothie

Makes 2 (12-ounce) smoothies
Prep time: 5 minutes   Cooking time: N/A   Passive time: N/A

I love this smoothie as my breakfast in the summer; it's hearty and high in protein. I tend to use whole strawberries, green tops and all. If you have a regular (not high-speed) blender, cut the strawberries into chunks before adding them to the blender. It might seem weird to include the organic strawberry tops, but as long as they are fresh and vibrant green, they add additional green nutrients to the smoothie. If you don't like the taste of raw beets, try cooked beets, which are sweeter. I often freeze chunks of leftover cooked beets to add to my smoothie. You can wear thin plastic gloves to keep your hands from getting stained.

1½ cups (375ml) organic whole milk, Hemp Milk (page 255), or coconut milk

2 tablespoons maca powder (optional)

2 tablespoons hemp seeds

2 tablespoons chia seeds

2 small or 1 large red or golden beet(s), peeled and cut into chunks

3–4 handfuls organic strawberries

3–4 mint leaves (optional)

Stevia to equal 2 teaspoons sugar (optional)

6–8 ice cubes

Budget friendly: Moderate

1. Add ingredients to the blender in the order listed. This will help ease the burden on your blender's motor, keeping it happy for many years.
2. Blend, starting on low and then turning up to high, until smooth and creamy. Use the tamper if you have a Vitamix.
3. Transfer to two glasses and serve right away, or store for up to 1 day in the refrigerator.

COOKS' NOTE: *While maca powder, hemp seeds, and chia seeds are pricey, they add wonderful protein and nutrients to this meal replacer. It's fine to skip one or all of them. If you don't care for the taste of raw beets, or if your strawberries aren't super sweet, feel free to add a little stevia to adjust the smoothie to your taste. Make sure any alternative milk you buy is free of guar gum (it can be irritating or an allergen for some people), xanthan gum, and carrageenan (a form of MSG derived from seaweed).*

Per 12-ounce serving: 15g protein, 36g carbohydrates, 17g fat, 3g saturated fat, 143mg sodium, 809mg potassium, 11g fiber

Creamy Not-ella Carob Butter

Makes about 16 ounces (450g)
Prep time: 10–15 minutes   Cooking time: 20–30 minutes   Passive time: 15 minutes

I created this recipe to give people an easy, luscious treat that still follows the Plan. While it doesn't taste exactly like Nutella, it's pretty darn close—even though I skipped the sugar, hazelnuts, chocolate, vegetable oil, soy lecithin, and milk powder. If you make up a jar of this, you'll have it to spread on gluten-free toast or apples when you want a sweet snack. Perfect for stashing in your desk at work along with an apple. A huge hit with my recipe testers, who called it creamy, dreamy, and addictive.

1 cup (230g) raw, unsalted sunflower seeds

1 cup (160g) hemp seeds

Stevia to equal 8 teaspoons sugar

½ cup (50g) carob powder

¼ cup (60mL) coconut oil

Budget friendly: Moderate (hemp seeds tend to be pricey)

COOKS' NOTE: *If you cannot get hemp seeds, you can substitute sunflower seeds for them.*

1. Preheat the oven to 300°F (150°C). Put the sunflower seeds on baking sheets lined with fresh parchment paper.
2. Toast the sunflower seeds for 10 minutes, then stir and return to the oven. Turn off the oven and toast the seeds another 5 to 10 minutes. You want them just golden brown but not dark brown or burnt. Taste a few if you aren't sure.
3. Transfer the baking sheet to a wire rack and let the toasted seeds cool for 15 minutes.
4. Put the toasted seeds in a food processor fitted with the S-blade or a high-speed blender and blend into a fine powder, about 1 minute.
5. Add the hemp seeds and stevia and blend for about 4 more minutes, stopping every minute to scrape down the sides. Eventually it will form a ball and become nut butter. Use the tamper if you have a Vitamix.
6. In a separate bowl, blend the carob powder with the oil, then add the mixture to the nut butter. (If you add the carob powder and oil directly to a food processor, you will have a powdery carob explosion that is not fun to clean up.)
7. Continue blending until you get the smooth consistency you want.
8. Serve right away or transfer to a glass jar and store in the refrigerator. It will be spreadable when refrigerated, and just a little thicker than Nutella at room temperature. Eat within a month.

Per 1-ounce serving: 5g protein, 9g carbohydrates, 11g fat, 3g saturated fat, 6mg sodium, 61mg potassium, 2g fiber

Herbed Cheese Spread

Makes 4 (1-ounce) servings
Prep time: 5 minutes   Cooking time: N/A   Passive time: N/A

When I first began on the Plan, I was always looking for snacks I could eat. I created this easy spread as an afternoon snack. It's perfect to take to work for that 3 p.m. "I need protein" craving. Each cheese and fresh herb pairing will provide a different taste. Ricotta is the lightest-tasting, mascarpone the richest. Cream cheese has the most tang. Avoid cream cheese if you have Meniere's or are very strict with your sodium intake.

1 tablespoon finely chopped fresh herbs such as parsley and thyme, oregano and basil, *or* cilantro and chives

4 ounces (115g) cream cheese, ricotta, or mascarpone

¼ teaspoon garlic powder

Budget friendly: Very

1. With a spoon or spatula, blend the fresh herbs with the cheese and garlic powder.
2. Serve right away or store in the refrigerator for up to 3 days.

COOKS' NOTE: *I like to eat this spread on hearty rice cakes, cherry tomatoes, or veggie sticks. It's also great tossed with hot gluten-free pasta for a quick dinner.*

Per 1-ounce serving (using cream cheese): 2g protein, 1g carbohydrates, 10g fat, 5g saturated fat, 89mg sodium, 40mg potassium, 0g fiber

---

STEPHANIE'S SPICE STAR: Garlic powder
While I am a huge fan of fresh garlic and use it in nearly all my savory cooking, there is a place for garlic powder (not garlic salt). Dried powdered garlic gives a savory flavor to many dishes, and it's far less assertive than fresh, raw garlic.

Roasted Chile Pepper Hummus ⊘ ⊘ ⊘ ⊘

Makes 2–3 cups, about 12 servings
Prep time: 10–15 minutes   Cooking time: 10 minutes   Passive time: 15 minutes

Store-bought hummus usually has lemon, might have onion, and often has sugars like dextrose. Make this on the weekend and then snack on it during the week. Bring some to work in an airtight container and store it in the fridge along with carrot or celery sticks, gluten-free crackers, or just a spoon, for your afternoon snack. One tester family called this simple to make and a great healthy after-school snack.

1 handful of fresh Italian flat-leaf parsley (optional)

2 Anaheim chiles or other mildly spicy peppers

2 medium red bell peppers

1½ cups (9 oz [275g]) cooked low-sodium chickpeas

1 tablespoon best-quality extra virgin olive oil

1–2 teaspoons smoked paprika, plus more to taste as needed

Budget friendly: Very

1. Wash and thoroughly dry the parsley, if using. Roll it up in a clean kitchen towel and set aside while you roast the peppers.
2. Cover a large baking sheet with aluminum foil and preheat the broiler. If your broiler is at the top of your oven, move the top oven rack to the highest position. You can also roast the peppers on a grill or a gas burner: Leave them whole and turn frequently until blackened.
3. Remove the cores from the chiles and bell peppers and cut each one in half, removing the seeds and ribs. If working with hot peppers, wear gloves. Flatten the peppers on the prepared baking sheet, cut side down. Cut slits in any curves, as needed, to get them as flat as possible. Larger pieces will be easier to peel later.
4. Transfer the baking sheet to the broiler or top rack of the oven, and broil for about 10 minutes, until the skins are blackened and puffy.
5. Remove the baking sheet from the oven and use tongs to drop the peppers into a paper bag. Roll the bag shut and set aside for 15 minutes, or until completely cool. This steams off the skins, making them easy to peel.
6. Rinse and drain the chickpeas. If using canned chickpeas, you can use an entire 15-ounce (425-g) can.
7. Put the parsley in a food processor and mince finely. Scrape it out into a bowl and set aside.
8. Once the peppers are completely cooled, remove from the bag and peel off the skins.

9. Add the peeled, roasted peppers, drained chickpeas, olive oil, and paprika to the food processor. Blend until very smooth, stopping occasionally to scrape down the sides. Taste and add additional smoked paprika if necessary.

10. Transfer the hummus to a serving bowl and gently stir in the parsley, leaving some aside to sprinkle on top. Top with an additional drizzle of olive oil and the reserved parsley. Store in a covered container in the refrigerator for up to 5 days.

COOKS' NOTE: *If you cannot find fresh chiles, you can use cayenne pepper. Start with ¼ teaspoon and add more as needed. Use low-sodium or salt-free canned beans. Note that smoked paprika and cayenne may be triggers for a few people. Serve with gluten-free crackers, unsalted tortilla chips, or veggie sticks.*

Per serving: 2g protein, 7g carbohydrates, 2g fat, 0g saturated fat, 2mg sodium, 111mg potassium, 2g fiber

Seedy Carrot Crackers

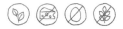

Makes 60–72 small crackers, about 12 servings
Prep time: 10–15 minutes   Cooking time: 15–20 minutes (oven version)   Passive time: 2–3 hours

It's hard to find crackers we can eat on the Plan. I developed these based on a raw cracker recipe from a restaurant called Café Gratitude. It's an easy recipe to make in the oven. If you have a food dehydrator, I've included instructions for that method, too. You can make them flatbread sized and load them up for more of a meal with bruschetta-style toppings. They're low in sodium, low-carb, grain-free, and also packed with potassium from the seeds. Flax seeds are one of the richest plant-based sources of omega-3 fatty acids and antioxidants. If you've never made crackers before, you might be surprised at how easy they are.

½ cup (60g) golden flax seeds

½ cup (60g) tan sesame seeds

2 large carrots, peeled and cut into chunks

1 teaspoon ground cumin

½ teaspoon smoked paprika

½ teaspoon garlic powder

¼ teaspoon white pepper

½ cup filtered water

¹⁄₁₆ teaspoon smoked salt, for sprinkling (optional)

Budget friendly: Moderate

TO BAKE IN THE OVEN:

1. Preheat the oven to 400°F (200°C).
2. Put the flax seeds into a food processor or blender and grind to a meal.
3. Add the carrots, cumin, paprika, garlic powder, white pepper, and water to the food processor or blender. Process, stopping to scrape down the sides twice, until it makes a uniform, sticky dough.
4. Line a baking sheet with parchment paper or a silicone sheet. Spray or oil lightly.
5. Spread the batter onto the sheet with a silicone spatula as evenly as possible, approximately ⅛ inch (3 mm) thick. The more even you can get it, the better.
6. Score into squares with a pizza cutter, paring knife, or butter knife. Sprinkle lightly with the salt, if using.
7. Bake for 15 to 20 minutes, until the edges are just turning brown.
8. Turn off the oven and let the crackers sit in there for about 2 hours, until completely cool. They should all be hard and crispy when you take them off the sheet. Some of the thin ones might be very brown but will taste OK.

TO MAKE IN A DEHYDRATOR:

1. Soak the sesame seeds in filtered water to cover for 4 hours. Drain and rinse.
2. Grind the flax seeds into meal using your food processor or blender. Soak in 1 cup filtered water for up to four hours. Do not drain.
3. Pulse the carrots in the food processor fitted with an S-blade until finely ground.
4. Blend all the ingredients, except the salt, including the carrot pulp and juice, together in a large bowl. You can use a stand mixer or the food processor for this. You should have a smooth, spreadable paste.
5. Spread on Teflex-lined sheets as evenly as possible.
6. Score into squares with a butter knife or steak knife. Sprinkle lightly with the salt, if using.
7. Dehydrate at 115°F (45°C) until they are dry to the touch.
8. Peel them off the Teflex sheet and continue to dry until they are completely crispy. This is usually overnight.
9. Store in an airtight container.

Per serving (5–6 crackers): 2g protein, 5g carbohydrates, 6g fat, <1g saturated fat, 11mg sodium, 130mg potassium, 3g fiber

COOKS' NOTES: *If any thicker ones are not completely dry after baking, do not store them with the others or they will make them all soft and possibly get moldy. Eat the thicker ones first and store them separately. Store dry crackers in an airtight container. Brown flax seeds also work; I like the taste of the golden ones better, as I find them milder and less overpowering. If you don't have a food processor, high-speed blender, or spice grinder, buying pre-ground meal is a better option. Smoked paprika may be a trigger for some people.*

Peach–Mango Power Smoothie

Makes 2 (14-ounce) smoothies
Prep time: 5 minutes   Cooking time: 1 minute   Passive time: N/A

This is my other favorite meal replacer. If you can't eat eggs, this makes a wonderful start to the day. If you are short on time in the mornings, make it the night before and store in the fridge for a grab-and-go breakfast. This one is a little sweeter because of the two types of fruit, so it is also good for an afternoon snack if you're used to something sweet then. Once you're used to less sweet foods, cut back on the fruit and add a cup of lightly cooked kale to balance it out.

1½ cups (375mL) organic whole milk, Hemp Milk (page 255), or coconut milk

2 tablespoons maca powder (optional)

2 tablespoons buckwheat or hemp seeds

2 tablespoons chia seeds

1 cup (154g) frozen peaches

1 cup (165g) frozen mango pieces

6–8 ice cubes

Budget friendly: Very

1. Add all the ingredients to the blender in the order listed. This will help ease the burden on your blender's motor, keeping it happy for many years.
2. Blend until smooth and creamy. Use the tamper if you have a Vitamix.
3. Drink immediately or store in the refrigerator for up to 1 day.

COOKS' NOTE: *You can use fresh peaches and mango if they are at peak sweetness. Omit the buckwheat for a grain-free smoothie. Make sure any alternative milk you buy is free of guar gum (it can be irritating or an allergen for some people), xanthan gum, and carrageenan (a form of MSG derived from seaweed).*

Per 14-ounce serving (using whole milk, without maca powder): 14g protein, 39g carbohydrates, 17g fat, 3g saturated fat, 77mg sodium, 559mg potassium, 8g fiber

Sunflower Seed Butter

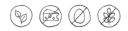

Makes about 8 ounces (225g)
Prep time: 5 minutes   Cooking time: 20 minutes   Passive time: 15 minutes

No, you don't have to make your own sunflower seed butter. But here's why you might want to: Commercially available sunflower seed butters either have added sugar or are made from raw seeds, giving them a taste and grayish-green color I find unappealing. Some brands of sunflower seed butter might contain another type of oil that's not on the Plan, like soybean or cottonseed oil. And they're more expensive. Making it yourself means you can make it as sweet as you like and use high-quality fat like ghee or coconut oil, which balances out the fat profile without adding additional omega-6 fats.

2 cups (230g) raw unsalted sunflower seeds

1–4 tablespoons ghee or coconut oil, as needed for creaminess

Stevia to equal 2 teaspoons sugar (optional)

Budget friendly: Very

1. Preheat the oven to 300°F (150°C). Spread the sunflower seeds on 2 baking sheets lined with fresh parchment paper.
2. Toast the sunflower seeds for 10 minutes, then stir. Turn off the oven and continuing toasting for another 5 to 10 minutes. You want the seeds just golden brown but not dark brown or burnt. Taste a few if you aren't sure.
3. Remove from the oven and let cool for 15 minutes.
4. Put the seeds in a food processor fitted with the S-blade or a high-speed blender and blend into a fine powder.
5. Continue blending for about 5 minutes, stopping every minute to scrape down the sides, until the powder forms a ball and becomes seed butter. Use a tamper if using a Vitamix. Stop a few times to let the machine rest so you don't overheat the blender's engine.
6. Transfer to a mixing bowl and blend in 1 tablespoon of the ghee or oil and the stevia, if using. Add additional ghee or oil, up to 4 tablespoons total, as needed to make the butter the creamy consistency you want. Some seeds have a higher oil content than others and will need less oil added, while some are drier and will need more.
7. Scrape into a clean glass jar and store in the refrigerator for up to 6 months. It will be very firm refrigerated but will soften to a spreadable consistency at room temperature.

Per 1-ounce serving (including 1 tablespoon coconut oil in the overall recipe): 5g protein, 7g carbohydrates, 14g fat, 3g saturated fat, 1mg sodium, 220mg potassium, 3g fiber

breakfast

———— ⋯ ————

Next on the Plan we switch over breakfast. If you're not used to eating in the morning, small portions are fine. But do eat something so you're not in a low–blood sugar fasting state, which can trigger a migraine attack. I've given you recipes for two kinds of breakfast meats: sausage and "bacon." Waffles, crepes, and French toast: all gluten-free. Granola is key for travel breakfasts. And a couple of egg recipes, including portable mini-quiches perfect for heating up at work.

Make Your Own Bacon

Makes about 24 pieces
Prep time: 5 minutes   Cooking time: 20 minutes   Passive time: N/A

Ask the butcher to slice the pork belly as thinly as possible ("like prosciutto") for the crispiest bacon. Because you control how much salt you add, you may decide to keep making your own, especially if you are sensitive to sodium.

1 pound pastured pork belly, sliced very thinly

1 teaspoon garlic powder

1 teaspoon smoked or regular paprika

1 teaspoon celery seed

¼ teaspoon white or freshly ground black pepper

¼ teaspoon dried sage

½ teaspoon smoked or regular fine sea salt

1 teaspoon coconut sugar or maple sugar (optional)

Budget friendly: Moderate

Per slice (24 slices per pound):
2g protein, 0g carbohydrates, 10g fat, 4g saturated fat, 55mg sodium, 40mg potassium, 0g fiber

1. Cut the thin slices of pork belly in half crosswise. You should end up with about 24 pieces. Wrap and freeze half of the pork so it stays fresh, as it has no preservatives.
2. To make the seasoning blend, grind the dry ingredients and the coconut or maple sugar, if using, in a spice grinder to a fine, uniform powder. Alternatively, use a mortar and pestle. Store in a jar with a fine shaker lid. (Save half the mixture to use when you thaw the frozen portion.)
3. Put the pork belly pieces in a nonstick or cast iron pan and lightly sprinkle the seasoning on top. Flip over immediately and sprinkle the other side so the seasoning cooks in.
4. Set the pan over medium–high heat.
5. Cook 6 to 10 minutes per side until crispy. Serve immediately.

COOKS' NOTE: *Reserve the rendered bacon fat in a jar; use it for cooking greens, stir-frying, or adding flavor in place of another oil. Rendered bacon fat is high in stearic acid, and saturated fats are excellent for migraine brains (just don't overdo it on saturated fats if you have not cut back on starchy carbohydrates).*

If you are sensitive to smoked paprika or smoked sea salt, use regular paprika and sea salt. Paprika adds a nice color to the bacon. Because the salt is finely ground, it adds just enough saltiness to the flavor and crispness to the bacon with a negligible amount of sodium per serving.

STEPHANIE'S SPICE STAR: Dried sage
Native to the Mediterranean, the leaves of the sage plant are dried and crumbled or powdered. The musty, savory flavor of sage pairs perfectly with pork dishes. It's an essential flavor for holiday stuffing recipes, especially at Thanksgiving.

Blueberry–Oat Waffles

Makes 6–7 square waffles
Prep time: 10 minutes   Cooking time: 20–25 minutes   Passive time: 5 minutes

These are a favorite weekend breakfast when I have more time to do something special. I love making extra waffles. Once cooled, I freeze them in zip-top bags for toaster waffles. Make these without the blueberries to use in place of gluten-free bread in sandwiches. Keep in mind that gluten-free flour absorbs a lot of liquid as it stands—so don't worry if you need the additional milk. You can also use strawberries, blackberries, minced apples, or pears instead of blueberries. One tester took them for breakfast on a long airplane flight, spread with Sunflower Seed Butter (page 195).

2 tablespoons gluten-free rolled oats, ground flax seed, cornmeal, or buckwheat flour

1 egg (see Cooks' Note for substitution)

¾–1½ cups (180mL–375mL) whole or 2 percent milk, rice milk, Hemp Milk (page 255), or coconut milk

¼ cup (60mL) grapeseed oil, ghee, or coconut oil, melted

1 teaspoon baking powder, or 2 teaspoons sodium-free baking soda

1⅓ cups (165g) all-purpose gluten-free flour blend

½ pint (250g) fresh blueberries

Unsalted grass-fed butter or ghee, for serving

1. Preheat a waffle maker.
2. If using rolled oats or flax seed, put them in a blender and pulse until finely ground. Dump them out into a bowl.
3. Put the egg, ¾ cup of the milk, the oil, and the baking powder or soda into the blender and pulse a few times until well blended.
4. Add the flour and ground oats and pulse just until well mixed. Let stand 5 minutes to thicken.
5. Add additional milk, 2 tablespoons at a time if needed, to create a pourable batter. The batter will continue to thicken as it stands.
6. Spray both surfaces of the waffle iron with cooking spray, or use a silicone brush to brush melted ghee or coconut oil on the waffle iron.
7. Following the manufacturer's instructions, fill the waffle iron, add a handful of blueberries on top of each waffle, and cook for about 5 minutes, or until golden brown and crispy. Be careful to spray or oil the iron with cooking spray between each batch. The blueberries tend to stick and burn. Don't overfill the iron. Repeat until you've used all the batter.
8. Serve right away with the unsalted butter or ghee and remaining blueberries. If serving a crowd, keep the waffles warm in a 200°F (95°C) oven.

Budget friendly: Very

COOKS' NOTE: *For an egg-free version, add 2 tablespoons ground flax seeds and ¼ cup (60mL) filtered water to a small bowl. Let it stand 5 minutes. If using this flax egg substitute, use oats, cornmeal, or buckwheat as the first ingredient to prevent the waffles from having a gluey texture. You may need additional milk, depending on the mix in your gluten-free flour. If you do not have a waffle iron, you can make these as pancakes on a hot griddle. Preheat until water droplets dance on the surface. If using a cast iron griddle, use a light coating of oil or cooking spray to keep from sticking. Thicker batter works better for pancakes. If using frozen blueberries, let thaw in the refrigerator overnight, then drain.*

Per waffle made with buckwheat flour, whole milk, and grapeseed oil: 5g protein, 25g carbohydrates, 10g fat, 2g saturated fat, 22mg sodium, 183mg potassium, 2g fiber

Crepes

Makes 10 crepes, about 5 servings
Prep time: 15 minutes   Cooking time: 20–25 minutes   Passive time: 20–30 minutes

Making these reminds me of my 50th birthday. We visited a Parisian neighborhood where all the restaurants made naturally gluten-free buckwheat crepes with rich fillings both savory and sweet. While they are a little futzy to get the hang of, you can make extra and freeze them.

⅓ cup (45g) sweet sorghum flour

¼ cup (30g) tapioca flour (starch)

¼ cup (40g) brown rice flour

¼ cup (50g) teff flour (or seeds)

1 cup (250mL) whole milk, coconut milk, or half-and-half

¼ cup (60mL) filtered water

3 eggs

3 tablespoons (45g) melted unsalted grass-fed butter, ghee, or coconut oil, plus more for frying

1 recipe Vanilla Ricotta Cream (page 263)

2 cups (296g) fresh berries (not raspberries), washed, drained, and sliced

Budget friendly: Moderate (if buying all the gluten-free flours)

1. Put the first 4 ingredients in a blender and blend into a fine powder. Add the milk, water, and eggs and blend for 1 minute. Let the batter stand for 20 to 30 minutes.
2. Melt the butter and, just before cooking the crepes, add it to the batter and blend.
3. Heat a large nonstick skillet or frying pan over medium heat. Try a small amount of test batter in the pan without adding the fat. If the batter sticks, add a small amount of butter, ghee, or coconut oil to the pan using a silicone brush. Alternatively, wipe it evenly around with a paper towel. You will have to re-oil the pan every couple of crepes.
4. Pulse the blender once or twice before pouring ¼ cup of the batter into the center of the pan, tilting the pan in a circle to spread the batter into a thin round as large as you can get it. Cook for 2 minutes, or until just set, then flip with a spatula or tongs, and cook another 30 seconds.
5. Transfer the crepe to a plate and set aside.
6. Pulse the blender each time to mix the butter back into the batter before pouring the next crepe. Repeat this process until the batter is gone.
7. As each crepe finishes, fill with a generous smear of the Vanilla Ricotta Cream and fresh berries, then roll up. Serve.

COOKS' NOTES: *Let extra crepes cool on separate plates (they stick together), then stack, separated by waxed paper, and wrap with plastic wrap, in a heavy freezer bag to freeze. They are also great for dinner with a savory filling like Breakfast Hash (page 281), topped with a simple gravy.*

Per serving (including Vanilla Ricotta Cream and strawberries): 9g protein, 18g carbohydrates, 16g fat, 10g saturated fat, 61mg sodium, 212mg potassium, 2g fiber

Denver Omelet

Makes 1 omelet, about 2 servings
Prep time: 10 minutes   Cooking time: 15 minutes   Passive time: N/A

This recipe is perfect to use up leftover cooked pork, as it stands in for the salty and aged ham that can be a migraine trigger. Traditional Denver omelets contain both red and green bell peppers. I personally don't care for the sharp taste of green peppers, which are unripened colored peppers. If you feel the same way, feel free to use a yellow and a red bell pepper, or just one whole red one. One tester called this affordable, fast, healthy, and a hit with her boys.

2 tablespoons unsalted grass-fed butter, ghee, or coconut oil

½ bunch green onions, white and green parts, thinly sliced

½ red bell pepper, chopped

½ green bell pepper, chopped

½ cup diced cooked pork loin, pork chop, or pork belly

4 eggs

1 tablespoon whole milk, half-and-half, or coconut milk

½ teaspoon freshly ground black pepper

Dash Chile Pepper Sauce (page 267) (optional)

Budget friendly: Very

1. Melt the butter in a large skillet or omelet pan set over medium heat.
2. Add the onions, red and green bell peppers, and pork and sauté until the onions start to become translucent.
3. In a small bowl, whip the eggs lightly with the milk, black pepper, and Chile Pepper Sauce, if using.
4. Add the egg mixture to the pan. Cook about 5 minutes until nearly set, tilting the pan if necessary to move unset eggs to the edges.
5. Slide a flexible spatula under the omelet, loosening it, then fold in half.
6. Cook another 5 minutes, or until completely set. Serve right away

COOKS' NOTE: *You could also add some mild hot pepper here, like a jalapeño or Anaheim.*

Per serving: 30g protein, 7g carbohydrates, 27g fat, 13g saturated fat, 180mg sodium, 574mg potassium, 2g fiber

Egg Mini-Quiches

Makes 8 mini-quiches, 1 per serving
Prep time: 10 minutes   Cooking time: 30 minutes   Passive time: N/A

I adapted this recipe from *The South Beach Diet*. These freeze beautifully, so you can make them on the weekend and then pop them in the microwave or toaster oven to heat up for breakfast at home or work. If you don't care for spinach, you can use chopped Swiss chard or kale.

10 ounces (285g) frozen or fresh chopped spinach or broccoli

4 eggs

¾ cup (180g) whole-milk ricotta cheese (optional)

½ cup (60g) diced red, yellow, or orange bell peppers

¼ cup (20g) diced green onions

3 drops Chile Pepper Sauce (page 267) (optional)

Budget friendly: Very

1. Preheat the oven to 350°F (180°C). Line a 12-cup muffin pan with 8 foil baking cups. Spray foil cups with cooking spray. If using silicone cups, no need to spray them; just set them on a baking sheet. Set aside.
2. If using frozen broccoli, microwave for 2 to 3 minutes on high until thawed. Squeeze dry with your hands or else the quiches won't set. Transfer to a large bowl.
3. Add all the remaining ingredients and mix well. Divide the mixture evenly among the cups, about half full.
4. Bake for 30 minutes, or until the quiches are firm to the touch and starting to brown a little. There may still be some bubbling, but they will set as they cool.
5. Eat warm. If freezing for later, transfer to a wire rack to cool. Wrap extras in plastic wrap once cool and store in a freezer bag.

Per serving (made with ricotta cheese): 8g protein, 3g carbohydrates, 6g fat, 3g saturated fat, 83mg sodium, 291mg potassium, 1g fiber

French Toast

Makes 4 servings
Prep time: 5 minutes   Cooking time: 20 minutes   Passive time: N/A

When we first got married, my husband used to be in charge of breakfast. He made great French toast. While on the Plan, you can still enjoy this favorite on the weekends once in a while. Just cut back on the syrup and have some protein with it. This is one of those dishes that is transformed by great spices. Splurge on a small bag of dried Vietnamese cinnamon and a whole nutmeg seed, and see what a difference it makes in a simple recipe like this. In addition to being delicious, cinnamon is a powerful antioxidant and anti-inflammatory.

1 cup (125mL) whole milk or coconut milk

2 eggs

1 teaspoon best-quality vanilla extract

1 teaspoon ground cinnamon

¼ teaspoon ground or freshly grated nutmeg

8 slices sturdy gluten-free, reduced-sodium bread

Fresh fruit and unsalted grass-fed butter, for serving

Budget friendly: Very

COOKS' NOTE: *Some testers added almond extract to this, which they loved. Be aware that almond extract might be a migraine trigger.*

1. Whisk together the milk, eggs, vanilla, cinnamon, and nutmeg in a shallow bowl and set aside for a few minutes to thicken.
2. Set a nonstick frying pan or griddle over medium heat until drops of water bounce off the top.
3. Spray the pan with cooking spray (for cast iron) or use coconut oil or butter just to coat the surface. (Do not use cooking spray on nonstick pans; it will ruin the surface.)
4. While the pan warms, place a slice of the bread in the milk mixture and let it soak into the bread. Then turn, allowing the other side to soak up the mixture.
5. When the pan is hot, add the slice of bread and start soaking another. Depending on the size of your pan, you can cook 2 to 4 slices at a time.
6. Cook each slice for 4 minutes on one side, or until golden brown, then flip and cook for 3 to 4 minutes more.
7. Transfer to an oven-safe plate and keep the finished French toast warm in a 200°F (95°C) oven while cooking the rest.
8. Serve right away with the fruit and butter.

Per serving: 12g protein, 27g carbohydrates, 7g fat, 2g saturated fat, 278mg sodium, 245mg potassium, 4g fiber

STEPHANIE'S SPICE STAR: Whole nutmeg
If you haven't tasted freshly grated nutmeg, you are in for a treat. Just buy one nutmeg seed from the bulk spice section and grate it on a fine grater or Microplane. It adds warm, sweet, spicy notes to baked goods and desserts.

Veggie Frittata

Makes 1 frittata, about 2 servings
Prep time: 5 minutes   Cooking time: 10–15 minutes   Passive time: N/A

You'll need an ovenproof pan for this recipe; a cast iron skillet is perfect. If you don't feel confident making and flipping omelets, the frittata is far easier, and it's another wonderful way to use up small amounts of leftover cooked veggies and meat. One tester loved making this for a weekend brunch for guests and had the leftovers for dinner with a side salad.

2 tablespoons unsalted grass-fed butter, ghee, or coconut oil

1 cup (250g) diced leftover cooked vegetables

4 eggs

1 tablespoon milk, half-and-half, or coconut milk

½ teaspoon freshly ground black pepper

Budget friendly: Very

1. Preheat the broiler. If your broiler is at the top of your oven, move the top rack to the highest position.
2. In a large ovenproof skillet or omelet pan set over medium heat, melt the butter.
3. Add the vegetables and sauté until they are golden brown.
4. Meanwhile, in a small bowl, whip the eggs lightly with the milk and pepper.
5. Pour the egg mixture into the skillet over the vegetables. Cook until set on the bottom and nearly set on the top.
6. Use an oven mitt or potholder to move the pan from the burner to the broiler or top rack of the oven. Broil for about 3 minutes, or until the top turns golden brown. If your broiler is too hot, you can bake the frittata for 12 minutes at 375°F (190°C) instead.
7. Cut into wedges and serve immediately. Leftover frittata wedges travel well for lunch or trips.

Per serving (using whole milk): 19g protein, 13g carbohydrates, 24g fat, 11g saturated fat, 427mg sodium, 343mg potassium, 2g fiber

Granola

Makes 14 servings
Prep time: 8 minutes   Cooking time: 25–30 minutes   Passive time: 30 minutes

My roommate Natalie used to make granola; she even had a special tall Tupperware container for it. I was never a fan back in the day, but I've learned to appreciate a cereal option that travels well. I make a batch of this before trips, then bag it up into individual servings. I can always find some kind of milk, a cup, and a spoon and have a migraine-friendly breakfast on the road. I haven't found a migraine-friendly granola at the grocery store; most contain nuts and/or a lot of sugar, even if they're gluten-free. Oats are high in magnesium and may enhance your immune response.

¼ cup (60mL) organic extra virgin olive oil

1 tablespoon pure maple syrup

Stevia to equal to 2 teaspoons sugar

½ teaspoon ground cinnamon

2 cups (200g) gluten-free rolled oats

1 cup (50g) unsweetened flaked coconut

1 cup (120g) raw pumpkin seeds

1 cup (130g) raw sunflower seeds

1 cup (15g) freeze-dried fruit, such as blueberries or strawberries (optional)

....

Budget friendly: Moderate

1. Preheat the oven to 300°F (150°C). Line a rimmed baking sheet with parchment paper and spray lightly with cooking spray. Set aside.
2. In a large bowl, whisk the olive oil, maple syrup, stevia, and cinnamon together.
3. Add the remaining ingredients, except the dried fruit, and toss well to coat.
4. Pour the mixture out onto the baking sheet, spreading evenly.
5. Transfer to the oven and bake for 15 minutes. Stir, then bake for another 10 minutes, or until the granola is golden brown but not too crispy. This may take up to 30 minutes total of baking.
6. Transfer the baking sheet to a wire rack to cool completely, about 30 minutes.
7. Add the dried fruit and mix well. Store in an airtight container for up to 3 weeks.

COOKS' NOTE: *One tester thought this was less like granola and more like muesli. Due to the lack of sugar, it doesn't make clumps like true granola does. If possible, use Vietnamese (Saigon) cinnamon for the best flavor.*

Per serving: 7g protein, 24g carbohydrates, 13g fat, 3g saturated fat, 19mg sodium, 241mg potassium, 4g fiber

Migas

Makes 4 servings
Prep time: 20 minutes   Cooking time: 35–40 minutes   Passive time: N/A

Migas, or "crumbs" in Spanish, is a breakfast dish that uses up stale corn tortillas. It's a wonderful, hearty breakfast that I make on the weekends when I have a little more time for prep. You could prep all the veggies and tortilla strips the night before and get this on the table in 15 minutes. One tester raved that this was as good as she gets in restaurants and loved serving leftover flank steak topped with fresh migas.

3–4 tablespoons (45–60g) extra virgin coconut oil, ghee, or unsalted grass-fed butter, divided

1 bunch green onions, sliced

2 red or yellow bell peppers, sliced

2 cloves garlic, minced

3–4 ounces cremini mushrooms, cleaned and sliced

4 (8-inch [20-cm]) corn tortillas, sliced into ¼-inch (1-cm) strips

1 cup (256g) chunky salsa, no-salt-added or low-sodium, onion-free

3 eggs

1 tablespoon half-and-half or coconut milk

½ teaspoon smoked paprika

¼ teaspoon ground cumin

½ bunch fresh cilantro, also called fresh coriander or Chinese parsley, minced

Budget friendly: Moderate (depending on price of bell peppers)

1. In a large nonstick frying pan set over medium–high heat, add 1 tablespoon of the coconut oil. Add the onions, stirring often.

2. Once the onions begin to turn translucent, add the peppers and garlic and continue stirring. Cook until peppers are browning and softened.

3. Set a cast iron frying pan over medium–high heat. When it's hot, add 1 tablespoon of the remaining coconut oil and ½ of the mushrooms. Stir or shake the pan until the mushrooms turn golden brown. Keep an eye on them; they cook quickly.

4. Add the cooked mushrooms to the nonstick pan with the vegetables, then cook the remaining mushrooms in more oil in the cast iron frying pan as needed. Leaving space in the pan allows the liquid from the mushrooms to evaporate without making them soggy. When cooked, transfer them to the nonstick pan.

5. Add more oil to the cast iron frying pan, if needed, and sauté the tortilla strips until crispy. Turn the heat off, but leave the pan sitting there to keep the tortillas crisp.

6. Add the salsa to the pan with the veggies and stir to combine. Reduce the heat to medium and cook until the mixture is hot.

7. Whisk the eggs in a bowl with the half-and-half or coconut milk, smoked paprika, and cumin. Pour into the pan with the vegetables and cook, stirring, until the eggs are set.

8. Stir the crispy tortilla strips and cilantro into the veggie pan. Serve right away.

COOKS' NOTE: *One tester substituted shiitake mushrooms, because she prefers them to creminis and pico de gallo (fresh salsa) instead of chunky cooked salsa. She loved the end result, too. Some people may be sensitive to smoked paprika. Salsa generally includes onions, which can be a migraine trigger. If you can't eat onions, or can't find low-sodium salsa, you can substitute fire-roasted canned tomatoes. Sometimes they include green chiles with the tomatoes, which is ideal for this recipe.*

Per serving: 10g protein, 20g carbohydrates, 17g fat, 9g saturated fat, 78mg sodium, 480mg potassium, 4g fiber

Pork Sausage Patties ⊘ ⊘ ⊛

Makes 12 patties
Prep time: 10 minutes   Cooking time: 8 minutes   Passive time: 15 minutes

Who knew that great-tasting breakfast sausage was so easy to make? Just whisk together a few spices, mix with the meat, and fry them up. I freeze extra cooked sausages so I can easily add some protein to our breakfast on busy mornings. If you love this spice blend, you can make it up in bulk and then easily make sausage whenever you like. If you haven't tried wild boar, it's available in the freezer case of many natural foods grocery stores. One tester declared it "the best sausage my husband and sons have ever had."

1 pound (450g) 85 percent lean fresh ground pork or frozen ground wild boar, thawed in refrigerator overnight

1 teaspoon dried thyme

1 teaspoon garlic powder

½–1 teaspoon dried sage

½–1 teaspoon smoked paprika

½ teaspoon ground or freshly grated nutmeg

¼ teaspoon ground white or black pepper

¼ teaspoon cayenne pepper

Budget friendly: Very to Moderate (depending on the meat)

1. Place the ground meat in a large bowl and allow it to reach room temperature.
2. Whisk all the herbs and spices together in a small bowl until they are a single color.
3. Sprinkle the spice mixture over the pork a little at a time, using a large-tined fork to turn and mix the meat. Use your hands if necessary (I wear food service gloves) to mix the spices through the meat without overworking the meat.
4. Set a large griddle or frying pan over medium–high heat.
5. Shape the pork into 12 equal patties. I use a food service scoop to make them evenly sized and then flatten each with my hand. Transfer each patty to a plate until ready to fry.
6. Add 6 patties to the griddle and pan-fry for at least 4 minutes per side, or until no longer pink in the center.
7. Transfer to a serving plate and serve immediately, or let cool slightly while frying the rest and then finish cooling in the refrigerator.
8. To freeze extra portions, allow to cool completely in the refrigerator, then place in freezer-safe containers.

COOKS' NOTE: *I like white pepper better with pork, as its milder, subtler flavor enhances this meat. Make this kid-friendly by using the smaller amounts of spices or omitting the cayenne altogether.*

Per serving (1 patty): 6g protein, 0g carbohydrates, 8g fat, 3g saturated fat, 21mg sodium, 117mg potassium, 0g fiber

Salmon, Asparagus, and Thyme Omelet

Makes 2 servings
Prep time: 10 minutes   Cooking time: 12–15 minutes   Passive time: N/A

You'll find that omelets are an easy way to get breakfast or dinner on the table. This simple recipe came about when I had just a small amount of baked salmon left over, and we didn't eat all the asparagus spears the previous night. I'm lucky to have fresh thyme growing in my garden, which adds lovely flavor, but dried thyme also works perfectly. Asparagus is high in inulin, one of the prebiotic fibers that feeds your good gut bacteria, and is another anti-inflammatory powerhouse.

4 ounces (120g) cooked salmon

3–4 spears fresh or frozen asparagus

12 sprigs fresh thyme, or ¼ teaspoon dried thyme (optional)

2 eggs

1–2 tablespoons (15–30mL) heavy cream, half-and-half, or coconut milk

1 tablespoon ghee, organic extra virgin olive oil, or extra virgin coconut oil

Budget friendly: Very

1. Flake the salmon into a bowl.
2. Cut the asparagus into bite-sized chunks and, if using fresh thyme, strip off the leaves (discard the stems).
3. Whisk the eggs with the cream and add the thyme leaves or dried thyme. Set aside.
4. Place a nonstick frying pan over medium heat, add the ghee, and swirl the pan to coat. Look for the ghee to start to shimmer before adding the asparagus.
5. Add the asparagus and sauté for 5 to 7 minutes.
6. Add the salmon and sauté another 2 to 3 minutes until the pieces start to turn golden.
7. Add the egg mixture to the pan. Cook about 5 minutes until nearly set, tilting the pan if necessary to move unset eggs to the edges.
8. Slide a flexible spatula under the omelet, loosening it, then fold in half.
9. Cook another 5 minutes, or until completely set. Serve right away.

Per serving: 21g protein, 2g carbohydrates, 21g fat, 5g saturated fat, 129mg sodium, 383mg potassium, 0g fiber

COOKS' NOTE: *This is the perfect way to use up leftover cooked salmon, which never tastes good microwaved. Canned, unsmoked salmon with no salt added is a fine substitute. Smoked salmon is not included on the migraine diet because smoked and preserved foods contain tyramine, a monoamine compound that triggers migraine attacks in some people. If using leftover pre-cooked asparagus, add it with the salmon during Step 6.*

lunch

For most of my life I worked in an office and brought my lunch, eating out only rarely. While you can still eat out on the Plan, learning to pack your own lunch will be most helpful for you to follow a migraine-friendly lifestyle. It will also save you a ton of money. I've included both hot and cold lunch recipes here, from soups to salads to sandwiches. Once you're eating dinner on the Plan, all dinner leftovers can become breakfast or lunch.

Chicken or Turkey Salad

Makes 4 servings
Prep time: 10 minutes   Cooking time: 5–8 minutes   Passive time: 10 minutes

If you have leftover cooked chicken or turkey, this is the perfect vehicle to transform it into lunch for several days. You can eat this on gluten-free bread or atop a bowl of greens. I add the carrot for sweetness and because I'm a fan of one-pot dishes that provide balanced nutrition. I'm always looking for ways to nudge a few more servings of veggies into my life.

½ cup (60g) raw pumpkin seeds

8 ounces (220g) cooked no-salt-added turkey or chicken

1 cup red grapes, sliced in half

2 stalks celery, thinly sliced

1 carrot, peeled and grated (optional)

¼ cup (55g) organic soy-free mayonnaise, plus more as needed

Budget friendly: Very

1. Toast the pumpkin seeds in a dry skillet set over medium heat for 5 to 8 minutes, or until golden. Remove from the heat and let cool for 10 minutes.
2. Dice the meat and place it in a medium bowl.
3. Add the toasted pumpkin seeds along with the rest of the ingredients and mix well. Add additional mayo if needed to get it to the consistency you prefer.
4. Serve immediately or refrigerate for up to 3 days.

COOKS' NOTE: *The ideal mayonnaise is made with light olive oil and contains no soybean oil or fillers like carrageenan. This salad is great over greens or on toasted gluten-free bread.*

Per serving (using chicken and no carrot): 16g protein, 13g carbohydrates, 7g fat, 1g saturated fat, 180mg sodium, 381mg potassium, 1g fiber

Farmers' Market Chilled Tomato–Basil Soup

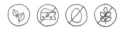

Makes 6 servings
Prep time: 10 minutes   Cooking time: 1 minute   Passive time: N/A

This is one of those recipes that, more than most, depends on peak, fresh ingredients. If you ignore this thoughtful note and use supermarket tomatoes, you'll think this recipe is terrible. You have been warned. Instead, use either homegrown peak summer tomatoes or organic tomatoes from the farmers' market. Same with the bell pepper. If you must make this when summer tomatoes aren't available, buy the reddest, happiest-looking organic cherry tomatoes you can find, as they have the best flavor year-round.

1 red, yellow, or orange bell pepper

3 large ripe heirloom tomatoes, about 1 pound (450g)

3 tablespoons (45mL) organic extra virgin olive oil

2 tablespoons white vinegar

2–3 fresh basil leaves, plus more for garnish

¼ teaspoon freshly ground black pepper

Heavy cream or coconut milk, for serving (optional)

Budget friendly: Very

1. Core the pepper and tomatoes.
2. Put everything, except the heavy cream and basil garnish, in the blender and blend until smooth.
3. Refrigerate the blender (with the cover on) until very cold.
4. Remove from the refrigerator and portion into serving bowls. Garnish with the reserved basil leaves and swirl in a spoonful of the heavy cream, if using.
5. Store in the refrigerator for up to 3 days. Do not freeze.

COOKS' NOTE: *Once you have tested white balsamic vinegar and find it's not a migraine trigger for you, use that in place of the white vinegar, which has a sharper taste.*

Per serving: 1g protein, 5g carbohydrates, 7g fat, 1g saturated fat, 6mg sodium, 260mg potassium, 1g fiber

Firehouse Turkey Chili

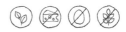

Makes 6 servings
Prep time: 15 minutes   Cooking time: 45 minutes   Passive time: N/A

I have made this chili so many times in so many variations, I don't even need the recipe any more. I've made it vegan, vegetarian, with meat, and with a variety of beans. I adapted it for the Plan by subbing in a bunch of green onions for the regular onion and omitting the salt. Kidney beans are traditional in chili, but you can also try Plan-approved black beans, which have a creamier texture. Adding the touch of sweetness does something magical to the chili, so don't skip that step. This is Husband Tested and Approved, perfect for a weeknight or fall dinner, and it packs well for lunch, too.

1 tablespoon organic extra virgin olive oil

1 bunch green onions, chopped

2 large carrots, diced

2 cloves garlic, minced

16 ounces (450g) ground turkey

2 tablespoons chili powder

½ teaspoon chipotle powder

28 ounces (800g) crushed or diced no-salt-added canned tomatoes

2 (15-ounce [425-g]) cans no-salt-added kidney or black beans, drained and rinsed

1 red bell pepper, diced

1 teaspoon pure maple syrup, or stevia to equal 1 teaspoon sugar

Budget friendly: Very

1. Warm the oil in a large lidded skillet set over medium–high heat. Add the green onions and carrots and sauté for 5 minutes, adjusting the heat if necessary so the vegetables don't burn.
2. Add the garlic and cook for 1 minute.
3. Add the ground meat and cook, breaking up the meat with a spoon, about 10 minutes, or until browned and no longer pink.
4. Stir in the chili powder and chipotle powder and cook 1 more minute.
5. Add the remaining ingredients and stir well. (You do not need to sauté the bell pepper.)
6. Raise the heat to high and bring the chili to a boil. Then reduce the heat to low and simmer, covered, for 30 minutes. Cook for up to 1 hour for even richer flavor.
7. Serve right away, store in the refrigerator for up to 5 days, or freeze in single-serving containers for lunch.

COOKS' NOTE: *You can use one can of each type of beans or two cans of one type. One tester substituted ground chicken for the ground turkey with excellent results. If you are vegan, just omit the meat; it still tastes great. I like to serve this with a green side salad. Omit the chipotle powder if you or your family don't like spicy food.*

Per serving: 28g protein, 44g carbohydrates, 10g fat, 2g saturated fat, 132mg sodium, 1,229mg potassium, 3g fiber

Spicy Fish Tacos

Makes 2 servings
Prep time: 15 minutes   Cooking time: 8 minutes   Passive time: N/A

I moved to San Diego from Chicago in 1997. I'd been here about six months when my friend Pete suggested going to Rubio's for lunch. I said, "What's Rubio's?" Pete said, "Wait a minute! You haven't had fish tacos?!?" I had to admit, I hadn't even heard of fish tacos. Decision made, we headed to the restaurant that brought fish tacos somewhat mainstream. Before that, they were mainly known to surfers visiting Baja California, who ate them on the beach. This version has a light gluten-free "breading," not a beer batter, and they're pan-fried, not deep fried. So you still get crispy fish with a little spice, the traditional cabbage topping, and a spicy mayo-based sauce. Surf's up, brah!

¼ cup (30g) sweet white rice flour or coconut flour

2 tablespoons canned light or full-fat coconut milk

1 teaspoon chili powder

¼ teaspoon chipotle or Anaheim chile powder

¼ teaspoon ground cumin

12 ounces (350g) firm white fish such as tilapia, halibut, cod, or tuna

2 tablespoons organic extra virgin coconut oil

¼ cup (55g) organic, low-sodium, soy-free mayonnaise

1 tablespoon Chile Pepper Sauce (page 267)

½ teaspoon garlic powder

1–2 tablespoons (15–30mL) whole milk, Hemp Milk (page 255), or coconut milk

4 small corn tortillas

1 cup (55g) finely shredded napa or savoy cabbage

1. Set out 3 shallow bowls or plates. Fill the first bowl with half of the flour, the second bowl with the coconut milk, and the last bowl with the remaining flour plus the chili powder, chipotle powder, and cumin. Mix flour and spices with a fork until it's a single color.

2. Cut the fish crosswise into 1-inch (2.5-cm) pieces. Pat the fish dry with a clean kitchen towel or paper towel.

3. Dip 1 piece into the unseasoned flour, dredging on all sides to give it a light coating. This helps the milk stick to the fish. Next, dip the floured fish piece into the coconut milk, then let it drip off. The coconut milk helps the breading to stick. Last, dip the fish piece in the seasoned flour mixture, coating each side evenly. Set the fully coated fish piece on a plate. Repeat this process until all the fish slices are coated.

4. Add the coconut oil to a large nonstick pan set over medium–high heat. Swirl to coat the pan and heat until shimmering.

5. Add the fish fillets and cook for 1½ to 2 minutes. When you see that the fish is cooked about halfway up, flip and cook for another 1½ to 2 minutes. For very thick fillets, give the other edges about 1 minute of cook time so all sides are golden and crispy. Keep warm.

Budget friendly: Moderate

6. While the fish is cooking, make the sauce: Whisk together the mayonnaise, Chile Pepper Sauce, and garlic powder. Add enough whole milk to make a pourable sauce; set aside.

7. While the fish is cooking, set a grill pan or cast iron pan over medium–high heat. Add the tortillas, and, using tongs, grill until lightly crisp on both sides. Alternatively, grill the tortillas over an open flame.

8. On serving plates, load each tortilla with one-quarter of the breaded fish and cabbage. Top each taco with the sauce and serve immediately.

COOKS' NOTE: *While traditional fish tacos are served with green or red cabbage, I prefer the lighter taste of napa or savoy cabbage. If you're looking for a grain-free and lower-carb option, use a whole napa or savoy cabbage leaf in place of a tortilla (no need to toast them). One tester marinated the shredded cabbage in the sauce while she was cooking the fish. Once you have tested lime and are certain it is not a migraine trigger for you, add a squeeze of lime juice to the sauce.*

Per serving (using tilapia, white rice flour, and full-fat coconut milk, excluding tortillas): 38g protein, 21g carbohydrates, 33g fat, 19g saturated fat, 347mg sodium, 725mg potassium, 2g fiber

STEPHANIE'S SPICE STAR: Chili powder

Chili powder is made from ground dried chiles (usually not spicy), with the additions of garlic, oregano, cumin, coriander, and/or cloves. Because it's not spicy, you use a large amount in a recipe (like 2 tablespoons in this recipe) to provide smoky, rich layers of flavor. Don't confuse chili powder with cayenne pepper or chipotle powder, both made from spicy dried chiles. Those are spicy and used in much smaller amounts, such as ¼ teaspoon.

Sloppy Joes

Makes 5 servings
Prep time: 15 minutes   Cooking time: 45 minutes   Passive time: N/A

My family always had Sunday dinner after church, a formal sit-down meal with a roast, vegetables, a starch, and dessert. Sunday nights were the only night of the week where we had a bit more freedom, making less-traditional and definitely less well-rounded meals. I'm talking hotdogs stuffed with Velveeta wrapped in crescent roll dough and baked in the toaster oven. Sloppy Joes were a favorite Sunday night dinner, which I learned to make in my early teens by adding ketchup to ground beef. This version adds mushrooms to extend the high-quality meat and includes almost no added sugar. Sloppy Joes have to be a little sweet or they're just not Sloppy Joes. Enjoy on any night with plenty of napkins. And a salad. Pack in a microwave-safe container for lunch; toast the bread just before eating. My recipe testers said this was "delicious healthy comfort food," "better than I remember as a kid."

16 ounces (450g) grass-fed, 85 percent lean ground beef

8 ounces (225g) cremini, button, or shiitake mushrooms

3 cloves garlic

1 bunch (125g) green onions, thinly sliced

6 ounces (115g) no-salt-added tomato paste

1 tablespoon molasses

2 teaspoons white vinegar

Stevia to equal 2 teaspoons sugar

1 teaspoon dried oregano

1 teaspoon smoked paprika

½ teaspoon freshly ground black pepper, or to taste

Dash hot sauce or Chile Pepper Sauce (page 267), or to taste (optional)

10 slices gluten-free bread, or 5 large savoy cabbage leaves, for serving

Budget friendly: Moderate

1. Set a large nonstick or cast iron skillet over medium heat.
2. Add the beef and cook until it's slightly browned and no longer pink, about 10 minutes.
3. Transfer the cooked beef to a plate lined with paper towels and set aside. Reserve the drippings in the pan and return it to the medium heat.
4. Clean the mushrooms using a damp towel to remove any soil. Quarter the mushrooms and add them, along with the garlic, to the bowl of a food processor with the S-blade attachment in place. Pulse a few times until the mushrooms and garlic are roughly chopped. Alternately, you can cut them by hand into a small dice.

5. Add the chopped mushrooms and garlic to the pan with the meat drippings and sauté for 10 minutes.

6. Add the sliced onions to the pan and cook, stirring frequently, for 5 minutes. When the vegetables are golden brown, add the cooked beef, tomato paste, molasses, vinegar, stevia, oregano, paprika, pepper, and Chile Pepper Sauce, if using. Stir well to combine. If the mixture seems dry, fill the entire tomato paste can with filtered water and add it to the pan, stirring well to combine.

7. Reduce the heat to low, partially cover, and cook 20 to 30 minutes. Taste and add more pepper and Chile Pepper Sauce as needed. Remove from the heat.

8. Serve between 2 slices of the gluten-free bread or wrapped with savoy cabbage leaves.

COOKS' NOTE: *One tester used ground chicken instead of ground beef. This is one of those recipes that uses a small amount of sugar in the form of molasses to achieve a specific flavor. If you wish to add sea salt, make your sandwich, then lightly sprinkle the top of the meat mixture with sea salt.*

Per serving (without bread or Chile Pepper Sauce): 20g protein, 15g carbohydrates, 14g fat, 5g saturated fat, 100mg sodium, 963mg potassium, 3g fiber

Provençal Chickpea Salad

Makes 8 servings
Prep time: 10 minutes   Cooking time: 40 minutes   Passive time: 12 hours

We spent my 50th birthday in Provence, a life-long dream. My friend Angela showed us the Tarascon farmers' market and made us an incredible lunch. This simple salad was one of many dishes that stand out in my memory from that bright, sunny day.

2 cups (250g) dried chickpeas

4 cups (1L) filtered water

3 stalks (65g) green onions

1 bunch (50g) fresh Italian flat-leaf parsley

1 clove garlic

½ cup (125mL) organic extra virgin olive oil

2 tablespoons white vinegar (see Cooks' Note)

1 teaspoon dried mustard powder

Freshly ground black pepper, to taste

Budget friendly: Very

Per serving (assuming ⅛ of the dressing is consumed with each serving): 4g protein, 12g carbohydrates, 15g fat, 2g saturated fat, 4mg sodium, 150mg potassium, 3g fiber

1. Soak the chickpeas in enough filtered water to cover them for 12 hours (overnight). Drain and rinse.

2. Add the chickpeas and 4 cups filtered water to a heavy cooking pot. Set it over high heat and bring to a boil. Reduce the heat to medium–low and simmer, covered, for 30 minutes. Taste; the chickpeas should be tender to the bite but not mushy. If they are not yet tender, continue cooking and taste after another 10 minutes.

3. Remove from the heat, drain, and rinse with cold water. Make sure the chickpeas are thoroughly drained before transferring them to a serving bowl. Set aside.

4. Remove the root ends and tips of the green onions and finely chop them. Soak the chopped onions in ice water for 10 minutes to remove the sharp bite, then drain thoroughly.

5. Stem and finely chop the parsley and set aside.

6. Use a garlic press or finely mince the garlic, and then add to a jar with a tightly fitting lid. Add the olive oil, vinegar, and mustard and shake until emulsified.

7. Add the chopped parsley and drained onion to the serving bowl with the chickpeas. Pour the dressing over and toss until combined. Taste and add the black pepper as needed.

COOKS' NOTE: *Once you have tested white wine vinegar and are certain it's not a migraine trigger for you, substitute that for the white vinegar for mellower flavor. Prepared mustard is not on the Plan because it's fermented and high in sodium, so dry mustard stands in. If you have never cooked dried beans before, please give it a try. It really improves the flavor of this salad to cook the beans from scratch. You can also cook the chickpeas in a pressure cooker for great results. If using canned chickpeas, use two (15.5-ounce [450-g]) cans, rinsed and drained well.*

Smoky Butternut Squash Soup ⊘ ⊘ ⊘ ⊘

Makes 4 servings
Prep time: 20 minutes   Cooking time: 50 minutes   Passive time: N/A

Roasted squash makes a tasty base for hearty, creamy soup. Roast it whole on a baking sheet to make this easier.

1 small (16-ounce [450-g]) butternut squash

Organic extra virgin olive oil, for brushing squash

1 medium white potato

2 cups (500mL) low-sodium vegetable or chicken stock

1 teaspoon smoked paprika

¼ teaspoon ground cumin

⅛ teaspoon chipotle powder

½ cup (60g) raw pumpkin seeds

8 fresh sage leaves

Budget friendly: Very

Per serving: 14g protein, 28g carbohydrates, 13g fat, 2g saturated fat, 50mg sodium, 967mg potassium, 5g fiber

1. Preheat the oven to 400°F (180°C).
2. To roast the butternut squash, cut off each end and halve it lengthwise. Using a grapefruit spoon, scoop out and discard the seeds.
3. Spray or brush the cut sides with the oil. Place the squash halves, cut side down, on a rimmed baking sheet. Poke each half with a fork 2 to 3 times.
4. Bake for 45 minutes, or until soft and tender.
5. Remove from the oven. Scoop out the flesh from the skin and transfer to a large bowl. Set aside.
6. Cut the potato into small cubes. Put in a microwave-safe container and cover with filtered water. Cook in the microwave on high until fork-tender, checking after 7 minutes. Drain.
7. Add the squash, potato, stock, paprika, cumin, and chipotle powder to the blender and blend until smooth. If using an immersion blender, put all the ingredients in a deep bowl and blend. Transfer the blended soup to a large pot set over low heat to warm.
8. While you are warming the soup, add the pumpkin seeds to a dry skillet set over medium heat and toast for 10 minutes, or until beginning to brown. Set aside.
9. Lightly spray or oil the skillet, then turn up the heat to medium–high, add the sage leaves, and lightly fry on each side until crispy. Remove from the heat.
10. When warm, ladle the soup into 4 individual bowls. Garnish with the crispy sage leaves and toasted pumpkin seeds and serve right away.

COOKS' NOTE: *Sub parsnips, sweet potatoes, or Honeycrisp apples for the white potato. One tester used curry powder instead of cumin.*

Spicy Kale and Split Pea Soup

Makes 8 servings
Prep time: 15 minutes   Cooking time: 2 hours   Passive time: N/A

For some reason, I have always hated green split pea soup and loved yellow split pea soup. No idea why. The taste is only slightly different, and the color of yellow split peas is only marginally better. But if you haven't had yellow split pea soup, give this recipe a try. It cooks up with very little hands-on time and makes plenty for freezing. While lentils are not on the Plan, split peas are, giving vegetarians and vegans a few more protein options until they can test more beans. Kale contains 45 different anti-inflammatory flavonoids, an omega-3 fat, and high levels of vitamin K. This soup can also be served over cooked brown rice, quinoa, or millet for a hearty meal.

16 ounces (450g) yellow split peas

1 tablespoon curry powder

1 teaspoon cumin seeds

1 teaspoon fenugreek seeds

1 teaspoon coriander seeds

½ teaspoon mustard seeds

½ teaspoon fennel seeds

½ teaspoon whole cardamom pods

1 tablespoon organic extra virgin olive oil

1 bunch (125g) green onions, thinly sliced

2 cloves garlic, minced

6 cups (1.5L) low-sodium vegetable or chicken stock

14 ounces (425g) no-salt-added fire-roasted canned tomatoes

16 ounces (450g) kale, stems attached, chopped into 1-inch (3-cm) pieces

1. Pick over the split peas to remove any pebbles or bruised peas. Rinse in a colander.
2. Add the spices to a small, dry skillet set over medium heat and toast for about 5 minutes, or until fragrant. Set aside.
3. In a large soup pot, warm the oil over medium heat. Add the onions and garlic and sauté for 5 minutes.
4. Add the toasted spices, stir, and cook for 2 minutes more.
5. If any spice powder is stuck to the skillet, use some of the broth to rinse it out into the soup pot. Add the tomatoes, remaining broth, split peas, and kale to the soup pot and stir to combine. Bring to a boil.
6. Stir again, cover, and reduce the heat to low. Simmer for about 2 hours, or until the peas are soft. If using pre-soaked peas (see Cooks' Note), check after 60 minutes. Remove from the heat.
7. Transfer to 8 individual soup bowls and serve right away, or let cool and store in the refrigerator. Freeze a few individual servings to use for lunches or dinners.

Budget friendly: Very

COOKS' NOTE: *If you cannot find fire-roasted tomatoes, regular diced canned tomatoes (no salt added) can be substituted. You can also substitute split mung beans for the yellow split peas. If you don't have all these spices, find a natural foods store that sells spices in bulk, and buy just a small amount of each. If you have these spices ground, use half as much of each. If you are missing one or two spices, it's okay. A recent nutritional analysis found that nearly all the potassium in kale is found in the stems. Our diets tend to be very low in potassium, so I include the stems in all my recipes. To further lower the sodium, use homemade salt-free stock. To shorten cooking time, soak peas overnight in filtered water, then drain and rinse.*

Per serving: 19g protein, 44g carbohydrates, 1g fat, 0g saturated fat, 455mg sodium, 1,122mg potassium, 17g fiber

STEPHANIE'S SPICE STAR: Coriander seed

It was years before I knew that coriander seeds, frequently used in Indian curries, grew into the plant we call cilantro. In other countries, they call cilantro fresh coriander, so there's no confusion. Coriander seeds have been used for centuries; some were discovered in Egyptian tombs dating back to 960 BCE. Cilantro haters alert! The seeds don't taste like cilantro, but instead impart a lemony-sagey-caraway flavor to foods.

Three Bean and Potato Salad

Makes 12 servings
Prep time: 10 minutes   Cooking time: 20 minutes   Passive time: 10 minutes

Served over greens, this dish makes a complete lunch. Add the optional stevia to get it to taste close to the deli version.

½ cup (120mL) no-sugar-added apple cider or apple juice

1 (15.5-ounce [450-g]) can no-salt-added red kidney beans

1 (15.5-ounce [450-g]) can no-salt-added wax beans

1 (15.5-ounce [450-g]) can no-salt-added chickpeas

1 red potato, plus more as desired

1 green onion, finely chopped

¼ cup (60mL) organic extra virgin olive oil

2 tablespoons white vinegar (see Cooks' Note)

1 teaspoon white pepper

Stevia to equal 1 teaspoon sugar (optional)

Budget friendly: Very

1. Add the apple cider to a small saucepan set over medium heat. Bring to a boil, then reduce the heat to low and simmer for about 10 minutes, or until the liquid is reduced to 2 tablespoons. Remove from the heat and let cool.
2. Rinse the canned ingredients well and leave in the colander to drain while you make the rest of the dish.
3. Finely dice the potato and rinse 3 times to remove the starch. Transfer to a microwave-safe dish and add filtered water just to cover. Cook on high in the microwave for up to 10 minutes, or until fork tender. Alternatively, you can boil the potato.
4. Drain immediately and rinse the potato with cold water to stop the cooking process.
5. Add the onion to 1 cup of ice water for 10 minutes to remove the bite. Drain well.
6. To make the dressing, add the reduced apple cider, oil, vinegar, white pepper, and stevia, if using, to a clean glass jar with a tight-fitting lid and shake well to emulsify.
7. Add the drained beans, chickpeas, potato, and onion to a large bowl and toss. Pour over about ½ of the dressing. Toss well; the flavors will intensify as it marinates.
8. Serve at room temperature or cold. Refrigerate up to 5 days

COOKS' NOTE: *If you have tested apple cider vinegar and it doesn't trigger you, feel free to substitute it for the white vinegar for mellower flavor. You can also use 15.5 ounces each of cooked beans, if you don't want to use canned. Store leftover dressing in the refrigerator; it keeps well for about five days and is delicious as a salad dressing.*

Per serving: 7g protein, 24g carbohydrates, 6g fat, 0g saturated fat, 5mg sodium, 385mg potassium, 6g fiber

Tuna or Salmon Salad

Makes 2 servings
Prep time: 2 minutes   Cooking time: N/A   Passive time: N/A

When I was first diagnosed, I had been eating a plant-based diet for four years. It was a difficult transition going back to animal products, one I didn't take lightly. We started with local eggs from a friend and canned wild-caught fish. There's some disagreement about whether canned fish is high in tyramine or is a migraine trigger. I haven't had problems with water-packed, no-salt-added albacore tuna or wild Alaskan pink salmon. This salad is a quick and easy lunch served over a big salad.

1 (4-ounce [115-g]) can no-salt-added albacore tuna or Alaskan pink salmon, rinsed and drained

3 tablespoons (45g) organic, low-sodium soy-free mayonnaise

1 teaspoon reduced-sodium Old Bay or seafood seasoning

Budget friendly: Very

1. Mix everything together in a bowl.
2. Serve right away or refrigerate for up to 2 days.

COOKS' NOTE: *My testers got creative with this recipe, adding finely chopped celery and red bell pepper. I like to eat this on a green salad or on top of a hearty rice cake or slice of toasted reduced-sodium gluten-free bread.*

Per serving (using salmon): 13g protein, 1g carbohydrates, 14g fat, 2g saturated fat, 121mg sodium, 218mg potassium, 0g fiber

STEPHANIE'S SPICE STAR: Old Bay or seafood seasoning
Old Bay seasoning is from the Chesapeake Bay area of Maryland. It's dynamite on seafood and is traditionally used for crab boils. Look for reduced-sodium versions of this spice blend to enjoy its unique flavor and amp up your salad, or to sprinkle over Fish Baked in Parchment Packets (page 228).

dinner

—— ⋯ ——

The final change in the Plan is to switch over dinners in Week 7. Any of these recipes can be eaten for breakfast or lunch, too. I've created several easy chicken dishes, two featuring fish, two pork, meatloaf, and a couple of vegetarian options as well as some hearty sides.

Maple Sesame Glazed Chicken

Makes 4 servings
Prep time: 25 minutes   Cooking time: 45–50 minutes   Passive time: ½–8 hours

This Asian-inspired glaze is close to teriyaki without being sticky-sweet. This dish is shown on the cover with Wild Rice and Carrots (page 246) and Spicy Kale and Swiss Chard Sauté (page 243).

1 bunch green onions

2 tablespoons white vinegar (see Cooks' Note)

2 tablespoons pure maple syrup

2 tablespoons toasted sesame oil

2 cloves garlic

1 teaspoon smoked paprika

1 teaspoon garlic powder

½ teaspoon ground ginger

1⅗–2 pounds (0.8–1kg) boneless, skinless chicken thighs (5–6 thighs)

1 tablespoon coconut oil

2 tablespoons dry toasted tan sesame seeds

Budget friendly: Very

1. Remove the roots and tips from the green onions. Cut the white parts into chunks and put them in a blender. Slice the green parts thinly and set aside.
2. To make the marinade, add the vinegar, maple syrup, toasted sesame oil, garlic, smoked paprika, garlic powder, and ginger to the blender and blend, along with the white parts of the onion, until smooth.
3. Put the chicken in a large bowl. Pour marinade over chicken. Cover the bowl with plastic wrap and marinate in the refrigerator for at least 30 minutes and up to overnight.
4. Heat the coconut oil in large nonstick lidded skillet set over medium heat until shimmering. Add the chicken pieces and cook for 5 minutes on each side, or until browned.
5. Drizzle any remaining marinade from the bowl over the chicken and sprinkle the reserved sliced green onions, stirring to coat chicken. Then, partially cover the pan and reduce the heat to medium–low. Cook for 10 minutes, turn the chicken, and cook for 10 minutes more. Leave a small opening between the cover and the pan so some of the steam can escape.
6. Remove lid from chicken pan to check chicken for doneness. Cook just until done, either by checking with a meat thermometer for 165°F (74°C), or by cutting open. Sprinkle sesame seeds over. Remove from the heat.
7. Serve right away or store in the refrigerator for up to 3 days.

COOKS' NOTE: *Use skinless chicken for this recipe, as this cooking method will not deliver crispy skin. If you're not sure about sesame oil, start with 1 tablespoon, then taste.*

Per serving: 46g protein, 11g carbohydrates, 18g fat, 3g saturated fat, 196mg sodium, 681mg potassium, 2g fiber

Chicken Cacciatore

Makes 8 servings
Prep time: 15 minutes   Cooking time: 45–90 minutes   Passive time: N/A

My testers and I worked hard on this one to get the savory flavor right without added salt. I made this five or six times before sending it off to the testers. We also wanted to keep the dish easy to make, so see my suggestions in the Cooks' Note for speeding things along. Gluten-free pasta is stickier than wheat pasta, so I add a small amount of olive oil to the cooking water. I find that adding the garlic and red pepper flakes infuses the pasta with wonderful flavor without salt. One tester made this in a slow cooker by following Steps 1 and 2, just browning the meat in Step 3, and then cooking the sauce for three hours on high. Another tester said, "My Italian husband, who is particular about Italian food, loved it!"

2 red bell peppers, roasted and peeled, or 1 (12-ounce [340-g]) jar roasted red peppers, drained and rinsed (see Cooks' Note)

1 (28-ounce [800-g]) can no-salt-added canned tomatoes

2 tablespoons organic extra virgin olive oil, plus more as needed for the pasta

8 ounces (225g) white button or cremini mushrooms, cleaned and thinly sliced

4 cloves garlic, finely minced

4 (5–6 ounce [141–169g]) uncooked boneless, skinless chicken breasts, diced

4 slices (150g) pork belly, diced (optional)

½ teaspoon freshly ground black pepper

½ teaspoon dried rosemary

½ teaspoon dried basil

½ teaspoon dried oregano

3 bay leaves

2 cloves garlic, smashed

½ teaspoon red pepper flakes

8 ounces (225g) gluten-free pasta

Shredded fresh basil leaves or finely chopped Italian parsley, for garnish (optional)

Budget friendly: Moderate

1. Roughly chop the roasted peppers and add them, along with the canned tomatoes, to a blender. Pulse on low a few times until the sauce is uniform but still has a rustic texture. Set aside.
2. Warm the olive oil in a heavy-bottomed saucepan or deep cast iron skillet set over medium heat. Add the mushrooms and minced garlic and sauté until golden brown, about 7 minutes.
3. Add the diced chicken breasts, pork belly, if using, black pepper, rosemary, basil, oregano, and bay leaves. Sauté until the meat is golden brown, about 8 minutes, stirring occasionally.

4. Pour the sauce into the saucepan and bring to a boil. Reduce the heat to low and simmer, uncovered, for at least 30 minutes (60 to 90 minutes is better). The sauce should be bubbling but not boiling. Remove and discard the bay leaves. Leave the sauce on low while you cook the pasta.

5. When the sauce is done, set a large pot of filtered water over high heat. Add a drizzle of olive oil, the smashed cloves of garlic, and the red pepper flakes. Bring to a boil. Add the pasta and cook until al dente. Drain and remove and discard the garlic cloves.

6. Rinse the pasta quickly with cool water, then toss with a drizzle of olive oil. Toss cooked pasta with the chicken and sauce in the saucepan.

7. Serve topped with the basil or parsley, if using.

COOKS' NOTE: *Check the ingredient list on the roasted red peppers. They should be low in sodium and without sulfites. Using jarred peppers greatly speeds up this recipe. For a grain-free option, serve over zucchini ribbons or cooked spaghetti squash strands. You can substitute 2 teaspoons of a salt-free Italian seasoning blend for the rosemary, basil, and oregano. Use pre-sliced mushrooms to make prep easier.*

Per serving (excluding pork belly): 12g protein, 20g carbohydrates, 22g fat, 3g saturated fat, 339mg sodium, 589mg potassium, 3g fiber

Fish Baked in Parchment Packets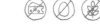

Makes 4 servings
Prep time: 5 minutes   Cooking time: 15 minutes   Passive time: N/A

One thing people worry about when cooking fish is either over- or under-cooking it. I wanted a foolproof fish recipe for this book to make it easy to include fish on your menu at least once a week, which fits the recommendation of the brain-protective MIND diet as well. I first learned about cooking fish in parchment paper packets from a magazine about 20 years ago. It worked beautifully. As I became more comfortable with baking, grilling, and pan-frying fish without ruining it, I forgot about this method. I went back to the method, remembering how easy it was. Every one of my testers loved this recipe, especially the nonexistent cleanup.

16–24 ounces (450–675g) tilapia, cod, turbot, or halibut fillets (4 equal pieces), fresh or frozen and thawed overnight

4 handfuls spinach leaves

Fine sea salt and freshly ground black pepper, to taste

4 tablespoons unsalted grass-fed butter, ghee, or organic extra virgin coconut oil, divided

½ teaspoon dried dill weed

1 carrot

1 zucchini

1 red bell pepper

Budget friendly: Very

1. Preheat the oven to 450°F (230°C).
2. Pat the fish dry with paper towels or clean kitchen towels and set aside.
3. Prepare the parchment packets by cutting four squares of parchment paper. Create squares by folding the parchment on the diagonal along the width of the roll into an even triangle and cutting along the remaining edge. Crease the diagonal fold well before opening.
4. Place 1 handful of spinach leaves to the left of the fold line. Top each bed of spinach with 1 fish fillet, laying the long edge of the fish along the fold. Sprinkle the fish with the sea salt and black pepper, then spread 1 tablespoon of the butter on each portion of fish. Sprinkle the dill weed over evenly over all.
5. Peel the carrot, then peel thin slices on top of the fish.
6. Thinly slice the zucchini, laying the slices on top of the carrot.
7. Core and thinly slice the red pepper, laying slices on top of the zucchini.
8. You should now have a pile of food in the center of the parchment to the left of the fold line. Fold the open side closed. Starting with the point nearest you, create the packet by folding the point over to the left and creasing. Continue folding and creasing around the food until you have a half-moon-shaped packet that is reasonably airtight.

9. Place the packets on a baking sheet.
10. Transfer the baking sheet to the oven and bake on the center rack for 15 minutes.
11. Transfer each packet to a plate and serve immediately, cutting open to eat and being careful of the steam as it escapes.

COOKS' NOTE: *Make the packets ahead and refrigerate until you begin preheating the oven. While you are welcome to substitute other vegetables, do not include potatoes in the packets; they need longer to cook. Mushrooms end up with a rubbery texture from steaming inside the packets, so they are not recommended. If desired, packets can also be microwaved on full power for 5 minutes in a lower-power microwave or for 4 minutes in a high-power microwave. The texture is not as pleasing, but it gets the job done. You can omit the dill and substitute mayonnaise mixed with a small amount of dry mustard for the butter or oil for a different flavor. This method is best suited for light white fish, not oily fish such as tuna, salmon, or swordfish.*

Per serving (using tilapia): 47g protein, 6g carbohydrates, 15q fat, 9q saturated fat, 158mg sodium, 1,091mg potassium, 2g fiber

Meatloaf

Makes 8 servings
Prep time: 20 minutes   Cooking time: 45–60 minutes   Passive time: N/A

I'm not sure what I love more: meatloaf, the sauce baked onto the top, or a cold meatloaf sandwich the next day. Since store-bought sauce tends to include migraine triggers like onion, this recipe includes homemade sauce. A portion of the sauce is reserved partway through cooking and added to the meat mixture, infusing the meatloaf with savory flavor without extra work. Testers called this "delicious and filling" and loved dipping gluten-free bread into the sauce.

SAUCE

1 tablespoon coconut oil

1 bunch green onions, thinly sliced

4 shallots, minced

2 cloves garlic, minced

8 ounces (225g) cremini or white button mushrooms, cleaned and thinly sliced

2 tablespoons extra virgin coconut oil

8 ounces (225g) cherry tomatoes, roughly chopped

1 cup (250mL) filtered water

1 (6-ounce [170-g]) can no-salt-added tomato paste

1 teaspoon dried basil

1 teaspoon dried oregano

MEATLOAF

16 ounces (450g) grass-fed ground beef, or a mixture of ground beef and ground pork, 85 percent lean

2 eggs

1 egg yolk

2 tablespoons ground flax seeds

Budget friendly: Moderate

FOR THE SAUCE

1. Melt the coconut oil in a heavy-bottomed saucepan set over medium heat. Add the onions, shallots, and garlic and sauté for 5 minutes, or until the vegetables are starting to turn gold.
2. Add the mushrooms and raise the heat to medium high. Sauté until the mushrooms turn golden brown, about 7 minutes.
3. Remove ½ cup of the vegetables and set aside to add to the meatloaf mixture.
4. Mix together the cherry tomatoes, water, tomato paste, and spices. Add to the saucepan. Reduce the heat to medium-low and simmer the sauce for 15 minutes.
5. Continue to simmer on low while the meatloaf is cooking. The sauce should reduce until it is very thick, almost a paste.

FOR THE MEATLOAF

1. Preheat the oven to 350°F (180°C). Line a loaf pan with parchment paper and spray the paper with cooking spray. Set aside.
2. In a large bowl, add the meat, eggs, egg yolk, flax seeds, reserved vegetables, and ½ cup of the simmering sauce. Mix with your hands or a large spoon just until well blended. (Overmixing toughens the meat.)
3. Fill the pan and smooth the top with a spatula.
4. Bake for 45 minutes
5. Spread the remaining thickened sauce evenly on the top of the meatloaf and bake another 15 minutes. The meatloaf should look golden on the edges and the sauce should be bubbling.
6. Remove from oven and let stand about 10 minutes to firm up before slicing. Serve hot. Refrigerate leftover meatloaf and eat hot or cold for lunch or dinner. It makes awesome cold sandwiches.

COOKS' NOTE: *The sauce base does double-duty as part of the ingredients in the meatloaf itself. You can use ground chicken, turkey, or any ground meat in this recipe. If using mini loaf pans, set them on a baking sheet and bake for just 15 minutes in Step 4. Continue with Steps 5 and 6 as directed.*

Per serving: 15g protein, 11g carbohydrates, 15g fat, 7g saturated fat, 82mg sodium, 649mg potassium, 3g fiber

Pasta with Vodka Chickpea Sauce ⊘ 🥛 ⊘ ✿

Makes 8 servings
Prep time: 10–15 minutes   Cooking time: 25 minutes   Passive time: N/A

The original recipe, sans vodka, came from my roommate Colleen years ago, who regularly cooked out of Jane Brody's *Good Food Book*. I've adapted it over the years, adding vodka to this version and replacing the regular onion with shallots. The chickpeas create a creamy sauce for pasta even without dairy, and the rosemary adds an herbal, Tuscan note to the sauce.

2 (15-ounce [425-g]) cans no-salt-added chickpeas, drained and rinsed, divided

2 large shallots

2 tablespoons organic extra virgin olive or coconut oil

4 cloves garlic, minced

1 (16-ounce [450-g]) no-salt-added chopped tomatoes

½ cup (125mL) vodka

½ cup (125mL) filtered water

1 tablespoon minced fresh rosemary, or ½ teaspoon dried rosemary

1 cup (250mL) cream, half-and-half, or coconut milk

1 teaspoon freshly ground black pepper, plus more to taste

1 clove garlic, smashed

16 ounces (450g) gluten-free pasta, preferably spaghetti

Organic extra virgin olive oil, for drizzling

1 sprig fresh rosemary, for garnish (optional)

Budget friendly: Very

1. In a blender or food processor, purée 1 can of the chickpeas with enough filtered water to make a smooth, pourable purée. Slice shallots in half, then thinly slice. Set the chickpea purée and the shallots aside.
2. Heat the oil in a large saucepan set over medium heat until it shimmers. Add the shallots and sauté for 5 minutes, then add the minced garlic. Continue sautéing just until the garlic begins to brown.
3. Add the tomatoes and their liquid, vodka, filtered water, rosemary, chickpea purée, and remaining can of chickpeas to the saucepan. Cook, stirring often, for about 15 minutes or until the mixture has thickened. Add the cream and black pepper and heat through. Leave on low until ready to serve.

4. While the sauce is cooking, set a large pot of filtered water over high heat and add the smashed garlic. When the water comes to a rolling boil, add the pasta. (I add a splash of olive oil when cooking gluten-free pasta, which makes it less starchy.)

5. Before draining the pasta, reserve ½ cup of pasta water. Add ¼ cup of the pasta water to the sauce and stir. Add more if it is still too thick to be a pourable sauce.

6. Drain the pasta when it is al dente, rinsing briefly with cool water. Drizzle with a little olive oil and toss. This greatly improves the texture of gluten-free pasta.

7. Toss the hot cooked pasta with the sauce in the saucepan. Garnish with the sprig of fresh rosemary, if using, a drizzle of the olive oil, and additional black pepper.

COOKS' NOTE: *If you'd like to use this recipe with dried chickpeas, start with 10 ounces (285g) of dried chickpeas, and use the cooking instructions on page 218. Vodka is one of the two alcoholic beverages (along with white wine) that's allowed in small quantities on the Plan. Most of the alcohol will cook off in this preparation, leaving the subtle vodka flavoring. For a grain-free option, serve the sauce over zucchini ribbons or cooked spaghetti squash strands.*

Per serving: 20g protein, 79g carbohydrates, 10g fat, 3g saturated fat, 33mg sodium, 651mg potassium, 9g fiber

Peachy Pulled Pork

Makes 16 servings
Prep time: 5–15 minutes   Cooking time: 6 hours, 15 minutes   Passive time: 15 minutes

I first tested this dish on a screaming-hot summer day. So hot that I banished the slow cooker to the laundry room, where it could emit its porky heat all day without making the house any hotter. I loved how fast the sauce came together, how little hands-on time it required, and how freaking delicious it turned out. I adapted it for the Plan after a few tries. If you add root vegetables to the slow cooker, this recipe provides meals for a week. One tester made "awesome" pork tacos from the leftovers.

10 ounces (285g) frozen or fresh ripe peaches, sliced

½ cup (125mL) unsalted chicken stock

¼ cup (60mL) molasses

5 cloves garlic

1 tablespoon white vinegar

1 tablespoon smoked paprika

1 teaspoon ground white pepper

¼ teaspoon dried mustard powder

¼ teaspoon red pepper flakes

3½–4½ pounds (1.6–2kg) pork shoulder roast (Boston butt), trimmed of excess fat

2 bunches green onions, thinly sliced

3 bay leaves

Large chunks of potato, sweet potato, carrots, parsnips, turnips, and/or rutabagas (optional, to fill up the slow cooker)

2 tablespoons filtered water

1 tablespoon arrowroot powder, tapioca flour, or cornstarch

Budget friendly: Moderate

1. Set a 6-quart slow cooker to low.
2. Put the first 9 ingredients—peaches through red pepper flakes—in a blender and blend until you have a completely smooth sauce. If using frozen peaches and you don't have a high-speed blender, let the peaches thaw first.
3. Pour enough of the sauce into the slow cooker to cover the bottom. Add the pork, turning to coat.
4. Add the green onions, bay leaves, and vegetables, if using. Pour the rest of the sauce over.
5. Cover and cook for 6 hours, or until the pork is very tender. Transfer the pork to a large cutting board. Strain the cooking liquid into a saucepan. Leave the vegetables in the slow cooker for now, discarding the bay leaves. Let the pork cool for 10 to 15 minutes.

6. Bring the cooking liquid to a boil and cook for 10 minutes, or until its volume is reduced by half.
7. Shred the pork with 2 forks, removing and discarding any pockets of fat.
8. Combine the filtered water and arrowroot powder in a small bowl, stirring with a whisk to create a slurry; whisk the slurry into the sauce, whisking constantly until the sauce is thickened.
9. Serve vegetables and pulled pork on a serving platter, drizzled with sauce.
10. Refrigerate for up to 3 days; freeze some in single portions for lunch.

COOKS' NOTE: *If you have a smaller slow cooker, choose a smaller piece of pork. A 1.5-pound roast will serve six. Sauce amount remains the same. There are several ways to remove some of the fat from the cooking liquid before making the sauce: (1) Place a large zip-top bag inside a 4-cup glass measuring cup. Pour the reserved cooking liquid into the bag after letting it cool for 10 minutes, and let stand 10 minutes so the fat can rise to the top. Seal the bag. Holding it over the saucepan, snip off one small bottom corner of the bag. Drain the cooking liquid into saucepan; stop just before the fat begins to drip out. Discard the bag. (2) Use a baster to remove the fat from the top. (3) Use a fat-separating measuring cup.*

Per serving (16 servings from 4.5 pounds pork, without root vegetables):
23g protein, 9g carbohydrates, 16g fat, 6g saturated fat, 83mg sodium, 597mg potassium, 1g fiber

Roasted Veggie Quinoa Casserole ⊘ ⊘ ⊘

Makes 8 servings
Prep time: 50 minutes   Cooking time: 60–75 minutes   Passive time: 10 minutes

It's not easy following the Plan if you are vegetarian or vegan, as so many of your protein sources are potential triggers. The quinoa and black beans in this dish are high in protein, making it a hearty vegetarian one-dish meal.

1 cup (175g) quinoa, any color

1 cup (250mL) filtered water

1 (1.5–2 pound [680–900g]) butternut or other fall squash

2 large carrots, peeled and cut into ½-inch dice

3 stalks celery, cut into ½-inch dice

½ cup chopped kale, stems included

½ cup cooked no-salt-added or low-sodium black beans, drained (optional)

6 cloves garlic, minced

¼ cup (60mL) organic extra virgin olive oil

2 tablespoons no-salt-added medium–hot curry powder

1½ cups (375mL) low-sodium vegetable stock

Budget friendly: Very

1. Put the quinoa and filtered water in a glass bowl and set aside to soak while you are prepping the vegetables.
2. Peel the squash, cut it in half, remove the seeds and strings, and cut into a ½-inch dice. Add to a large mixing bowl, along with the carrots, celery, kale, black beans, if using, and garlic.
3. Drizzle the oil over the vegetables and toss. Sprinkle with the curry powder and toss until evenly coated. Set aside.
4. Preheat the oven to 400°F (200°C). Spray or oil a large lidded casserole dish. If you don't have a lid, cut a piece of aluminum foil to cover. Set aside.
5. Drain and rinse the quinoa.
6. Add the drained quinoa and stock to the casserole dish. Gently agitate the dish to distribute the quinoa evenly, while keeping it submerged in the liquid.
7. Carefully add the vegetables evenly on top, spreading with a spatula and keeping as much of the quinoa in contact with the liquid as possible.
8. Bake, covered or wrapped tightly in foil, for 35 to 45 minutes, or just until the vegetables are fork-tender.
9. Remove from the oven, uncover, and let rest for a few minutes before serving.

COOKS' NOTE: *You must use a casserole dish with a lid, or cover your dish tightly with foil, or the quinoa will dry out and not cook properly. Choose pre-prepped or frozen butternut squash to shorten prep time. You can prep all the vegetables a day ahead. It's important to cut them uniformly; the small dice allows them to cook through.*

Per serving (excluding black beans): 6g protein, 36g carbohydrates, 9g fat, 1g saturated fat, 202mg sodium, 868mg potassium, 6g fiber

Salmon–Potato Cakes

Makes 4 servings

Prep time: 20 minutes   Cooking time: 10–20 minutes   Passive time: 20 minutes

These hearty cakes have enough veggies in them to qualify as a meal. Perfect for using up grilled or canned salmon. See page 283 for more patty ideas.

6 ounces (170g) canned no-salt-added Alaskan pink salmon

1 cup (90g) grated potatoes

1 small or ½ large carrot

¼ red bell pepper

1 egg

4 tablespoons (25g) ground flax seeds

2 tablespoons half-and-half or coconut milk

1 teaspoon reduced-sodium seafood seasoning

1 teaspoon garlic powder

½ teaspoon dried dill

¼ teaspoon freshly ground black pepper

1 recipe Smoky Mustard Sauce (page 273) or another creamy sauce, for serving

Budget friendly: Moderate

Per serving: 13g protein, 12g carbohydrates, 11g fat, 2g saturated fat, 59mg sodium, 463mg potassium, 3g fiber

1. Drain the salmon and flake it into a large mixing bowl. Add the potatoes.
2. Put the carrot in a food processor and pulse until roughly chopped. Add the red bell pepper and pulse until both are finely chopped, but do not overwork it. Add the mixture to the bowl with the salmon.
3. Add the remaining ingredients, except for the mustard sauce, to the bowl and mix with a spatula until evenly distributed. Use the spatula to smoosh everything together, so that the starches from the potatoes and flax seeds make it very sticky. Set aside and let rest for 20 minutes.
4. Preheat an electric grill to medium high or set a grill pan or nonstick frying pan over medium–high heat. Brush the grill, grill pan, or pan with high-heat oil such as grapeseed oil.
5. Using a measuring cup, egg ring, or ice cream scoop, portion out the patties evenly, about a ½ cup per patty. (You can make 2 patties per person or 1 large one.)
6. Cook the patties in 2 batches for 5 to 8 minutes per side, or until golden. Flatten with a spatula after flipping them. Transfer cooked patties to a serving platter or individual plates.
7. Serve right away with Smoky Mustard Sauce. Store covered in the refrigerator for up to 3 days, or freeze in individual portions for lunch.

COOKS' NOTE: *You can use frozen shredded potatoes for this recipe, but they do include dextrose and a preservative. If you don't care for canned fish, you can prebake fresh or frozen salmon for dinner one night, reserving enough leftovers for this the next night. If you don't have a large pan or grill surface, cook the patties in several batches.*

Scallop Corn Chowder

Makes 4 servings
Prep time: 20 minutes   Cooking time: 50 minutes   Passive time: N/A

If I could only eat one kind of seafood for the rest of my life, scallops would win, shells down. Perfectly cooked scallops are a luxury item to me. I've also always loved rich, New England–style clam chowder. This recipe combines my love of both in a migraine-friendly version that can easily be dairy-free. I make the scallops go farther in the dish while reducing the sodium they contribute by cutting them in half, capturing all the juice they release to flavor the rich broth.

1 cup (120g) fresh or frozen corn kernels, divided

½ cup (125mL) heavy cream or coconut milk

2 tablespoons unsalted grass-fed butter or extra virgin coconut oil

1 (8-ounce [225-g]) package frozen jumbo sea scallops, thawed and liquid reserved

½ teaspoon smoked paprika

½ teaspoon freshly ground black pepper

8 green onions, thinly sliced

1 large shallot, diced

1 russet or Yukon gold potato, scrubbed, diced, and covered in filtered water

1 large carrot, diced

2 cups (250mL) low-sodium chicken stock

½ teaspoon dried dill

½ teaspoon liquid smoke (optional)

½ red or orange bell pepper, diced

¼ cup chopped fresh Italian flat-leaf parsley, for garnish

Budget friendly: Moderate

1. Add half of the corn and all of the heavy cream to a blender; blend until smooth. Do not over-blend. Set aside.
2. In a large skillet set over medium–high heat, warm the butter until it melts and shimmers. Swirl the pan to coat evenly.
3. While the butter melts, pat the scallops dry. They should be very dry, otherwise moisture might cause the oil to splatter and burn you. Then cut each in half crosswise. If they have partially split in half, cut them that direction instead. Sprinkle each scallop with the paprika and black pepper.
4. Add all the scallops to the skillet and cook 1 to 2 minutes per side, or until golden brown, using tongs to flip. Transfer to a plate and set aside. Reserve the drippings in the skillet.
5. Add the green onions and shallot to the drippings in the skillet and cook over medium heat for 5 minutes, or until translucent.

6. Drain the potatoes and add to the skillet with the carrots. Sauté for 5 minutes.
7. Add the stock, reserved scallop liquid, dill, and liquid smoke, if using. Bring to a boil over high heat. Once boiling, partially cover and reduce the heat to low. Simmer for 10 minutes.
8. By now, liquid from the resting scallops will have collected on the plate. Add this liquid, the remaining ½ cup of corn, and the bell peppers to the skillet. Simmer on low for another 10 to15 minutes, or until all the vegetables are tender.
9. Add the scallops and cream–corn mixture and simmer gently to heat through. Sprinkle with the parsley.
10. Serve immediately. Refrigerate extra portions for up to 2 days.

COOKS' NOTE: *Since scallops are naturally high in sodium, these are used sparingly. I slice large sea scallops in half to extend the scallop flavor and the pleasure in eating them. You can use less expensive bay scallops; sprinkle with spices and sauté them quickly. If using fresh scallops, you won't have any scallop juice in Step 9. One tester loved it so much she made it again with double the corn and cream. Prep all the vegetables and put them in separate bowls. This makes cooking go faster and can be done the night before. Liquid smoke may be a trigger, so test it before using. Choose a brand of liquid smoke that includes only smoke and water as ingredients. Chop the parsley right before serving to maintain freshness, and sprinkle on top of each serving.*

Per serving: 15g protein, 29g carbohydrates, 13g fat, 7g saturated fat, 159mg sodium, 829mg potassium, 4g fiber

Spice-Rubbed Seared Pork Chops with Oven-Baked Sweet Potatoes and Cranberry–Pear Sauce

Makes 2 servings
Prep time: 10 minutes   Cooking time: 30–35 minutes   Passive time: 5 minutes

While I didn't love red meat as a kid, Shake 'n Bake pork chops were my favorite meal. This is an upscale version, making an elegant dinner while being easy to prepare. The dry rub makes enough for about six pork chops; store extra spice rub in a clean glass jar. The sauce cooks on the stove while the chops and potatoes roast in the oven. I like to serve this meal with a side salad. Testers loved the autumn flavors in this one-dish meal, calling it "really lovely," while one plans on using the spice rub for grilled pork chops in the summer.

2 teaspoons ground cumin

2 teaspoons smoked paprika

2 teaspoons freshly ground black pepper

2 teaspoons garlic powder

2 teaspoons dried tomato (optional)

½ teaspoon chipotle powder

2 large (1-inch- [3.5-cm-] thick) pork chops

3 tablespoons (45mL) extra virgin olive oil or coconut oil, divided

1 large sweet potato or yam

½ teaspoon freshly ground black pepper

2 pears

1 cup fresh or frozen cranberries

Stevia to equal 2 teaspoons sugar

3 tablespoons toasted unsalted pumpkin seeds

Budget friendly: Moderate

1. Preheat the oven to 350°F (180°C).
2. To make the dry rub, mix together the first six ingredients, through chipotle powder, in a bowl until it becomes a single color.
3. Use a spoon to sprinkle the dry rub fairly thickly over the pork chops on each side, rubbing it in with your fingers, then wash your hands.
4. In an ovenproof cast iron skillet set over medium–high heat, warm 1 tablespoon of the oil until it is shimmering. Put in the chops and cook for 5 minutes on each side, turning only once with tongs, until each side has a brown crust.
5. While the chops are cooking, peel the sweet potato, halve it lengthwise, and then cut it evenly into slices about ⅛ inch (3 mm) thick, or as thin as you can get them. This will speed

up the cooking time. Use a mandolin on the thinnest setting if you have one. Toss with the remaining 2 tablespoons olive oil or melted coconut oil to coat potatoes evenly, and sprinkle with black pepper.

6. When the chops are seared with a brown crust on each side, spread the sweet potatoes over them in an even layer. If using a traditional meat thermometer, place it in the thickest part of 1 chop now.

7. Place the skillet on the center rack of the oven for 25 to 35 minutes, or until the thermometer reads 140°F (60°C).

8. While the meat and sweet potatoes are cooking, peel and core the pears and cut into chunks. Place the pear chunks, cranberries, and stevia in a food processor and pulse until the mixture is chunky and the cranberries are broken up. Pour into a saucepan set over medium heat. Cook the sauce until just boiling, then reduce the heat to low and simmer, partially covered, until the meat and sweet potatoes are rested.

9. Remove pork from oven and let rest for 10 minutes. The pork's temperature should rise with carryover cooking to 145°F (63°C).

10. Stir the toasted pumpkin seeds into the sauce just before serving.

11. Place one chop on each plate with a generous serving of potatoes. Pour the sauce over each chop and serve.

COOKS' NOTE: *If your chops are thinner, this method won't work; your meat will overcook and your potatoes will be underdone. For thinner chops, precook the potatoes in the microwave until not quite done. Sear the chops for only 3 minutes per side on the stovetop, spread the precooked potatoes over, and use the meat thermometer to determine doneness in the oven. They might only need 10 minutes.*

Per serving: 9g protein, 60g carbohydrates, 34g fat, 6g saturated fat, 421mg sodium, 1,570mg potassium, 13g fiber

STEPHANIE'S SPICE STAR: Dried tomato
This spice is not widely available, but if you can find it online, it adds an incredible flavor to the spice rub and a savory crust to the meat.

Scalloped Potatoes with Roasted Chiles

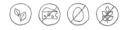

Makes 10 servings
Prep time: 30 minutes   Cooking time: 70–75 minutes   Passive time: 15 minutes

Make this with coconut milk; no one will ever know it's non-dairy! It's perfect for a brunch or potluck.

1 tablespoon extra virgin olive or coconut oil

2 bunches green onions, thinly sliced

5 fresh Hatch or Anaheim chiles, or 2–3 red or yellow bell peppers, roasted and thinly sliced (see instructions on page 190), divided

3 cups (750mL) coconut milk

1 teaspoon freshly ground black pepper

1 teaspoon smoked paprika

¼ teaspoon chipotle powder

6–8 (3 pounds [1.4kg] total) large Yukon gold potatoes

Budget friendly: Very

Per serving: 6g protein, 34g carbohydrates, 4g fat, 2g saturated fat, 41mg sodium, 858mg potassium, 5g fiber

1. In a large skillet set over medium–high heat, warm the oil until it shimmers. Reduce the heat to medium and add the onions. Cook, stirring occasionally, for 10 to 15 minutes, or until the onions are golden. Stir in half of the sliced chiles, remove the skillet from the heat, and set aside.

2. Preheat the oven to 400°F (180°C) with a rack adjusted to the middle position. Spray or oil a large rectangular baking dish and set aside.

3. In a large, heavy saucepan set over medium heat, warm the milk, black pepper, paprika, and chipotle powder. Meanwhile, using a mandolin or sharp knife, cut the potatoes crosswise into ¹⁄₁₆-inch- (2-mm-) thick slices. As you slice, add as many of the potatoes as will fit in the pan. Bring the liquid just to a boil, stirring every few minutes so the mixture doesn't burn. This helps release the starch from the potatoes to thicken the milk. Remove from the heat after it has come to a boil.

4. If some of the potato slices don't fit, put them in the prepared baking dish and stir in the chile–onion mixture. Pour the milk–potato mixture over all and stir to combine.

5. Sprinkle the reserved sliced chiles on top. Cover with foil.

6. Bake for 45 minutes, or until the potatoes are tender when poked with a fork. Remove the foil and bake for another 10 minutes, or until the top is nicely browned. Remove from the oven and let stand for 15 minutes before serving.

COOKS' NOTE: *You can make this with sweet bell peppers or spicy peppers; it's good both ways. Do not use coconut cream, as it may include migraine triggers. Be sure to use starchy Yukon gold potatoes; they're key to the sauce thickening properly.*

Spicy Kale and Swiss Chard Sauté

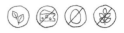

Makes 4 servings
Prep time: 15 minutes   Cooking time: 20 minutes   Passive time: N/A

I did not grow up eating greens. I had to learn how to cook them, and truthfully, it took a while for me to develop a taste for them as an adult. They're incredibly nutritious, so I now try to make some once a day, and I rotate which types we eat to balance out the nutrients they provide. This recipe is a wonderful introduction to greens, as it combines two types of flavorful oils to complement the greens, while the seeds provide textural crunch and extra protein. Cooked greens combined with a healthy fat make the nutrients more bio-available, too. #winning

1 tablespoon extra virgin coconut oil or ghee

1 bunch green onions, thinly sliced

3 cloves garlic, minced

1 jalapeño, thinly sliced (optional)

1 bunch (500g) Swiss chard, stems removed, thinly sliced, and reserved and leaves thinly sliced

1 bunch (500g) kale, stems and leaves thinly sliced

1 tablespoon hot sesame oil

1 tablespoon dark toasted sesame oil

1 tablespoon raw sunflower seeds

1 tablespoon raw pumpkin seeds

1 tablespoon raw sesame seeds

Budget friendly: Very

1. In a large frying pan or sauté pan set over medium–high heat, melt the coconut oil. Add the onions, garlic, and jalapeño, if using, and sauté for 5 minutes, or until golden.
2. Add the chard stems and cook for another 3 to 4 minutes. Add the rest of the chard and the kale. Cover the pan with a lid to help the greens wilt, about 5 minutes. Once they have wilted a bit, add the hot and dark toasted sesame oils, stirring to coat.
3. Add the sunflower, pumpkin, and sesame seeds and continue to sauté, uncovered, for 10 minutes, or until cooked through.

COOKS' NOTE: *After washing greens, I roll them up in a clean kitchen towel to absorb moisture. For the Swiss chard, stack the leaves, then cut off the stems using a deep V cut. Thinly slice the stems and set them aside separately. Thinly slice the green leaves. If you do not like spicy food, skip the jalapeño and the hot sesame oil. Wear gloves while handling the jalapeño. You can use all Swiss chard or all kale for this recipe if you prefer. Bunches of greens tend to weigh 16 ounces in the United States.*

Per serving: 6g protein, 13g carbohydrates, 15g fat, 4g saturated fat, 108mg sodium, 607mg potassium, 4g fiber

Steak and Roasted Vegetable Salad ⊛ ⊛ ⊘ ⊛

Makes 2 servings
Prep time: 30 minutes   Cooking time: 35 minutes   Passive time: 10 minutes

A while back I bought a special issue of *Shape* magazine with a 21-day New Year's eating plan. A lot of the recipes became part of my repertoire, getting renovated along the way as my diet changed. I came back to this one for my blog and this Plan, as it's a hit with both carnivores and vegetarians. Omit the steak altogether for a hearty vegan lunch or dinner. The salad dressing was a bit of a challenge, as it was full of potential triggers, but I was able to keep the spirit and flavor profile of the original with a few migraine-friendly tweaks. I make this as a hearty dinner salad or for lunch on the weekend when I have a little more time. We love the contrast of the warm ingredients with the chilled greens.

8 ounces (225g) lean pastured or grass-fed sirloin steak

1 clove garlic

1 teaspoon freshly ground black pepper, divided

1 teaspoon smoked paprika, divided

⅛ teaspoon fine sea salt, divided (optional)

6 large cremini or button mushrooms, cleaned and halved

3 small carrots, cut on the diagonal

1 summer squash or zucchini, cut into large chunks

8 fingerling or baby new potatoes

1 red or yellow bell pepper, cored and cut into chunks

2 tablespoons plus ¼ cup (60mL) organic extra virgin olive oil, divided

1 small shallot, finely minced

1 pint (300g) cherry tomatoes

1 teaspoon white vinegar

2 tablespoons filtered water

1 teaspoon dried mustard powder

1 sprig fresh tarragon or savory, or ¼ teaspoon dried tarragon

½ (5- to 6-ounce) package mâche, baby spinach, baby arugula, or mesclun blend

Budget friendly: Moderate

1. Preheat the oven to 450°F (230°C). Line a large baking pan with parchment paper and set aside.
2. Pound the steak using a mallet or rolling pin so that it is all the same thickness. Cut the clove of garlic in half and rub the cut side over each side of the steak, then season both sides with ½ teaspoon of the black pepper, ½ teaspoon of the smoked paprika, and ¹⁄₁₆ teaspoon of the salt, if using. Discard the garlic. Rub the seasoning into the meat with your fingers, then wash your hands. Set the meat aside for 30 minutes, while you are prepping and roasting the veggies.

3. Combine the mushrooms, carrots, squash, potatoes, bell pepper, and 2 tablespoons of the olive oil in a deep bowl and toss. Season with the remaining ½ teaspoon of black pepper, ½ teaspoon of smoked paprika, and ¹⁄₁₆ teaspoon of salt, if using, to coat them all evenly. This creates the lovely brown crust. Transfer the vegetables to the prepared baking pan and roast for 30 to 35 minutes, or until the vegetables are golden and the potatoes are fork-tender.

4. While the vegetables are roasting, make the dressing. First, soak the minced shallot in ice water for 10 minutes. This helps take the edge off the raw shallot. Drain. Chop 6 of the cherry tomatoes and set aside. Start with 1 teaspoon of the shallot and add it, along with the vinegar, the ¼ cup of olive oil, the filtered water, the dry mustard, the tarragon, and the 6 chopped cherry tomatoes to a large jar. Using an immersion (stick) blender, blend until very smooth. If you have a smoothie blender (like a Magic Bullet), that will also work. The small volume of ingredients makes it difficult to blend in a regular blender. Let the dressing sit for a while and taste. If it needs more shallot, add a bit more and blend to incorporate. Some testers found it too strong to add the entire shallot. Set the dressing aside.

5. When the vegetables are done, remove them from the oven and turn on the broiler. Broil the steak about 4 inches (10cm) from the heating element for 5 to 6 minutes per side. Turn once with tongs, not a fork. (If you use a fork, it may release the juice from the meat, causing it to dry out.) The steak should reach 140°F (60°C) on an instant-read thermometer for medium–rare or 155°F (68°C) for medium. Remove the steak from the broiler and let it rest for 5 to 10 minutes before cutting. This allows the meat to reabsorb the juices. Trim off any fat, then cut the steak crosswise into ¼-inch- (6-mm-) thick slices.

6. To assemble, divide the greens evenly on 2 separate plates. Slice the remaining cherry tomatoes and divide among the plates, along with 1 to 2 large spoonfuls of roasted vegetables and half of the steak slices. Dress lightly and serve.

COOKS' NOTE: *Don't use delicate greens like spring mix, which can't stand up to the heat of the other ingredients. If you avoid white potatoes, sub parsnips, turnips, rutabagas, or sweet potatoes (or a mix) for them. Make sure that all the cut pieces of vegetables are about the same size, roughly 2 inches (5 cm) across. If I'm going to roast vegetables, I like to roast a large pan of them. They're easy to reheat for dinner or blend with chicken or vegetable stock and coconut milk for a quick soup. You can use leftover steak for this recipe; just warm slices under a broiler before adding to the plate.*

Per serving (salad with no dressing, including 4 potatoes): 48g protein, 145g carbohydrates, 22g fat, 4g saturated fat, 387mg sodium, 6,001 mg potassium, 23g fiber

Per tablespoon of dressing: <1g protein, <1g carbohydrates, 4g fat, <1g saturated fat, <1mg sodium, 19mg potassium, <1g fiber

Wild Rice and Carrots

Makes 4 servings
Prep time: 15 minutes   Cooking time: 55 minutes   Passive time: 10 minutes

Many people haven't tried wild rice, which is a nutritious grass that grows only in North America. It's harvested by hand using canoes, and often its purchase supports the Native American cooperatives who produce it. It has an earthy, hearty flavor. If you're not sure you'll like it, bring a measuring cup to a natural foods store and buy just 1 cup from the bulk bin to make this recipe. I think I'll make you a fan. One tester called this "hearty, unique, and easy."

2 cups (500 mL) filtered water or unsalted chicken or vegetable stock

1 cup (150g) wild rice, rinsed and drained

1 tablespoon organic extra virgin olive oil or unsalted grass-fed butter

2 large carrots, thinly sliced on the diagonal

2 ribs celery, finely minced

1 handful fresh Italian flat-leaf parsley, finely chopped

½ teaspoon freshly ground black pepper

Budget friendly: Very

1. In a medium saucepan set over high heat, combine the filtered water and rice. Cover and bring to a boil, then reduce the heat to low and cook for 45 minutes. Turn off the heat and leave the cover on for at least 10 minutes.
2. In a large skillet set over medium heat, warm the olive oil. Add the carrots and celery and cook, stirring frequently, for 6 to 8 minutes, or until tender. Stir in the rice, parsley, and black pepper. Cook 1 minute more until everything is warmed through.
3. Serve right away or refrigerate, covered, for up to 5 days.

COOKS' NOTE: *Wild rice is only grown in North America and may not be available overseas. You could substitute a hearty brown rice instead. I wash the parsley, then roll it up in a clean kitchen towel to help absorb extra moisture. Finely chop just before adding to the recipe.*

Per serving: 6g protein, 35g carbohydrates, 4g fat, 0.5g saturated fat, 54mg sodium, 381mg potassium, 4g fiber

---

STEPHANIE'S SPICE STAR: Freshly ground black peppercorns
If you're used to ground black pepper in the shaker, you're probably used to stale black pepper. Try buying a pepper grinder and a small amount of whole black peppercorns. You'll be amazed at the zippy kick it adds to dishes. In addition, fresh spices are more likely to include beneficial phytonutrients, which add additional nutrition to your meal.

desserts, drinks, and treats

———···———

Dessert is very important. I repeat, very important. I don't want you to feel deprived on the Plan, as it adds stress and crankiness to your life. The trick with Plan-approved desserts is to utilize the natural sweetness of fruit, enhancing it with a small amount of stevia. Here you'll find pie-like cobbler, brownie-like carob squares, custardy cherry clafoutis, a show-stopping trifle for special occasions, three drink options, pudding, upside-down cake, and a frozen fruit granita.

Berry Cobbler

Makes 6 servings
Prep time: 10 minutes   Cooking time: 35–40 minutes   Passive time: N/A

It's important for you to feel like you can still enjoy meals and desserts, or else you won't stay on the Plan very long. This cobbler is a great starting recipe, as it can be made with fresh or frozen berries, and the crust comes together easily in the food processor. It's a homey, summery dessert that focuses on the natural goodness of fruit.

½ cup (70g) all-purpose gluten-free flour blend

¼ cup (35g) sweet sorghum flour

2 tablespoons cold unsalted grass-fed butter or organic extra virgin coconut oil (see Cooks' Note)

1 teaspoon sodium-free baking soda substitute, or ½ teaspoon regular baking powder

½ cup (125mL) heavy cream or coconut milk, or as needed

2 tablespoons arrowroot powder

Stevia to equal 2 teaspoons sugar

1 teaspoon ground cinnamon

½ teaspoon white vinegar

4 cups (1kg) fresh or frozen and thawed mixed berries (no raspberries)

Coconut Whipped Cream (page 254) or Vanilla Ricotta Cream (page 263), for serving

1. Preheat the oven to 375°F (170°C). Grease a 6-cup (1.6-L) ovenproof baking dish with cooking spray, coconut oil, or butter and set aside.
2. Start the crust. In the bowl of a food processor, add the flour blend, sorghum flour, butter, and baking soda. Pulse a few times on a low setting until the mixture looks like crumbly small peas.
3. With the machine running, add the cream a little at a time, just until the mixture forms into a ball. You will likely not use the full amount.
4. Wrap the dough in plastic wrap and store in the freezer while you prep the filling.
5. Start the filling. In a large bowl, combine the arrowroot powder, stevia, cinnamon, and vinegar with the berries. Mix well.
6. Pour the fruit into the prepared baking dish.
7. Remove the dough from the freezer and press it by hand into a rough circle or square, using the plastic wrap to keep it from sticking to the counter, or roll it between 2 sheets of waxed paper until it's the size that will just fit into the baking dish. It's fine if it cracks. Unwrap the dough and set it on top of filling.
8. Bake for 35 to 40 minutes, or until the filling is bubbly and the crust is golden brown.
9. Remove from the oven. Serve warm or cold. For an additional treat, top with the Coconut Whipped Cream or Vanilla Ricotta Cream.

Budget friendly: Moderate

COOKS' NOTE: *If you are strictly watching your sodium, use EnerG baking soda substitute, which is sodium-free. You can use any type of berries except raspberries, which may be a migraine trigger. Fresh or frozen peaches are also excellent in this. Make sure your gluten-free flour blend does not contain fava bean or garfava flour. If using coconut oil, you want it solid (not liquid). In the summer it may be liquid at room temperature. Measure out 2 tablespoons, then refrigerate just until it firms up.*

Per serving (using butter and heavy cream): 3g protein, 29g carbohydrates, 8g fat, 5g saturated fat, 6mg sodium, 242mg potassium, 3g fiber

Berry Sauce

Makes about 2 cups, 8 servings
Prep time: 5 minutes   Cooking time: 1 minute   Passive time: N/A

This recipe originated with my sister, Melinda, and I still have it in my desserts binder in her handwriting. I swapped a small amount of stevia for the sugar. This is great on gluten-free cheesecake, coconut milk ice cream, Vanilla Ricotta Cream (page 263), or Cherry Clafoutis (page 252) made without fruit as a simple vanilla cake. It's also an ingredient in my Berry Trifle (page 253). One tester was "shocked it tasted this good made with frozen fruit. I used it on brownies, in smoothies, with yogurt, and ate it straight from the jar at 3 a.m."

2 cups (200g) fresh or frozen and thawed blueberries, strawberries, or blackberries, or a mixture

Stevia to equal 4 teaspoons sugar

3 tablespoons filtered water

1 tablespoon organic arrowroot powder or cornstarch

Budget friendly: Very

1. If using strawberries, remove and discard the green tops, then slice them thinly.
2. In a medium saucepan set over medium heat, add the berries and stevia.
3. Combine the filtered water and arrowroot powder in a small bowl, stirring with a whisk to create a slurry; stir the slurry into the berry mixture.
4. Bring just to a boil, then cook for 1 minute, mashing the berries with a fork as it cooks. Remove from heat.
5. Use an immersion blender, food processor, or blender to give the sauce a slightly chunky consistency.
6. Transfer to a serving pitcher and let cool. Use immediately or store in a covered glass container in the fridge for up to 5 days.

COOKS' NOTE: *This is a perfect recipe for frozen fruit, which is available year round and generally picked at peak flavor, but doesn't need to look perfect. Don't use raspberries until you test them; they may be a migraine trigger. Frozen sweet cherries are also excellent. If using blackberries, press the sauce through a fine-mesh sieve to remove the seeds.*

Per ¼ cup serving (with blueberries): 0g protein, 8g carbohydrates, 0g fat, 0g saturated fat, 0mg sodium, 28mg potassium, 0g fiber

Carob Squares

Makes 8 servings
Prep time: 10 minutes   Cooking time: 30–45 minutes   Passive time: N/A

When I saw that chocolate could be a migraine trigger, I was an unhappy camper. Enter carob, chocolate's sorta cousin. It's another ground, dried pod, a bit sweeter than chocolate, with fewer bitter notes. This recipe sounds super weird, but if you follow the directions exactly (no substitutes on this one), you'll be rewarded with a pan of cake-style goodies that fooled many taste testers, who couldn't believe they had no chocolate in them. I don't call them brownies, because then you'll be comparing them to their sugary chocolate kin. Let them fly their carob flag proudly.

1 (14-ounce [425-g]) can no-salt-added black beans, rinsed and drained

¾ cup (175g) mashed cooked sweet potato

¼ cup (25g) carob powder

2 eggs

Stevia to equal 8 teaspoons sugar

2 tablespoons extra virgin olive oil

2 teaspoons sodium-free baking soda (see Cooks' Note)

2 teaspoons best-quality pure vanilla extract

1 recipe Coconut Whipped Cream (page 254), for serving (optional)

Budget friendly: Very

Per serving: 5g protein, 22g carbohydrates, 6g fat, 1g saturated fat, 27mg sodium, 387mg potassium, 6g fiber

1. Preheat the oven to 350°F (180°C). Spray or lightly oil 8 ramekins or an 8-inch (20 cm) square baking dish. Set aside.
2. Combine all the ingredients, except for the whipped cream, in a food processor or blender and pulse in short pulses 10 to 15 times just until smooth, stopping occasionally to scrape down the sides. You should still see small flecks of black bean but not large pieces. Do not over blend or you will end up with a gluey texture from the beans.
3. Transfer to the baking dish(es) and bake for 30 to 35 minutes (if using ramekins) or 30 to 40 minutes (if using the baking dish), until the tops are dry and cracked and there is no jiggling in the center when you shake the pan a little. The edges should start to pull away from the sides.
4. Remove from the oven and transfer to a wire rack to cool for 10 minutes before serving, if you want them warm. Otherwise, cool completely.
5. Slice into 8 squares, if using the baking dish. Top with a dollop of the Coconut Whipped Cream, if using, and serve. Store in a sealed container on the counter or tightly wrap squares in plastic wrap and freeze in a zip-top bag.

COOKS' NOTE: *To reduce extra sodium in my diet, I use EnerG baking soda substitute, a mixture of calcium carbonate and magnesium carbonate. Do not use regular baking powder in this recipe (sodium bicarbonate); trust me, an unfortunate chemical reaction renders the result inedible. You can sub unsweetened applesauce; the result is better with sweet potato.*

Cherry Clafoutis

Makes 8 servings
Prep time: 10 minutes   Cooking time: 35–40 minutes   Passive time: 10–15 minutes

A true clafoutis (pronounced kla-foo-TEE) is made with fresh black cherries and rich custard, and dusted with powdered sugar. They originated in the Limousin region of France. I use frozen sweet cherries, which are already pitted. When made with fruit other than black cherries, this dessert is properly called a flaugnarde (flo-nyard). One tester said it made both a lovely dessert *and* breakfast.

1 cup (250mL) whole milk or coconut milk

4 eggs

2 tablespoons unsalted grass-fed butter or extra virgin coconut oil, melted

1 tablespoon best-quality pure vanilla extract

Stevia to equal 2 teaspoons sugar

½ cup (70g) all-purpose gluten-free flour blend

2 cups (370g) fresh or frozen and thawed pitted sweet cherries

1 recipe Coconut Whipped Cream (page 254) or Vanilla Ricotta Cream (page 263), for serving (optional)

Budget friendly: Moderate, depending on price of fruit

1. Preheat the oven to 325°F (165°C). Oil or butter a cast iron skillet or pie pan and set aside.
2. In a blender, combine the milk, eggs, butter, vanilla, and stevia and blend until frothy. Add the flour and pulse a few times until smooth.
3. Pour the batter into the prepared pan and scatter the cherries onto the batter.
4. Bake for 35 to 40 minutes, or until puffed and golden.
5. Remove from the oven and transfer to a wire rack to cool for 10 to 15 minutes before cutting into 8 slices. Top each slice with the Coconut Whipped Cream or Vanilla Ricotta Cream, if using. Serve warm or at room temperature.

COOKS' NOTE: *During summer cherry season, use a chopstick to pit fresh sweet cherries. Do not use canned cherries, which are too sour for the sweetening power of the amount of stevia in this recipe. You can also use in-season stone fruit, like peaches, purple (not red) plums, or blackberries, blueberries, or strawberries. If you don't have a blender, whisk the ingredients together in the order listed. One tester recommended increasing the stevia to the equivalent of 1 tablespoon sugar. Make sure your gluten-free flour blend does not contain fava bean or garfava flour.*

Per serving (using whole milk and butter): 5g protein, 13g carbohydrates, 7g fat, 3g saturated fat, 48mg sodium, 137mg potassium, 0g fiber

Berry Trifle

Makes 10 servings
Prep time: 30 minutes   Cooking time: 35–40 minutes   Passive time: 30 minutes

OK, this isn't a quick "whip up a dessert" recipe. I wanted to give you one showstopper recipe that you can make for special occasions. The components can all be made a day ahead: Coconut Whipped Cream (page 254), Berry Sauce (page 250), fresh berries, and cake. For optimal visual impact, borrow a glass trifle dish from someone.

1 pint (350g) each blueberries, strawberries, and blackberries

3 tablespoons best-quality pure vanilla extract, divided

Stevia to equal 6 teaspoons sugar, divided

2 cups (500mL) whole milk or coconut milk

8 eggs

4 tablespoons (60g) unsalted grass-fed butter or extra virgin coconut oil, melted

1 cup (140g) all-purpose gluten-free flour blend

1 recipe Berry Sauce (optional)

2 recipes Coconut Whipped Cream (page 254)

Budget friendly: Moderate

Per serving (without the Coconut Whipped Cream or Berry Sauce): 8g protein, 18g carbohydrates, 10g fat, 5g saturated fat, 77mg sodium, 173mg potassium, 1g fiber

1. Preheat the oven to 325°F (165°C). Oil or butter 2 cast iron skillets or pie pans of roughly the same size.
2. To make the berry layer, remove the green tops and thinly slice the strawberries; halve the blackberries. Add the cut berries and blueberries to a medium bowl, along with 1 tablespoon of the vanilla and the stevia to equal 2 teaspoons of sugar. Stir to combine and set aside.
3. To make the batter, in a blender, combine the milk, the eggs, the melted butter, the remaining 2 tablespoons of vanilla, and the remaining stevia to equal 4 teaspoons of sugar and blend until frothy. Add the flour and pulse a few times until smooth.
4. Pour the batter into the prepared pans, dividing evenly.
5. Bake for 35 to 40 minutes, or until puffed and golden.
6. Remove from the oven and transfer to wire racks to cool completely, about 30 minutes.
7. To assemble, use a pretty glass bowl, trifle bowl, or individual wine glasses. Tear the cooled cake into chunks. Start with a layer of cake, then add some of the berry mixture and the juice that has accumulated in the bottom of the bowl, Berry Sauce, if using, and finally the Coconut Whipped Cream. Repeat, making 2 to 3 layers, ending with whipped cream on the top. Reserve a small amount of Berry Sauce to drizzle on top just before serving. Refrigerate until ready to serve.

COOKS' NOTE: *I cut the blackberries in half for three reasons: They are easier to eat, you get more out of a pint, and they also absorb more of the vanilla and stevia flavor when cut. They will stain, so watch your clothing and counters. Make sure your gluten-free flour blend does not contain fava bean or garfava flour.*

Coconut Whipped Cream

Makes about 2 cups, 8 servings
Prep time: 5 minutes   Cooking time: N/A   Passive time: 30 minutes

When I first went on the Plan, I made this All. The. Time. It seemed like a necessary treat for me during my transition period: lightly sweet, super creamy, rich, decadent. Now I make it for special occasions or holidays. But, do what you gotta do. It's fantastic on berries or other Plan-approved fruit, it's a key ingredient in the Berry Trifle, you can use it as pretty frosting, top Blueberry–Oat Waffles (page 198) with it, fill Crepes (page 200) with it . . . you get the idea.

1 (13.5-ounce [400-mL]) can full-fat Thai Kitchen coconut milk (*not* light), chilled overnight

Stevia to equal 2–3 teaspoons sugar

1 teaspoon best-quality pure vanilla extract

¼ teaspoon cream of tartar (optional)

Budget friendly: Very

Per serving: 1g protein, 3g carbohydrates, 10g fat, 9g saturated fat, 6mg sodium, 105mg potassium, 0g fiber

1. Chill your mixer's beaters and bowl for 30 minutes.
2. Open the chilled can of coconut milk and use a spatula to scrape out all the fat at the top of the can into the chilled mixer bowl. Strain the clear liquid into a jar and reserve it for another use, such as smoothies. Scrape the remaining contents of the can into the bowl, along with any chunks caught in the strainer. Add the rest of the ingredients.
3. Start beating the coconut cream on low speed, then slowly move the speed up to high, beating for 2 to 4 minutes or until soft peaks form.
4. Transfer to a lidded container and store in the refrigerator for up to 5 days. It gets firmer as it chills.

COOKS' NOTE: *Some coconut milks, although they do not say "light" on the can, do not have enough fat in them to turn into whipped cream. The only brand I have had consistent results with is Thai Kitchen. If you open the can and there is not a heavy layer of thick cream on top, it will not whip. I store my cans in the back of the fridge so I always have some ready to go if I want a treat. I find the cream of tartar helps keep the coconut cream in the whipped emulsion state. Guar gum is frequently added to coconut milk as a thickener and should be OK for the migraine diet. Some people may be sensitive to cream of tartar or guar gum. Do not use canned coconut cream, which has sugar and other ingredients that are not on the Plan. If you are sensitive to coconut or guar gum and not sensitive to dairy, you can make whipped cream using organic heavy whipping cream and the same amounts of stevia and vanilla extract. Omit the cream of tartar. If for some reason your whipped cream fails, don't throw it out. Store it in a glass jar in the refrigerator and use in smoothies.*

Hemp Milk

Makes 5 servings
Prep time: 3 minutes   Cooking time: N/A   Passive time: N/A

Hemp seeds are super high in protein, and while hemp is a nickname for marijuana, they are not precisely the same plant. While both are types of cannabis, hemp grows tall outdoors, doesn't have buds (plants are usually male), and is low in THC, the active compound that provides the high in marijuana. Hemp has been used by humans to create fabric, paper, and rope for millennia. George Washington and Thomas Jefferson both grew it. The plant lasts longer than cotton and is produced using far less water per acre. It's a more sustainable source of paper and cardboard than trees. Hemp oil can also be used for a variety of industrial applications, including making nontoxic diesel oil.

Hemp milk is one of the few non-dairy milks allowable on the Plan (as nuts and soy are triggers). Commercial hemp milks often contain fillers and thickeners that may be triggers, so making it at home is a good option, especially since it's simple to do. One tester called this "creamy and mellow, with versatile flavor."

3 cups (750mL) filtered or spring water

1 cup (160g) hemp seeds

1 teaspoon best-quality pure vanilla extract

Stevia to equal 2 teaspoons sugar

Budget friendly: Moderate

1. Combine all the ingredients in a high-speed blender. Start on low, then shift to high speed for 1 minute. If you are using a regular blender, blend for 2 minutes.
2. Store in a covered container in the refrigerator for up to 5 days.

COOKS' NOTE: *Choose organic hemp seeds (also called hemp hearts) if you can. For the best flavor, use filtered or spring water, not tap water.*

Per serving: 16g protein, 5g carbohydrates, 21g fat, 2g saturated fat, 0mg sodium, 1mg potassium, 2g fiber

Grilled Peaches with Cardamom–Maple Cream Sauce ⊗ ⊗ ⊘ ⊛

Makes 4 servings
Prep time: 15 minutes   Cooking time: 5–10 minutes   Passive time: 5 minutes

If you've never had grilled peaches or nectarines, you're welcome. Once you taste how incredible this fruit becomes when grilled, you'll be firing up the grill at random times to get this smoky sweetness fix. One tester was blown away: "Wow, so tasty. I figured it would be good, I didn't think it would be spectacular! The coconut cream sauce was the highlight of this dish. It made it amazing."

2 tablespoons unsalted grass-fed butter, ghee, or extra virgin coconut oil

1 tablespoon pure maple syrup

¼ teaspoon ground cardamom

4 medium ripe peaches

½ cup (85g) coconut cream (from the top of the can of full-fat coconut milk), room temperature

1 teaspoon best-quality pure vanilla extract

1 cup (120g) strawberries, hulled and sliced

Leaves from 1 sprig fresh mint

Budget friendly: Very

1. In a medium saucepan set over low heat, combine the butter, maple syrup, and cardamom, and warm until everything is melted. Mix well. Remove from the heat.
2. Using a paring knife, cut the peaches in half along the seam. Twist the halves in opposite directions until the peaches open. Remove the pits with your knife.
3. Add the peaches to the pan and toss to coat. Let stand for 5 minutes before grilling. When you're ready to grill, hold each peach section over the pan and allow any extra sauce to drip back into the pan. Reserve the sauce in the pan.
4. Set a grill pan over medium heat, set an electric grill to medium, or prepare an outdoor grill. Coat the pan or grill grate with cooking spray. Arrange the peaches on the grill pan or grill and cook for 2 minutes on each side, or until grill marks appear and the flesh is soft and starting to caramelize. If using an outdoor grill, grill over medium heat (not over direct coals) in the same fashion. Transfer the peaches to serving plates, cut sides up.
5. Add the coconut cream and vanilla to the pan containing the remaining cooled sauce and whisk to combine.
6. Top the peaches with the strawberries, drizzle on the cream sauce, and top with mint leaves. Serve right away.

COOKS' NOTE: *Some coconut milks, while not labeled "light," do not have enough fat in them to separate into a layer of coconut cream. For this recipe, use the coconut milk at room temperature in order to whisk with the other ingredients. The cardamom–maple cream sauce is tasty over any type of fruit. You can also grill nectarines. Refrigerate and then whip leftover coconut cream to make extra Coconut Whipped Cream (page 254), smoothies, or curry. One tester suggested sprinkling some toasted sunflower seeds or Granola (page 205) on top for crunch.*

Per serving: 2g protein, 22g carbohydrates, 12g fat, 9g saturated fat, 6mg sodium, 433mg potassium, 3g fiber

STEPHANIE'S SPICE STAR: Cardamom

Cardamom is used in Scandinavian baking as well as in Indian food. Native to India, it's grown throughout the tropics. Cardamom has a warm, spicy-sweet flavor that people tend to love or hate. Buy just a small amount from a natural foods store that sells spices in bulk to try it out. It pairs beautifully with baked goods and really sings in spicy masalas. For that use, I buy green cardamom pods and crush them just before cooking, to maintain the essential oils. The pods usually break down while cooking and the seeds within soften enough to eat.

Cucumber–Basil Water

Makes 4–5 servings
Prep time: 2 minutes   Cooking time: N/A   Passive time: N/A

If you were a big fan of soda, finding another drink will be important for you to be happy on the Plan. You can certainly make herbal iced tea, so long as all the ingredients are Plan-approved. Another option is making infused water, which tastes incredibly fresh. You may have had this type of infused water at a spa or restaurant but never considered making it at home. It's critically important to use organic ingredients in this recipe (as well as in the Strawberry–Mint Water recipe, page 259), as the water will draw any pesticides out of the produce. One tester loved how refreshing this was, and added that it's a perfect way to use up leftover cucumbers with fresh herbs.

1 large organic cucumber, or 3 organic Persian cucumbers

1 large handful (3–6 sprigs) organic basil leaves

8 cups (2 quarts [2L]) filtered or spring water, or as needed

Budget friendly: Very

1. Peel the regular cucumber or wash the Persian cucumbers. Cut into medium slices and add to a pitcher.
2. Wash the basil, bruise the leaves a bit, and add them to the pitcher. Add the water and infuse for at least 4 hours before drinking.
3. Store in the refrigerator for up to 5 days. You can add more water on the first 2 days. Remove the cucumbers after 2 days.

Strawberry–Mint Water

Makes 4–5 servings
Prep time: 2 minutes   Cooking time: N/A   Passive time: N/A

For the best flavored water, do not use tap water. If you have a 2-quart (2-liter) pitcher, just fill to the top after adding the flavorings. This recipe looks just like that super-sweet kid's strawberry drink after a day of infusing.

1 large handful (about 1 cup) organic fresh or frozen strawberries

1 large handful (3–6 sprigs) organic mint leaves

8 cups (2 quarts/2L) filtered or spring water, or as needed

Budget friendly: Very

1. Wash the strawberries, remove and discard the green tops, cut the fruit in half, and add to a pitcher. Frozen strawberries don't have to be thawed.
2. Wash the mint, bruise the leaves a bit, and add them to the pitcher. Add the water and infuse for at least 4 hours before drinking.
3. Store in the refrigerator for up to 5 days. You can add more water on the first 2 days. Remove the strawberries after 2 days.

Pear Upside-Down Cake

Makes 8 servings
Prep time: 30–35 minutes   Cooking time: 60 minutes   Passive time: 15 minutes

My mother used to make pineapple upside-down cake for my older brother Jim. I have a popular blood orange upside-down cake on my blog RecipeRenovator.com: gorgeous and surprisingly easy to make. I adapted that recipe for the Plan, using some of the pears to sweeten the batter. You can substitute seasonal stone fruit for the pears. This was one tester's favorite recipe.

1½ cups (200g) raw sunflower seeds

2 tablespoons white or black chia seeds

4 tablespoons (60 mL) filtered water

½ cup (65g) all-purpose gluten-free flour blend

½ cup (65g) stone-ground white corn grits, gluten-free cornmeal, or polenta

2 teaspoons sodium-free baking powder

1 teaspoon ground allspice

2 tablespoons pure maple syrup

1 tablespoon unsalted grass-fed butter, ghee, or extra virgin coconut oil

1 pear, peeled, stemmed, cored, and cut into ¼-inch-thick slices

1 cup peeled chopped pears

1 cup (245g) unsweetened applesauce

½ cup (125mL) extra virgin olive oil

Stevia to equal 4 teaspoons of sugar, or less as needed

Budget friendly: Moderate

1. Preheat the oven to 325°F (160°C) with a rack adjusted to the middle position. Line a 9-inch (22-24-cm) round cake pan with parchment paper cut to fit the bottom. Spray or oil the pan and set aside.
2. While the oven preheats, put the sunflower seeds on a baking sheet and toast for about 10 minutes, or until golden brown. Remove from the oven and set aside to cool. (Keep the oven on.)
3. Put the chia seeds in a small bowl with the filtered water. Set aside to gel.
4. Whisk the flour, cornmeal, baking powder, and allspice in a medium bowl until the mixture is a single color. Set aside.
5. In a small saucepan set over medium heat, add the maple syrup and butter and bring just to a boil. Swirl the pan a few times to mix. Pour the sauce into the prepared pan, tilting the pan to cover the bottom evenly.
6. Fit the pear slices closely together into the pan, creating a pretty pattern.

7. Add the toasted sunflower seeds to a food processor and pulse until finely chopped but not a powder. Add the cup of chopped pears, applesauce, olive oil, and the chia seed mixture. Pulse until everything is well incorporated. Taste. If the mixture is not very sweet (some pears are very sweet, others less so), add the stevia in small increments, pulsing and tasting until you reach the desired level of sweetness.
8. Add the flour mixture and pulse a few times to combine.
9. Pour the batter on top of the pear slices in the pan and smooth the top with a spatula. Bake for 55 to 60 minutes, or until the cake is evenly golden, firm when pressed in the center, and a toothpick inserted into the center comes out with just a few crumbs attached, no goo.
10. Remove from the oven. Holding carefully with hot pads, tilt the pan and drain any excess liquid into a jar, then set on a wire rack to cool for 10 to 15 minutes. Draining the excess liquid keeps the cake from getting too gooey. Reserve the liquid to pour over the cake slices if serving the next day.
11. Run a knife or thin spatula around the edge to release it. Place a serving plate face down on top of the pan, then flip the whole thing over and wait for that satisfying thunk as it drops onto the plate. Remove the pan and peel off the parchment paper.
12. Cut into slices and serve. Wrap remaining cake tightly with plastic wrap and store on the counter for 1 day, pouring over reserved liquid before serving.

COOKS' NOTE: *Choose fruit depending on the season: purple (not red) plums, peaches, or nectarines can all sub for the pears. While you can use black chia seeds in this recipe, the resulting cake is prettier using white or tan seeds. When slicing fruit, the most important thing is to make all the slices a consistent thickness. Make sure your gluten-free flour blend does not contain fava bean or garfava flour.*

Per serving (using butter and cornmeal): 8g protein, 40g carbohydrates, 29g fat, 4g saturated fat, 5mg sodium, 493mg potassium, 8g fiber

Rice Pudding

Makes 6 servings
Prep time: 5 minutes   Cooking time: 35–40 minutes   Passive time: 10 minutes

Rice pudding is one of my homey, comfort-food desserts. I call for Arborio rice in this recipe, the same type of starchy rice used to make risotto. You can use regular white or brown rice, although short-grain, glutinous rice will yield the best sticky dessert consistency.

1 cup (190g) Arborio rice

4 cups (1 quart [1L]) whole milk, coconut milk, or Hemp Milk (page 255), divided

¼ teaspoon freshly grated nutmeg

Stevia to equal 4 teaspoons sugar, or to taste

½ teaspoon ground cinnamon

Coconut milk and ground cardamom, for serving

Budget friendly: Very

1. Rinse the rice until it runs clear. Drain well.
2. In a medium saucepan set over medium heat, combine the rice and 2 cups (500mL) of the milk and bring to a boil. Add the grated nutmeg.
3. Reduce the heat to low, cover, and simmer, stirring frequently for 15 to 20 minutes.
4. Heat 1 cup (250mL) of the remaining milk in a separate saucepan or in the microwave, stir it into the rice mixture. Cook for 10 minutes.
5. Add 1 more cup of hot milk and stir. (Continue to cook and stir until the pudding is creamy and the rice is completely cooked.
6. Stir in the stevia and cinnamon. Remove from the heat. Let rest for 10 minutes and taste. You can add a bit more milk if you want it creamier and with a looser texture.
7. Portion the pudding into 6 bowls. Top each with a small amount of the coconut milk and a pinch of the cardamom. Serve right away, or store covered in the fridge for up to 5 days.

COOKS' NOTE: *If you wish to add fruit in Step 5, try sliced strawberries, blueberries, blackberries, or diced apples or pears. You can also use leftover cooked plain rice to make rice pudding. Simply put cooked rice in a saucepan and add enough milk just to cover, stirring in nutmeg, stevia, and cinnamon. Heat until it reaches a thick pudding consistency, adding more milk if needed.*

Per serving: 7g protein, 38g carbohydrates, 5g fat, 3g saturated fat, 65mg sodium, 259mg potassium, 1g fiber

Vanilla Ricotta Cream

Makes 4 servings
Prep time: 5 minutes   Cooking time: N/A   Passive time: N/A

When I had my spinal fusion surgery in 2003, I asked my surgeon what I could do to prepare for the best possible outcome. He suggested that if I was carrying any extra weight, it would put additional pressure on my spine that could hamper my healing. My husband and I went on the South Beach Diet so I could slim down. I ate a lot of the book's Vanilla Ricotta Crème, sweetened with aspartame. When I was creating my Plan, I went back to *South Beach* for inspiration, adapting its recipe to be migraine-friendly. It turns out I'm now sensitive to dairy, so I don't eat this anymore. But as long as you can tolerate dairy, this makes a luscious treat, especially with organic whole-milk ricotta.

1 (15-ounce [425-g]) tub organic whole-milk ricotta

1 tablespoon best-quality pure vanilla extract

Stevia to equal 2 teaspoons sugar

½ teaspoon ground cinnamon

⅛–¼ teaspoon freshly grated nutmeg

Budget friendly: Moderate

1. Use a spatula to mix all the ingredients together in a glass bowl, then return to the ricotta tub.
2. Store, covered, in the refrigerator for up to 4 days.

COOKS' NOTE: *Using Vietnamese (Saigon) cinnamon brings this simple dessert to another level of taste. Trust me. Great as a filler for Crepes (page 200). Decadent on its own. Wonderful topped with fruit.*

Per serving: 12g protein, 6g carbohydrates, 14g fat, 9g saturated fat, 89mg sodium, 117mg potassium, 0g fiber

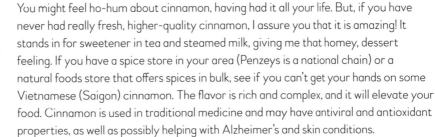

STEPHANIE'S SPICE STAR: Vietnamese cinnamon
You might feel ho-hum about cinnamon, having had it all your life. But, if you have never had really fresh, higher-quality cinnamon, I assure you that it is amazing! It stands in for sweetener in tea and steamed milk, giving me that homey, dessert feeling. If you have a spice store in your area (Penzeys is a national chain) or a natural foods store that offers spices in bulk, see if you can't get your hands on some Vietnamese (Saigon) cinnamon. The flavor is rich and complex, and it will elevate your food. Cinnamon is used in traditional medicine and may have antiviral and antioxidant properties, as well as possibly helping with Alzheimer's and skin conditions.

Watermelon–Mint Granita

Makes 12 servings
Prep time: 10 minutes   Cooking time: N/A   Passive time: 4 hours

I first learned about granita from a magazine article showcasing the technique and a variety of recipes. I had never heard of it, and it truly seems like magic. All I need is a wide flat pan, a fork, and a freezer, and I can make frozen dessert? It's true alchemy. You just have to be around to rake it every 30 minutes or so once it starts freezing. Great fun to make with kids. One tester planned on "eating a ton of this while sitting on the porch on a hot summer evening."

5 cups (1250mL) watermelon juice, made in a blender from seedless watermelon chunks

1 handful fresh mint leaves

Stevia to equal 4 teaspoons sugar

Budget friendly: Very

1. Finely chop the mint leaves and stir them into the watermelon juice along with the stevia.
2. Clear space in the freezer for a 9 × 13–inch (23 × 33–cm) baking dish. Pour the mixture into the dish and set it flat in the freezer. Freeze for 1 hour.
3. After 1 hour, break up any ice with a fork.
4. Freeze for 4 more hours, raking with a fork every 30 minutes until you have fluffy snow.
5. Transfer the granita to an airtight container and store in the freezer for up to 1 week. To serve, rake lightly into bowls.

COOKS' NOTE: *If your watermelon isn't very sweet, add more stevia to taste. If watermelon isn't in season, try cantaloupe or honeydew melon instead. Other suggestions: Sub ½ teaspoon ground cinnamon, ginger, or cardamom instead of the mint. One tester preferred bruising the mint leaves and infusing the watermelon juice, then removing the mint leaves before freezing. Use any Plan-approved fruit juice to make granita with this method. You can add 1 to 2 tablespoons of vodka to spike the recipe for adults.*

Per serving: 0g protein, 6g carbohydrates, 0g fat, 0g saturated fat, 1mg sodium, 80mg potassium, 0g fiber

condiments, sauces, and salad dressings

One of the challenges of living on the Plan is that most store-bought condiments are out. Yet spice rubs, creamy sauces, and salad dressings are important for both flavor and enjoyment. One especially tricky aspect of recipe development for these is that they normally rely on vinegar or citrus to provide acidity. I've turned to Plan-approved naturally acidic fruits and vegetables to provide that tang.

Bacon Salad Dressing

Makes ½ cup (125mL), about 8 (1-tablespoon) servings
Prep time: 5 minutes   Cooking time: N/A   Passive time: N/A

Inspired by the Cobb salad, a small amount of crumbled crispy bacon adds texture to this rich, mustardy dressing. I loved the tester comments on this recipe, as it was universally loved. "To quote my husband, 'This is better than almost every other salad dressing I've tried in my life.' I was a little bummed as I've made some pretty good ones in my time, but I got over it, because I agree!"

¼ cup (60mL) half-and-half or coconut milk

2 tablespoons organic, low-sodium soy-free mayonnaise

1 teaspoon smoked paprika

½ teaspoon dried mustard powder

¼ teaspoon garlic powder

1 slice crisply cooked Make Your Own Bacon (page 197), drained well and finely minced

Budget friendly: Very

1. Add all the ingredients to a glass bowl and whisk together until smooth.
2. Use right away or store refrigerated in a clean glass jar or squeeze bottle for up to 2 days.

COOKS' NOTE: *Store-bought bacon is a potential trigger, being cured and salty. After testing for myself for a week, I am able to use small amounts of uncured, reduced-sodium bacon that is free of nitrates and nitrites, is low in sugar, and is made from humanely raised meat. Some people are sensitive to smoked paprika. If you aren't sure whether you will like the mustard, start with ¼ teaspoon, mix well, and let it sit for about 30 minutes before tasting. Dry mustard packs a lot of punch.*

Per 1-tablespoon serving: 1g protein, 2g carbohydrates, 1g fat, 1g saturated fat, 17mg sodium, 24mg potassium, 0g fiber

---

STEPHANIE'S SPICE STAR: Dry mustard
You might never have used or seen dry mustard, since you've likely always bought the prepared condiment. Mustard seeds are ground into this powder, which is very strong. Very. Don't overdo it. When added to a recipe, it gets stronger over time as well. If you're missing condiments, you can easily whisk some dry mustard into Plan-approved mayo and get your fix.

Chile Pepper Sauce

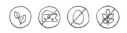

Makes 1 cup (250mL), about 16 (1-tablespoon) servings
Prep time: 5 minutes   Cooking time: 20 minutes   Passive time: N/A

When I was diagnosed, I spent about a month reading labels at the grocery store. One of the first items I found was a sweet and spicy chile pepper sauce from Trader Joe's. I wanted to create a similar recipe for the book, as the one from the store contains sugar and not everyone has access to it. Avoid fermented chile pepper sauces like Sriracha, as they might be triggers due to high tyramine content. We have a neighbor who loves this sauce so much that he trades us freshly caught tuna for it.

8 ounces (225g) red bell pepper plus red or green jalapeño or other hot red chile, stemmed, seeded, and chopped (see Cooks' Note)

½ cup (120mL) filtered water

¼ cup (60mL) white vinegar

Stevia to equal 2 teaspoons sugar (optional)

....

Budget friendly: Very

1. In a small saucepan set over medium heat, combine the peppers, water, and vinegar. Bring to a boil, then reduce the heat to low and simmer for 15 minutes. Remove from the heat and let cool.
2. Using an immersion (stick) blender, blend until very smooth, adding the stevia, if using. Alternatively, use a blender. Transfer to clean glass jars and store in the refrigerator for up to 3 months.

COOKS' NOTE: *If you don't have a home kitchen scale, weigh the peppers at the grocery store before buying. The total weight should be 8 ounces (225g). This is approximately ½ cup chopped peppers. For a spicier sauce, try two or more habaneros plus bell peppers to make 8 ounces. Wear gloves while handling the habaneros or jalapeños. Some people are sensitive to the capsaicin in hot peppers, while others find it pain relieving. If you are sensitive to stevia, substitute 2 teaspoons of coconut sugar.*

Per 1-tablespoon serving: 0g protein, 1g carbohydrates, 0g fat, 0g saturated fat, 0mg sodium, 20mg potassium, 0g fiber

Cilantro Mayonnaise

Makes 1 cup (250mL), about 16 (1-tablespoon) servings
Prep time: 5 minutes   Cooking time: N/A   Passive time: N/A

Cilantro is a love-it or hate-it herb. That's because some people have a gene that makes cilantro taste like soap. It's highly cleansing, so if you love it, try to eat some on a regular basis. This is a recipe I adapted from *The South Beach Diet*, as it's excellent on fish, patties, chicken, and vegetables. So easy to make, and I love that it uses up the entire bunch of cilantro. If you have another recipe that uses only a partial bunch of cilantro, make a half batch of this mayo to use up the rest of the bunch.

¾ cup (175g) organic, low-sodium soy-free mayonnaise

Up to 1 bunch organic cilantro

1 small clove garlic

1 teaspoon ground cumin

½ teaspoon ground white pepper

½ teaspoon distilled white vinegar

1. Add all the ingredients to a blender and blend until smooth.
2. Transfer to a clean glass jar and store in the refrigerator for up to 1 week.

COOKS' NOTE: *You can substitute freshly ground black pepper for the white pepper, but I like the smoother taste of white pepper in this recipe. If you're a cilantro-hater, sub Italian flat-leaf parsley or basil for the cilantro.*

Per 1-tablespoon serving (using low-sodium mayonnaise): <1g protein, <1g carbohydrates, 3g fat, <1g saturated fat, 19mg sodium, 37mg potassium, <1g fiber

Budget friendly: Very

STEPHANIE'S SPICE STAR: Cumin
Cumin is a key spice in savory dishes, adding a warm, nutty flavor that's synonymous with chili and Mexican food.

Italian Dressing

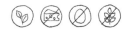

Makes 1 cup (250 mL), about 16 (1-tablespoon) servings
Prep time: 5 minutes   Cooking time: N/A   Passive time: 10 minutes

One thing that's kind of a pain when you're following any special eating plan is all those food items you take for granted, like salad dressings and condiments, which may be off your plan. While it means a little extra work, making fresh versions of these foods can be a flavor revelation. One big challenge for me as I developed recipes to fit with my Plan was the very limited acidic ingredients (no citrus or vinegar except white vinegar), which are key to a balanced salad dressing. I found that the natural tartness of cream of tartar could stand in, plus it helps the dressing hold the creamy emulsion. One tester said, "I used this on chicken, pasta salad, as a dip for everything, and as a mix-in with mayo for a tasty sandwich spread. So many possibilities!"

4 cloves garlic, roughly chopped

1 shallot, roughly chopped

½ cup (125mL) organic extra virgin olive oil

¼ cup (60mL) white vinegar

¼ cup (60mL) filtered water

2 teaspoons dried oregano

¼ teaspoon cream of tartar (optional)

⅛ teaspoon fine sea salt (optional)

⅛ teaspoon freshly ground black pepper

Budget friendly: Very

1. Soak the chopped garlic and shallot in ice water for 10 minutes, then drain well.
2. Place the soaked garlic and shallot, along with all the remaining ingredients, in the blender. Blend until smooth.
3. Transfer to a clean glass jar and store in the refrigerator for up to 2 weeks.

COOKS' NOTE: *Soaking the garlic and shallot helps remove some of the strong bite that can be overpowering. While cream of tartar adds tartness and helps keep the emulsion, some people may be sensitive to it. If you notice any gastrointestinal distress, omit it the next time. Use this dressing sparingly, as even white vinegar can be a trigger. Once you have tested vinegar, a white balsamic or apple cider vinegar will give mellower flavor.*

Per 1-tablespoon serving: <1g protein, <1g carbohydrates, 7g fat, 1g saturated fat, <1mg sodium, 11mg potassium, 0g fiber

Pomegranate Marinade for Beef or Chicken

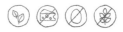

Makes enough to marinate 3–5 pounds (1.4–2.25kg) of meat
Prep time: 5 minutes   Cooking time: 5 minutes   Passive time: N/A

Another category that's tough to create without acidic foods? Marinades. Usually they are wine and oil, vinegar and oil, or citrus and oil. After requests from my Plan testers for marinades, I hit upon some naturally tart fruit juices to provide the balance. This one was a huge hit with the recipe testers, too, who gave it "rave reviews!" and said, "My four-year-old said, 'I would eat this every day.' My whole family went back for thirds!"

2 tablespoons whole cumin seeds

2 tablespoons whole coriander seeds

¼ teaspoon red pepper flakes

2 cups (500mL) unsweetened pomegranate juice

½ cup (125mL) organic extra virgin olive oil

½ teaspoon ground allspice

Budget friendly: Very

1. Add the spices to a small, dry skillet set over medium heat and toast for about 5 minutes, or until fragrant Remove from the heat and let cool, then grind the toasted spices and the red pepper flakes with a mortar and pestle or spice grinder.
2. Add the ground spices, along with all the remaining ingredients, to a bowl and stir to combine. Use right away. Make sure to let the meat marinate for at least 30 minutes, up to overnight.
3. Cook meat as you wish, by grilling or roasting.

COOKS' NOTES: *This is tasty on chicken but does stain it a dark red. Red pepper flakes may be a migraine trigger for some people. You can use pre-ground spices if you don't have whole spices, use 1 tablespoon each of the cumin and coriander. If you don't have time for the toasting in Step 1, you can skip it, but toasting brings out the full flavor of the spices. If you wish to make sauce, pour off the marinade when you begin cooking the meat and bring to a boil in a pan for at least five minutes. Cook at a simmer until reduced by half. Thicken the sauce further by combining 2 tablespoons filtered water and 1 tablespoon arrowroot powder in a small bowl, stirring with a whisk to create a slurry; whisk the slurry into sauce, whisking constantly until sauce is thickened.*

For the entire recipe (not including meat): 4g protein, 77g carbohydrates, 114g fat, 16g saturated fat, 78mg sodium, 1,433mg potassium, 6g fiber

Quick Alfredo-Style Pasta Sauce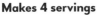

Makes 4 servings
Prep time: 5 minutes   Cooking time: N/A   Passive time: N/A

Back when I was teaching low-fat eating in a hospital program, we discovered that cottage cheese plus a blender made an incredible creamy sauce. I recommend using full-fat cottage cheese for this. If you're watching your sodium closely, use salt-free cottage cheese, which is usually low-fat. One tester loved how easy this was, a "wonderful alternative to cooking tomato sauce or just using olive oil."

16 ounces (450g) organic cottage cheese (4 percent milkfat is best)

1–2 cloves garlic, roughly chopped

¼–½ teaspoon white pepper

Budget friendly: Very

1. Add all the ingredients to a blender. Blend until smooth, stopping as necessary to scrape down the sides.
2. Use right away.

COOKS' NOTE: *Cottage cheese is fairly salty, so avoid it if you have Meniere's, or use low-sodium cottage cheese if available. You can substitute black pepper for white pepper. Several testers lightly sautéed the garlic in olive oil before blending to mellow the flavor. If you are making this as you cook pasta, add 2 to 4 tablespoons (30-60mL) pasta cooking water in Step 1. If you're following a grain-free diet, try this on zucchini ribbons or cooked spaghetti squash strands, top with minced fresh Italian flat-leaf parsley.*

Per ¼ cup serving (with 4 percent milkfat cottage cheese, without pasta):
52g protein, 20g carbohydrates, 20g fat, 8g saturated fat, 1660mg sodium, 640mg potassium, 0g fiber

Per ¼ cup serving (with low-sodium, lowfat cottage cheese, without pasta):
56g protein, 16g carbohydrates, 4g fat, 4g saturated fat, 72mg sodium, 556mg potassium, 0g fiber

Ranch Dressing

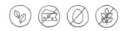

Makes 1 cup (250mL), about 16 (1-tablespoon) servings
Prep time: 5 minutes   Cooking time: N/A   Passive time: 5–10 minutes

This is a favorite salad dressing for so many people, but most people have probably never made it fresh. True ranch dressing is made with buttermilk, which gives it that tangy flavor. I replace buttermilk with coconut milk that has been curdled with vinegar. Testers loved this recipe, finding a variety of uses for it: on spinach-mushroom salad, as a dip for pizza crusts, and mixed into Chicken Salad (page 211).

½ cup (125mL) coconut milk

2 teaspoons white vinegar

½ cup (125mL) light olive oil or grapeseed oil

1 teaspoon garlic powder

1 teaspoon cream of tartar

1 teaspoon dried, or 1 tablespoon minced fresh Italian flat-leaf parsley

1 teaspoon dried, or 1 tablespoon minced fresh dill

½ teaspoon dried, or 1 teaspoon minced fresh chives

Budget friendly: Very

1. Add the coconut milk and vinegar to a blender and let stand 5 to 10 minutes to curdle.
2. Add the oil, garlic powder, and cream of tartar and blend until smooth and creamy.
3. Pour into a clean glass jar and add the herbs. Shake to blend. (If you add the herbs to the blender, you get green dressing.) Store in the refrigerator for up to 1 week.

COOKS' NOTE: *Don't use extra virgin olive oil in this recipe; the grassy taste will overpower the delicate herbs. Once you have tested apple cider vinegar, use that in this recipe. Note that even small amounts of any vinegar can be a trigger. You can skip the blender altogether if you're willing to shake the jar really hard. If your coconut milk has any chunks of coconut fat in it, you'll need to use the blender.*

Per 1-tablespoon serving: <1g protein, <1g carbohydrates, 8g fat, 2g saturated fat, 1mg sodium, 51mg potassium, 0g fiber

Smoky Mustard Sauce

Makes about ⅓ cup (90mL), about 5 (1-tablespoon) servings
Prep time: 5 minutes   Cooking time: N/A   Passive time: N/A

I first tasted Joe's Mustard Sauce when we were following the South Beach Diet. The original recipe is from Chef Andre Bienvenue for Joe's Stone Crab restaurant in South Beach. I took the spirit of the recipe—the creaminess and mustard flavor—and have adapted it for the Plan, because it's an incredibly versatile, quick sauce that can stand in for condiments. One tester called it, "Quite delicious on crab cakes, and good on fish in general. It might be nice on potatoes, or to make potato salad."

4 tablespoons (60mL) half-and-half or coconut milk (see Cooks' Note)

2 tablespoons organic, low-sodium soy-free mayonnaise

1 teaspoon smoked paprika

½ teaspoon dried mustard powder

Budget friendly: Very

1. Add all the ingredients to a small bowl and whisk together until smooth.
2. Transfer to a clean glass jar or squeeze bottle and store in the refrigerator for up to 2 weeks.

COOKS' NOTE: *If you use coconut milk instead of half-and-half, start with 1 tablespoon, whisking and adding a little at a time until you achieve the pourable consistency you want. Some people might be sensitive to smoked paprika, so test it for yourself. This is perfect on Patties (page 283) or Salmon–Potato Cakes (page 237).*

Per 1-tablespoon serving: <1g protein, <1g carbohydrates, 4g fat, 1g saturated fat, 21mg sodium, 17mg potassium, 0g fiber

STEPHANIE'S SPICE STAR: Smoked paprika

If you've tasted regular paprika (often called Hungarian paprika) and thought, "what's the point," you're not alone. I never understood it either. But smoked paprika is a whole 'nother ballgame. Also called pimentón, it's made from a special type of red pepper pod that's native to Spain and slowly smoked and dried over an oak fire. It adds incredible depth of flavor and smoky, meaty notes to dishes, especially useful if you're eating plant-based cuisine.

Salsa Verde

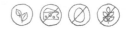

Makes 1 cup (250 mL), 16 (1-tablespoon) servings
Prep time: 15 minutes   Cooking time: 15 minutes   Passive time: 15 minutes

Most store-bought salsa contains onions, a migraine trigger for many. I wanted to provide one salsa recipe, in case you love Mexican flavors as much as I do. Roasting the vegetables adds deep, smoky notes to the salsa. Use it in Migas (page 206), on top of an omelet, with salt-free tortilla chips, and to make slow-cooker pulled pork or chicken.

10 ounces (285g) tomatillos, husked and washed well

4 green jalapeños

1 bunch green onions

3 cloves garlic, unpeeled

1 teaspoon ground cumin, or as needed (optional)

¼ teaspoon liquid smoke (optional)

1 bunch cilantro

Budget friendly: Very

1. Turn the broiler to high and move the rack to its highest position under the broiler. Lightly spray or oil a shallow ovenproof dish.
2. Add the tomatillos, jalapeños, onions, and garlic cloves to the prepared pan. Broil for 4 minutes, then, using tongs, remove any garlic and onions that look brown. Return the pan to the broiler and broil for another 5 minutes.
3. Check the veggies again. Take care opening the oven door, as the pepper fumes can be strong. After 10 minutes total, the tomatillos should be starting to brown, and the peppers might be blackened on the top. Flip everything over and return to the broiler for another 5 minutes.
4. Remove the pan from the broiler and set tomatillos, onions, and garlic aside to cool.
5. Transfer the jalapeños to a paper bag and roll down the top. This steams the peppers so the skins are easy to remove. (You can leave the skins on, but you'll find little hard bits of skin in the salsa, which are not ideal.)
6. Add everything to the blender as it cools: Squeeze out the garlic centers into the blender and discard the papery husks. Add the tomatillos and green onions.
7. When the jalapeños have cooled enough to handle, about 15 minutes, remove the outer skin, seeds, ribs, and stems and discard. Add the remaining cooked pepper flesh to the blender. Wear gloves when handling hot peppers.

8. Add the cumin and liquid smoke, if using, to the blender. Begin with ¼ teaspoon cumin and add more to your taste.
9. Roughly chop most of the cilantro, reserving about ¼ cup (a large handful). Finely mince the reserved cilantro.
10. Add the chopped cilantro to the blender. Blend until smooth, then stir in the minced cilantro by hand before transferring to clean glass jars. Use within 5 days or freeze a portion for up to 6 months.

COOKS' NOTE: *If you are a cilantro hater, skip it. It's still a tasty salsa minus the cilantro. Liquid smoke may be a trigger, so test it before using. I love the smoky taste it imparts to this salsa, making up for the missing salt. Choose a brand of liquid smoke that includes only smoke and water as ingredients.*

Per 1-tablespoon serving: <1g protein, 2g carbohydrates, <1g fat, 0g saturated fat, 3mg sodium, 112mg potassium, 1g fiber

Spice Rub for Chicken and Fish

Makes ⅓ cup
Prep time: 5 minutes   Cooking time: N/A   Passive time: 10 minutes

If you don't own an electric coffee grinder, it's a tool I wish I had bought years before. I don't drink coffee, and I foolishly thought I would rarely use it as a spice grinder. Instead, I use it at least once a week to create fresh-tasting spice blends and dry rubs. This blend perfectly complements both chicken and fish. Adapted from a recipe by Chef Christian Plotczyk in *The South Beach Diet*. One batch will flavor three whole chickens.

1 tablespoon whole cumin seeds

1 tablespoon whole black peppercorns

1 tablespoon whole fennel seeds

1 tablespoon whole coriander seeds

1 tablespoon whole fenugreek seeds

2 teaspoons ground white pepper

Budget friendly: Very

1. Combine all the spices, except for the white pepper, in a small, dry skillet set over medium heat and toast for about 5 minutes, or until fragrant. Remove from the heat and let cool completely, about 10 minutes.
2. Transfer the cooled seeds and white pepper to a spice grinder and blend until finely ground. Alternatively, use a mortar and pestle.
3. Store in a clean glass spice jar for up to 6 months.

COOKS' NOTE: *This rub is great on grilled chicken breasts, whole chickens, or fatty fish like tuna steaks. If you cannot find whole seeds, you can substitute ¾ tablespoon ground seeds for each of the whole seeds.*

For the entire recipe: 6g protein, 22g carbohydrates, 4g fat, 0g saturated fat, 27mg sodium, 435mg potassium, 11g fiber

Tart Cherry Marinade for Beef or Pork

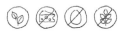

Makes enough for 1 large roast or 8 pork chops
Prep time: 5 minutes   Cooking time: N/A   Passive time: N/A

Tart cherry juice has many health benefits, including reduced muscle damage, quicker recovery from exercise, and cancer-fighting anthocyanin compounds, as well as adding acidity to this marinade.[212] Enjoy this marinade, and cook your red meat low and slow (such as braising) to reduce the potential cancer-causing issues with red meat. Testers loved the ease of this recipe and reported it was kid-friendly.

2 cups (500mL) unsweetened tart cherry juice

½ cup (250mL) organic extra virgin olive oil

1 teaspoon ground allspice

1 teaspoon freshly ground black pepper

½ teaspoon ground cloves

Budget friendly: Very

1. Add all the ingredients to a bowl and mix to combine.
2. Use right away; make sure to marinate the meat for at least 30 minutes or up to overnight.

COOKS' NOTE: *The acidity in the cherry juice stands in for vinegar in this marinade. Cook meat according to your recipe. If you wish to make sauce, pour off the marinade when you begin cooking the meat and bring it to a boil in a pan for at least five minutes. Cook at a simmer until the sauce is reduced by half. Thicken the sauce further by combining 2 tablespoons filtered water and 1 tablespoon arrowroot powder in a small bowl, stirring with a whisk to create a slurry; whisk the slurry into the sauce, whisking constantly until the sauce is thickened.*

For the entire recipe: 4g protein, 65g carbohydrates, 109g fat, 15g saturated fat, 20mg sodium, 642mg potassium, 8g fiber

STEPHANIE'S SPICE STAR: Allspice
This dried berry is native to South America and the West Indies. It's called "allspice" because it tastes like a combination of cinnamon, nutmeg, and cloves. It's frequently included in autumn baking and spice blends like pumpkin pie spice. It adds lovely sweet notes to a meat marinade, especially combined with the cherry juice here.

Tomato–Herb Salad Dressing

Makes about ⅓ cup (90mL), about 5 (1-tablespoon) servings
Prep time: 5 minutes   Cooking time: N/A   Passive time: N/A

I used the natural acidity of tomatoes to bump up the acidity in this salad dressing, which blends together in just a minute or two and tastes incredibly fresh.

3 large or 6 small cherry tomatoes, cut into chunks

2 tablespoons organic extra virgin olive oil

2 tablespoons filtered water, or as needed

1 tablespoon organic, low-sodium soy-free mayonnaise

½ tablespoon fresh tarragon, thyme, or savory leaves, or ¼–½ teaspoon dried tarragon

½ teaspoon white vinegar

½ teaspoon dried mustard powder

Budget friendly: Very

1. Add all the ingredients to the blender, starting with only 1 tablespoon water. Blend, stopping to scrape down the sides as needed, until very smooth. Add additional water if needed to achieve a pourable consistency.
2. Transfer to a clean glass jar and store in the refrigerator for up to 3 days.

COOKS' NOTE: *Once you have tested apple cider vinegar, white balsamic vinegar, and white wine vinegar, use any of them in this recipe for mellower flavor.*

Per 1-tablespoon serving: <1g protein, <1g carbohydrates, 6g fat, 1g saturated fat, 24mg sodium, 30mg potassium, 0g fiber

recipes that use leftovers

———— ••• ————

I am the queen of using up leftovers. It all stems from my extremely thrifty German American mom, who lived through the Depression as well as post-war Germany with my Army-officer dad. She never, ever threw anything out. However, she wasn't great about using things up. After learning more about food waste (see page 91), I have vowed never to waste food again. I wanted to give you a few starter recipes to help you make use of all those wonderful ingredients you'll be buying. As you get more comfortable cooking, I hope you'll feel braver about experimenting as well.

Frittata

Makes 2–4 servings

Frittatas are the perfect vehicle for leftovers, as you can transform just about anything into a meal. Even tiny scraps of meat, a sprig of herbs, some cooked veggies you might otherwise toss . . . make a frittata! You can eat it hot or cold, make it for breakfast, take it for lunch, or make a quick hot dinner in a flash.

1–2 tablespoons extra virgin olive or coconut oil

¼–½ cup diced leftover cooked vegetables, or <1 full serving of diced takeout (such as Italian, Mexican, or Thai)

3–4 eggs

1 tablespoon milk of your choice

Fresh herbs to match flavor profile (page 90), minced

1. Preheat the broiler. If your broiler is at the top of your oven, move the top rack to the highest position.
2. In a large skillet or omelet pan set over medium heat, warm the oil.
3. Add the vegetables or leftovers and sauté until they are golden brown.
4. In a small bowl while the vegetables cook, whip the eggs lightly with the milk. Sprinkle the fresh herbs on top.
5. Pour the egg mixture into the skillet over the vegetables. Cook until set on the bottom and nearly set on the top.
6. Use an oven mitt or potholder to move the pan from the burner to the broiler or top rack of the oven. Broil for about 3 minutes, or until the top turns golden brown. If your broiler is too hot, you can bake the frittata for 12 minutes at 375°F (190°C) instead.
7. Cut into wedges and serve immediately. Leftover frittata wedges travel well for lunch or trips.

COOKS' NOTE: *Use the Flavor Profiles (page 90) to explore a variety of herb and spice combinations. If you don't have fresh herbs, use ½ teaspoon of dried herbs to start.*

Breakfast Hash

Makes 1–2 servings

This is my go-to breakfast most days—a wonderful way to start the day with vegetables. If you're not used to eating vegetables for breakfast, give this a try. I make enough for four days at once, then store the extras, so breakfast is still quick and easy. Add an egg with a soft-cooked yolk for instant sauce, or use leftover gravy if you have it.

½–1 cup cooked, ¼-inch-diced potato, sweet potato, French fries, or other cooked root vegetables

Diced cooked meat (any amount)

2 strips uncooked Make Your Own Bacon (page 197) (optional)

Leftover fresh herbs such as rosemary, thyme, savory, or tarragon, minced

1. Set a nonstick or cast iron frying pan over medium–high heat.
2. Cook bacon, if using, until fat is rendered out. Pour off all but 1 tablespoon of the fat and reserve it in a glass jar for another use.
3. If not using bacon, add 1–2 tablespoons extra virgin olive or coconut oil to the pan, swirling to coat.
4. Sauté all the other ingredients in the remaining bacon fat or oil until hot and crispy.
5. Serve at once. If making extra for additional breakfasts, refrigerate in a covered glass container for up to 4 days.

COOKS' NOTE: *For a vegan or vegetarian version that's a full breakfast, add up to 1 cup per person cooked Plan-approved beans to the hash. If serving with eggs, push the cooked hash to the edge of the pan, add a small amount of additional fat if needed, and cook one to two eggs per person over easy. Serve the eggs on top of the hash, then break the yolks for a decadent sauce. If using fresh rosemary, use just a few needles, finely minced, so its strong flavor doesn't overpower the dish.*

Pasta with Vegetables

Makes 1 serving

Sometimes you just need a quick dinner for one. If cooking for more people, just multiply the amounts by the number of servings. This recipe does not provide leftovers. The general rule is 2 ounces of dry pasta per serving. If you don't have a kitchen scale, you can guesstimate using the bag or box. An 8-ounce bag would provide four servings, so you would use one-quarter of the bag for one person. Instead of just eating plain pasta, I sneak vegetables into the cooking water for a one-pot dinner that's amped up with veggie nutrition in under 15 minutes.

1 clove garlic, smashed

1 pinch red pepper flakes

2 ounces gluten-free dried pasta

½ tablespoon extra virgin olive oil

1 carrot, peeled into thin strips

1 stalk broccoli, chopped

1 handful fresh baby spinach leaves or thinly sliced hearty greens

Fine sea salt, to taste

Freshly ground black pepper, to taste

1. Add garlic and red pepper flakes to a large pot of filtered water. Bring to a rolling boil. Add pasta and a splash of olive oil. Return to a boil, stirring regularly.
2. When you are 5 minutes from pasta being done (gluten-free pasta takes 9 to 15 minutes), add the vegetables to the boiling water.
3. Continue to stir until pasta is cooked.
4. Drain, then toss with extra virgin olive oil in your serving bowl. Add sea salt and freshly cracked black pepper.
5. Serve at once.

COOKS' NOTE: *If you have migraine-friendly cheese, herb pesto, or leftover Herbed Cheese Spread (page 189), stir it in at the end. Yum!*

Patties

Makes 1 or more servings

When I was a kid, we had our big Sunday dinner after church. On Sunday nights we were able to eat non-traditional dinners like pizza, toaster oven items, and something my mom called Thick Fritters using canned tuna. I have adapted that concept here. If you like the Salmon–Potato Cakes (page 237), then expand your patty horizons. Patties are the perfect vehicle to use up leftover cooked grains like brown rice, teff, millet, quinoa, or amaranth; cooked fish that's less than a full serving; and cooked vegetables. Serves one or more, depending on the amount of leftovers used. Use the recipe as a starting point, then get creative. The main goal is to make sure the patties hold together.

1 cup (approx. 150g) cooked grains

1 cup (approx. 150g) chopped cooked veggies

2–3 ounces (60–90g) cooked fish, flaked

1–2 eggs

1 tablespoon Italian herb seasoning

Up to 2 tablespoons ground flax seeds, or as needed

1. Combine all the ingredients, except for the flax seeds, in a large bowl; mix well. Smoosh the mixture with the back of the spoon so it gets tacky. If you need more stickiness to get it to form patties, add the ground flax seeds, 1 tablespoon at a time, stirring well. Stop when it sticks together and will easily hold the shape of a patty.

2. Preheat an electric grill, grill pan, or nonstick frying pan to medium high. Spray or oil the pan with high-heat oil such as grapeseed. (Do not use spray on a nonstick pan or you will ruin the finish.)

3. Use a measuring cup, egg ring, or ice cream scoop to portion out the patties evenly, about ½ cup per patty. (You can make 2 patties per person or 1 large one.)

4. Cook for 5 to 8 minutes per side, until golden. Flatten with a spatula after flipping them.

5. Serve with Smoky Mustard Sauce (see recipe on page 273) or another creamy sauce.

COOKS' NOTE: *Experiment with Flavor Profiles (page 90), substituting other spice blends for the Italian blend, such as curry powder, garam masala, Herbes de Provence, or one of the spice blends in this book.*

Pizza

Makes 2 servings

You can buy frozen gluten-free pizza crusts in many grocery stores, or order them online from Venice Pizza; most include eggs, but a few are vegan. With a few migraine-friendly tweaks, you can still enjoy pizza and stay on the Plan. These crusts tend to be on the smaller side, serving two people comfortably.

1 gluten-free frozen pizza crust, thawed

1 (6-ounce [180-g]) can no-salt-added organic tomato paste

1–2 teaspoons no-salt-added Italian herb seasoning

1–2 cups (approx. 150–300g) precooked vegetables, such as zucchini, bell peppers, or mushrooms

1–4 ounces crumbled goat cheese or ricotta cheese (optional)

1–2 eggs (optional)

1. Preheat the oven to 425°F (220°C). Line a baking sheet with parchment paper and set aside.
2. If your crust requires prebaking, follow the package directions now.
3. To assemble the pizza, place the crust on prepared baking sheet. Add the tomato paste and spread thinly. Sprinkle the Italian herb seasoning evenly over the tomato paste. Sprinkle the vegetables evenly on top and then add the goat cheese, if using, over that. Break the eggs, if using, on top of the pizza.
4. Transfer to the oven and bake for about 10 minutes, or until the crust is brown, the cheese is melty, and the eggs are set. (If the package directions indicate that the pizza needs longer than 10 minutes to bake, add the eggs to the top when you have 10 minutes remaining on your timer.)
5. Remove from the oven, slice, and serve.

COOKS' NOTE: *If you own a pizza stone, cut a piece of parchment paper to fit the stone, then reserve the paper and put the stone on the center rack of the oven to preheat. Place the parchment paper on a large cutting board (you'll use the board to transfer the pizza to the stone). Assemble the pizza as directed in Step 3. Pull the pizza stone out of the oven and set it on a heatproof surface. Slide the pizza and the parchment paper directly onto the stone. Bake the pizza as directed in Step 4. You could also use leftover Herbed Cheese Spread (page 189) in place of the goat cheese.*

Quiche

Makes 6–8 servings

I have a favorite memory of making quiche with a college friend named George. I was visiting him in Washington, DC. We spent the day sightseeing, walking and talking, then came home famished. We made a quiche together without a recipe, which is not the quickest way to get dinner on the table! It tasted so delicious that I wrote up the recipe to take home. I still have the hand-written card in my recipe box. Quiche is far simpler than it might seem, as it's just ingredients baked in custard: milk whisked with eggs. Turning leftovers into a quiche always provides a result that's better than the sum of its parts. It's oven alchemy, pure and simple. You can purchase gluten-free pie crusts in the frozen section of many grocery stores. Or find my recipe on RecipeRenovator.com.

1 store-bought gluten-free pie crust

1 cup (approx. 150g) cooked ground or chopped meat, or less as available

1 cup (approx. 150g) chopped cooked vegetables, or less as available

1 bunch green onions, or less as available, thinly sliced and sautéed until golden

1–2 cloves garlic and/or shallots, minced and sautéed until golden

4–6 ounces (115–175g) goat cheese or ricotta (optional)

6 eggs

½ cup (125mL) milk of your choice

¾ teaspoon freshly ground black pepper

¼ teaspoon fine sea salt

1. Preheat the oven to 350°F (180°C) with a baking sheet set the center rack of the oven. Baking the quiche on a hot baking sheet helps crisp up the bottom crust.
2. Put pie crust in a pie dish, or thaw the frozen crust.
3. Sprinkle the meat, vegetables, and sautéed onions, garlic, and shallots over the pie crust. Crumble the cheese, if using, over as evenly as possible.
4. In a small bowl, whisk the eggs with the milk, black pepper, and sea salt.
5. Pour the egg mixture over the pie filling.
6. Bake for 50 to 60 minutes, or until the top is golden and completely set. It should not jiggle when shaken.
7. Remove from the oven and transfer to a wire rack to cool for at least 10 minutes. Slice and serve. Refrigerate extra quiche for up to 3 days. This travels well and makes an excellent lunch.

COOKS' NOTE: *Quiche is another blank slate to play around with herbs. If you have a few sprigs of fresh thyme, strip the leaves off the stems into the bowl in Step 4. Minced fresh chives, parsley, basil, and oregano would all be lovely in quiche. I would not suggest cilantro or rosemary in quiche, as they could both overpower the delicate flavors.*

Rice Bowl

Makes 1 serving

A rice bowl is one of those quick meals that's so easy I tend to forget about it. It was a staple during my years as a vegetarian. While it seems simple, it's comforting, filling, and another way to use up small amounts of leftover precooked food. What happens if you look in the fridge and you only have a small amount of sauce, cooked chicken or beans, and a little cooked rice, quinoa, or millet? Rice bowl!

½ cup (approx. 75g) cooked rice (or other grain), or more as desired

½ cup (approx. 75g) sautéed or steamed vegetables, or more as desired

½ cup (approx. 75g) cooked beans

½ cup (approx. 75g) chopped cooked chicken (optional)

1 tablespoon Smoky Mustard Sauce (page 273)

1. Place all the ingredients, except for the mustard sauce, in a bowl with the rice on the bottom. Microwave until hot. If you don't wish to use a microwave, then heat all the ingredients on the stove first.
2. Drizzle the bowl with the Smoky Mustard Sauce and serve right away.

COOKS' NOTE: *The Rice Bowl is great with the Smoky Mustard Sauce, but if you want to mix it up, try any of these condiments instead: dark toasted sesame oil and Chile Pepper Sauce (page 267), Italian Dressing (page 269), or Salsa Verde (page 274). If making for more than one person, just evenly divide your leftovers between the bowls and top with a drizzle of sauce or dressing.*

Chopped Salad

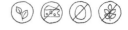

Makes 1 serving

Obviously, you know how to make a salad. Duh. But you might think salad has to have lettuce in it. Nope. A chopped salad is simply a whole bunch of uniformly chopped raw or par-cooked vegetables, maybe some toasted seeds, and chopped meat or beans for protein. And it's a perfect place to mix in small amounts of leftover deli salad items like coleslaw or chicken salad, as they'll add wonderful flavor and seasoning. I've made chopped salad from celery leaves, zucchini, cucumber, radishes, and leftover chicken salad. Use this recipe as a starting point the first time, then feel free to experiment.

1 cup shredded lettuce

½ cup (approx. 75g) raw fresh vegetables, whatever you have on hand

½ cup (approx. 75g) chopped meat such as chicken, turkey, or steak (optional)

½ cup (approx. 75g) cooked or canned beans

¼ cup (approx. 35g) leftover deli salad, such as chicken salad, potato salad, or coleslaw

1–2 tablespoons dressing of your choice (see Cooks' Note)

1. Chop all the vegetables and meats into uniformly sized pieces.
2. Toss everything together in a large bowl with the dressing of your choice. Serve in an individual bowl right away.

COOKS' NOTE: *Use any of my dressings on this, such as Ranch Dressing (page 272), Italian Dressing (page 269), or Cilantro Mayonnaise (page 268). If making more than one serving, toss all the ingredients in a large salad bowl with the dressing of your choice, starting with 1 tablespoon per person. Note that lettuce tossed with dressing will get wilted if stored, so only make enough for one meal.*

Creamy Soup

Makes 2 to 4 servings

I have some version of this soup in my fridge almost daily. Overcook some vegetables in the pressure cooker? Make soup. Have some leftover roasted vegetables? Make soup. Don't know how to use up the last of those vegetables you bought with good intentions? Roast, steam, or nuke them and make soup. Freeze soup in 1-cup servings to take for lunch or for a hearty afternoon snack.

1 cup (approx. 150g) cooked vegetables, such as roasted root vegetables, steamed broccoli, oven-roasted cauliflower, or steamed or grilled asparagus

1½ cups (375ml) low-sodium vegetable or chicken stock

1 teaspoon spice blend of your choice

1. Add all the ingredients to a blender. Blend until smooth and creamy.
2. Transfer to a medium saucepan set over medium heat. Cook, stirring occasionally, until warmed through. Alternatively, use a microwave.
3. Transfer to serving bowls and serve immediately.

COOKS' NOTE: *This soup tastes best with one primary vegetable flavor. If the vegetables already have Italian seasoning, add ¼ teaspoon Italian seasoning blend to start, then taste. See Flavor Profiles (page 90) for more ideas. For a creamier soup, use 1 cup stock and 1 cup full-fat coconut milk. If you're not sure what spice blend to use, try up to 1 tablespoon mild curry powder, which melds with nearly every flavor that might already be on the vegetables. If you are using mostly beets, stir in ½ teaspoon dried dill weed and use mostly coconut milk. Try serving cold, stirring in some minced cucumber.*

conclusion

———— ··· ————

One year almost to the day after my first visit with Dr. Y, I was back in his office, waiting to take a test called electronystagmography. I had put this test off for a few months. I didn't want to get more bad news until I felt emotionally ready. And I wanted more information before undergoing the test.

I had never asked a doctor in advance how my test results would affect my treatment plan. I wanted to understand if the test results would change my medication or potential procedures, or if they were just gathering data for the future.

The PA told me on the phone that they were suspicious that I had Meniere's disease but couldn't be sure without doing these tests. The tests would determine how my inner ears were functioning, give a baseline for how badly damaged they might be, and give them more information about my prognosis. Since the test wasn't time-sensitive, I opted to put it off until I felt better emotionally, in case it was more bad news. But I was hoping that the test would show that my ears were basically OK. I also didn't want to learn later that they could have done something to save my hearing, if only I had taken this test.

I had gone online, done some research, and asked in a forum whether people had any long-term negative effects from the test itself. Part of the test, called the caloric test, involves pouring "warm or cool" water into the ear. It didn't sound fun, but no one had any long-term problems afterwards.

So that's how I found myself sitting on an exam table wearing crazy black goggles, waiting for the electronystagmography technician to come in. I had meditated for a few days beforehand about it going well, and I was feeling calm. It seemed that my meditation practice would come in handy, as every section of the test involved holding my eyes open—without blinking—for interminable periods of time. Eye movement is connected to our balance system, and tracking this movement would tell Dr. Y what was happening deep inside my head. Before we started, the technician told me that if I blinked a lot, I would fail that portion of the test, and I would have to do it over again. If I did a good job, I would be done in an hour. I was determined not to fail.

Part one: I stared at a red dot seemingly forever without blinking. Between the goggles and the not blinking, it was part sci-fi torture scene, part claustrophobia.

Part two: I followed red dots as they tracked faster and faster across the screen without moving my head or blinking.

Part three: I held my head rock steady at a specific angle while the technician poured water into my ear. If I flinched, moved, or blinked, I would fail the test. He told me that it was normal for the test to make people really dizzy. He told me what temperature the water would be. It sounded innocuous: 85 degrees for the cool water and 110 degrees for the warm water. He said that once he sat me back up he would ask me some questions to help my brain reset as the final part of the test. He gave me a towel to wedge under my left ear.

First came the cool water in my left ear, which felt ice cold. It escaped the towel and started running down my back, a tiny rivulet of chilled water, over my shoulder blade, past my bra strap. It was really cold. I worked hard to think about something other than the icy drip: my yoga teacher, Deepak Chopra's soothing voice, a candle flame. Anything to distract me from the water. I breathed as deeply as I could without moving. I squeezed my husband's hand, hard. Once the cool water portion was completed for that ear, he sat me back up. I was wicked dizzy. He asked me to name as many states as I could until he told me to stop. My head was spinning and I couldn't think. I stumbled over words.

"Ohio. Mich-i-gan. Illi-nois." Wait, states? Why can't I think of states? "Nebraska. Nevada." I could picture the map in my mind, but my brain couldn't seem to form any words. The room spun around. Where do I live now? "California. Arizona." My sister lives in Arizona, doesn't she? What's next to Arizona? "New Mexico. Um . . . Iowa. Illinois. Indiana." I knew I was repeating them, but I couldn't think of anything else.

I finally passed that section. Next the right ear. More cold water, more holding my head still. More spinning. More questions.

"Name as many cities as you can think of."

Cities? Cities. Cities are where people live. I live in a city. "San Diego. Las Vegas. New York." What's near New York? "Boston." My sister used to live in Boston. "New York." I knew I repeated it, but my brain simply wasn't working. I tried not to giggle, as I knew I must look and sound ridiculous: a speech-challenged woman wearing Stanley Kubrick goggles. My brain landed on the rust belt. "Chicago. Detroit. Kalamazoo." Pass again.

Then there was only one part left. The "warm" water. I placed the towel firmly under my left ear to catch any drips. I took a deep breath. He started pouring. It was freaking hot water. It hurt. A lot. I squeezed my husband's hand as hard as I could, digging my nails into his palm. I was determined to do this only once.

"Name as many animals as you can think of."

"Golden retriever. Labrador retriever. Chocolate lab. Yellow lab. Shi-tsu." I was looking at a dog park in my mind as the room spun around. "Border. Collie. Australian. Shepherd." What's that big huge dog that I love? "Bernese mountain dog." I couldn't think of another dog so I started on the zoo animals I remembered. "Koala. Panda. Kudu. Panther. Tiger."

Finally, it was the last test on the final ear. Deep breath. Boiling water. Trying not to move or yell. The room started spinning.

"Name as many drinks as you can think of."

"Iced tea. Water. Filtered. Water. Mint. Water. Strawberry. Water. Cucumber. Water. Fizzy. Water." I could tell my husband and the technician were trying not to laugh. I was trying not to laugh, too. All I could think of were iterations of water. I knew there were more. "Hot. Water. Earl Grey tea. English breakfast tea."

"Okay, you can stop. You're all done!"

After my brain reset, I did another hearing test before I left. One of the earplugs came loose midway through, and I couldn't hear much of anything. I felt like I totally failed it. Over the years I have come to hate this computer program and its flat, robotic male voice repeating simple words, words I should easily be able to hear, whose results are so critical to my life. Since there wasn't an option to redo just one portion of the program, and I was tired, I tried to let it go.

I made an appointment the next week to come back and get my results.

The following Tuesday, I was back in Dr. Y's office, waiting in the exam room. I deliberately avoided thinking about this moment in advance. On the way there, I told my husband, "This test doesn't define me. These results, good or bad, don't define me. I am still a healthy person, a strong person, a person who is getting better. These results are just another piece of information. I am not my results."

When Dr. Y came in, he seemed happy to see me. He looked at my labs.

"Whatever you are doing, just keep doing it. Your test results are great. Really great. Your hearing is really good. Your inner ear balance structures are really good. Your follow-up MRI leads me to believe that you may not have Meniere's, but a benign tumor called a schwannoma. And it seems to be a little smaller than last year. That anti-inflammatory stuff you're doing is probably helping a lot. We'll keep watching it.

"You are not a typical person I see."

"What do you mean?"

"Based on how you presented last year, from then to now, in my experience I've only seen 3 to 5 percent of people with these kinds of results. You are doing great."

He asked about my medications, did I need refills? He confirmed that my potassium level was back up in the normal range, a very good thing. When you take a diuretic, it pulls the sodium and the potassium out of your system. Low potassium levels can cause heart failure. So that tiny peach-colored pill I take every morning is far more powerful than its size suggests. But my levels were good, all those high-potassium foods I had been eating seem to be helping.

"Come back in four months unless something changes. Keep up the good work."

On the way home I tried to keep the visit in perspective. It was great news, but it could just as easily have been more sobering.

> I am not my test results or my condition.

My hope for you is that over time you hear the same encouraging feedback from your doctor by following the Plan, and that you are able to remember that, whatever the news, you are not your test results. If you have other health challenges like diabetes or obesity, I hope you'll start to see improvement in those, too.

You will know long before your doctor that you are doing better because you live in your body every day.

One year before this visit, I was given a scary diagnosis. Since then I've had some rough days, some frustrating days. I had to be chauffeured around for the first few months.

I've missed some social engagements. It was more than a year before I went back to LA, and the first trip back I got a migraine. The second time, three days later, I took my meds before I left and did much better.

I still get migraine attacks during our hot-bright Santa Ana weather conditions when the humidity drops and the barometric pressure changes, no matter how closely I follow the Plan. Those attacks used to lay me out for at least a day. Now, I can usually manage them much better and still function. I have gotten a migraine almost every time I have flown so far. But my balance is much better. I haven't had a vertigo attack in more than two years. I have been able to add back a whole bunch of my favorite foods. I gave a keynote address in Australia. I wrote a book. My husband and I went to Italy. I am incredibly lucky.

What has this experience taught me? First, that I can greatly impact my health by choices I make on a daily basis. Second, that my highly educated, caring, and well-intentioned specialist doesn't necessarily know everything, and that educating myself and advocating for myself was and is empowering. This diagnosis gave me a new purpose in life: to use my specific skills to create this Plan and help others to heal.

And finally, I was reminded that life is a crapshoot. We do our best; bad things can still happen. I was eating what I thought was the healthiest possible diet. I exercised. I took care of myself. This still happened to me.

One of my author friends—who gave me wonderful feedback about this book in our writing workshop—got cancer and died within six months. We lost her long before I ever finished this book, and before she finished her beautiful memoir about growing up in France.

I don't know what will happen to me tomorrow, next month, or next year. No one does. But I do know, now more than ever, to seize the day. Be present. Serve others. Make the best choices I can today.

And to slowly savor every delectable bite that life has to offer. I encourage you to do the same.

acknowledgments

Thanks to . . .

Bob, who has partnered with me every single step of the way, tasted all the recipes, and willingly gone along with every diet change I have had to make with nary a complaint. I love you.

My beta testers, who pioneered this Plan with me:

Christie, Jenna, Jo, Lexie, Noelle, Sandy, and Sarah. You inspire me every day, and your success keeps me going.

My content contributors:

Sarah Achleithner, BS, for recipe analysis; Ulka Agarwal, MD; Jonathan Borkum, MD; KC Brennan, MD; David Buchholz, MD; Kelly Clancy, PhD; Robert Cowan, MD; Mustafa Ertas, MD; Peter Goadsby, MD; Trupti Gokani, MD; Ricki Heller, PhD; Kathrynne Holden, MS, RD; Joanna Kempner, PhD; Cynthia Lair; Susan Mathison, MD; Jean McFadden Layton, ND; Alec Mien, PhD; Sabrina Modelle; Martha C. Morris, PhD; David Perlmutter, MD; Laura Plumb; Nathan Phillips and Tommy Gomes from Catalina Offshore Products; Ian Purcell, MD, PhD; Elizabeth Seng, PhD; Clea Shannon; Kenneth Shulman, MD; Justin Sonnenburg, PhD; Chef Joanne Stabile; EA Stewart, RD; Stewart Tepper, MD; Jennifer Weinberg, MD, MPH, MPE; Ayla Withee, MS, RDN, LDN, CLT; Caroline Wolfe, MD.

My intrepid recipe testers, who gave me incredible feedback along the way:

Brie Alissa, Beth Anderson, Sara Biffer, Jacki Bigas, Diane Bucka, Christie Bunch, Carolina Contreras, Faith Currant, Drew Ann Daniels, Nikke DeYear, Tiana Dodson Renard, Helene Dujardin, Lisa Falk, Julie Flahive, Eugenia Hall, Amanda Horton, Jessica A. Jiménez, Kyla Lupo, Noelle McClure, Bill Melli, Laura Plumb, Carolyn Sanders-Kull, Marc Simpson, Nancy Sobel Butcher, EA Stewart, Christine Szweda, Jennifer Weinberg, and Caroline Wolfe.

And the following lovely people who read the manuscript, gave me support, and otherwise helped this project come into the world:

Vicki Abelson and her Women Who Write workshop; Laura Bashar for the beautiful photography; Casey Benedict and Robyn Webb at Eat Write Retreat; Joan Borysenko, PhD; Dreena Burton; Carl Cincinnato of the World Migraine Summit; Carol Elliott; Ellen Dolgen; Patrick Dorman, DC; Alisa Fleming; Kathleen Flinn; Jessica Goldman Foung; Donald Gazzaniga; Dallas Hartwig; Holly Herrick; Mark Hyman, MD; Denise Lee Yohn; Kim Lutz; Tess Masters; Anne McLaughlin; Carole Murko; Sharon Palmer, MS RD; Chef Mary Papoulias-Platis; Kaya Purohit; Wendy Polisi; Teri Robert; Kristina Sloggett; and Lisa Wells. To my agent Sally Ekus plus Jaimee Constantine, Sara Pokorny, Christine Bennet, and Lisa Ekus of The Lisa Ekus Group, having your support has meant the world to me. And finally, to Doug Seibold; my stellar editor, Jessica Easto; my designer, Morgan Krehbiel; and the entire team at Agate Publishing—I feel so blessed to have collaborated with all of you to bring this book to life in such a beautiful way.

GLOSSARY
unfamiliar ingredients

———— ••• ————

Choose organic versions whenever possible.
Visit MigraineReliefPlan.com for brand-name lists, sources, and how-to videos.

ARROWROOT POWDER: A finely ground white powder made from the tuber of the arrowroot plant. Used as a starch or thickener in both gluten-free and Paleo baking and cooking. Can substitute one for one in recipes for cornstarch if you are avoiding corn. If thickening a sauce or making a filling that will be baked—like pie—use tapioca flour/starch instead.

BAKING SODA SUBSTITUTE, SODIUM-FREE: A mixture of calcium carbonate and magnesium carbonate. Use double the amount called for of regular baking powder or baking soda when substituting this ingredient into regular recipes.

CAROB POWDER: The ground pods of an evergreen tree. Naturally sweet, low in fat, high in calcium, caffeine-free. Used as a chocolate-like substitute, as it's not known to be a migraine trigger. Better if you don't expect it to taste exactly like chocolate, but rather chocolate-esque.

CHIPOTLE CHILE POWDER: Ground, smoked, dried jalapeños. Might be a migraine trigger, so use sparingly. Doesn't take much to add spicy, smoky flavor to foods like chili. Start with ⅛ teaspoon.

COCONUT OIL: Rich in healthy medium-chain triglycerides as well as being anti-inflammatory, antibacterial, and antifungal. Organic extra virgin coconut oil is best; you can use **REFINED COCONUT OIL** for high-heat frying or if you don't want to add coconut flavor.

COCONUT MILK: Canned light coconut milk works in my recipes unless specifically noted, but feel free to use the full-fat version if you have lowered your carb intake. Ingredient list should be coconut and water; many use gums and other thickeners that might be triggers. Guar gum should be OK for migraine.

DRIED MUSTARD POWDER: Yellow powder made from ground yellow mustard seeds. Mustard in a jar of any type is fermented, high in sodium, and may contain other triggers. Dried yellow mustard powder stands in for this great condiment in my recipes.

EXTRA VIRGIN OLIVE OIL: From the first press of the olives, usually dark green or yellow–green in color. Buy in smallish quantities, from an olive oil store if possible, and store in the refrigerator. Use it raw to maintain the highest health benefits from the polyphenol compounds. **LIGHT OLIVE OIL** is refined olive oil and is clear light yellow in color. I use it for making mayonnaise; it's also good for cooking if you don't care for the taste of coconut oil or animal fat.

FILTERED WATER: Filtered water is all I use for cooking. Spring water also works. This offers three benefits: (1) It removes any harmful minerals or chemicals that might be in your tap water. (2) It makes the end result taste better. (3) It removes any sodium from the water. Depending on your budget, you can use a filtering pitcher, a tap filter, or a more expensive installed system.

GHEE: Clarified butter (which means the milk proteins have been removed) used in Indian cooking, does not need refrigeration. Good for high-heat cooking and for people with milk protein allergies or sensitivities. Choose grass-fed organic ghee if available. Available at some national specialty grocers in addition to natural grocery stores.

GLUTEN-FREE FLOUR BLEND: A flour blend usually made from rice flour and tapioca starch. For best baking results, choose a blend with at least four flours, such as brown rice, white rice, bean or sorghum flour, and tapioca starch. If the blend already includes xanthan gum, omit the psyllium husk powder in the baking recipe. Some people are sensitive to xanthan gum.

MILLET: High-protein, gluten-free grain; light yellow. Cook with water or stock at a 1:1 ratio. A good substitute for couscous. Rinse and drain before using.

QUINOA: High-protein, gluten-free grain; black, tan, or red. When cooked, grains have a tiny, curly tail. Cook with water or stock at a 1:1 ratio. Another good sub for couscous or bulgur wheat. Rinse and drain before using.

PSYLLIUM HUSK POWDER: A high-fiber seed that absorbs water at a magical rate, helping gluten-free dough hold together and not crumble. I use it, with great results, substituted one for one in recipes that call for xanthan gum. If you can't find it in the grocery store, you can purchase plain Metamucil or its generic counterpart.

SEA SALT: Salt produced from evaporating sea water, comes in fine and coarse grains. Natural sea salt contains as many as 80 elements in trace amounts. Look for natural sea salt in any color (pink, gray, blue) and use sparingly at the table. Commercial white table salt contains potassium iodide, dextrose, and sodium bicarbonate; bleach is used during the refining process, and it may also contain sugar. Commercial salt may be implicated in auto-immune conditions.

SMOKED PAPRIKA: Also called *pimentón*, it's a type of sweet red pepper that is smoked and dried, providing delicious smoky flavor. Be aware that peppers and smoked foods are triggers for some. I use it in small amounts, as it adds amazing flavor.

STEVIA: A natural sweetener from the leaves of the stevia plant, far sweeter than sugar. For the best taste, choose an organic brand without added fillers like erythritol or xylitol. I use NatVia from Australia, which does not have an aftertaste to me. Most stevia packets are the equivalent of 2 teaspoons of sugar, but it varies by brand and whether they have fillers. Five drops of liquid stevia is usually equal to 1 teaspoon of sugar. If you cannot use stevia, substitute coconut sugar, which is lightly processed and low-glycemic. You might find that growing the plant itself will improve your experience of stevia. Use fresh leaves to sweeten iced tea, and dried powdered leaves in recipes in very small amounts.

TAHINI: Sesame seeds crushed into a creamy paste. Used in hummus, also great in marinades or salad dressings to amp up the sesame flavor. Usually has no additional ingredients. Store in the refrigerator.

TAPIOCA STARCH: Also labeled "tapioca flour." Get the finest grind you can; you want it powdery like flour, not grainy.

TOASTED SESAME OIL: Also labeled "dark toasted sesame oil." Adds Asian flavor to marinades and stir-fry dishes, especially in the absence of soy.

Additional information from Cynthia Lair's classic book, *Feeding the Whole Family: Down-To-Earth Cookbook and Whole Foods Guide.*

APPENDIX A
checklists

––––––––– ... –––––––––

FOOD

☐ Reduce carbohydrates under 150 grams per day

☐ Switch to extra virgin olive oil, coconut oil, or pastured animal fat

☐ Add homemade chicken stock or grass-fed gelatin to your diet each day

☐ Add 1 tablespoon of organic, extra virgin coconut oil daily (once you've gotten off sugar and starchy carbs)

☐ Add organ meats once per week

☐ Eat vegetables in equal ratios each day: brightly colored, sulfur-containing, greens

HEALTHCARE

☐ Discuss getting off medications that might be causing medication overuse headache with your doctor; download the Dr. Buchholz medications list from MigraineReliefPlan.com to share with your doctor in case you need acute care during this weaning-off period

☐ Visit a chiropractor if you think your spine or neck might be out of alignment

☐ Get a referral for biofeedback sessions

☐ Visit an acupuncturist for pain management

☐ Get a deep tissue massage on a regular basis

AUTOIMMUNE ISSUES

☐ Get tested for delayed-reaction food allergies

☐ Follow the autoimmune protocol diet (AIP) for a month or two

☐ Try the plan in *Living Candida-Free* if you have issues with yeast infections

LIFESTYLE

☐ Try dry brushing and oil pulling

☐ Listen to a meditation once per day

☐ Try the eight-week meditation program detailed in *You Are Not Your Pain*

☐ Write out what is going well each week

APPENDIX B
recommended supplements

———— ⋯ ————

KEY SUPPLEMENTS FOR MIGRAINE

———— • ————

I take Migraine Prevention Formula, which provides the perfect balance of these migraine-friendly supplements.

Supplement	Daily recommended dose
Riboflavin (vitamin B2)	400mg (200mg in morning and 200mg at night)
Magnesium	360mg (180mg in morning and 180mg at night)
Feverfew*	100mg (50mg in morning and 50mg at night)
Butterbur**	150mg (75mg in morning and 75mg at night)

* standardized to 0.5% parthenolide [500mcg]

** standardized to 15% petaisin [22.5mg] and PA free. Many MDs no longer recommend butterbur because of issues with standardization.

KEY SUPPLEMENTS FOR BRAIN HEALTH

———— • ————

Supplement	Daily recommended dose
Coconut oil	1 tablespoon
Alpha-lipoic acid	600mg
Docosahaexaenoic acid (DHA)	1,000mg*
Probiotics**	10 billion active cultures from at least 10 different strains (up to 3 times per day on an empty stomach)
Resveratrol	200mg (100mg in morning and 100mg at night)
Turmeric	700mg (350mg in morning and 350mg at night)
Vitamin D3	5,000 IU

* It's fine to buy a fish oil supplement that includes DHA

** These must be kept refrigerated; very important for balancing your gut microbiota; fermented foods can be powerful migraine triggers. If you are able to eat daily servings of fermented foods, you might not need to supplement.

ADDITIONAL SUPPLEMENTS

Supplement	Recommended daily dose
SAMe*	200mg twice daily to start, then increase by 200mg every 3 days until you reach 1,000 to 1,200mg per day
Melatonin**	3mg, 2 hours before bedtime

* Suggested for arthritis, fibromyalgia, and chronic pain. May help with depression. Note: If you have any symptoms of depression, please see a doctor right away.

** One study showed that after three months of use, melatonin reduced the number of migraine attacks by almost two-thirds and the severity by half.

APPENDIX C
plan overview

———•••———

MONTH 1: Begin tracking; reduce salt and caffeine; slowly increase movement

Week	Assignments	Daily Steps	Daily Active Minutes	Daily Sodium (mg)	Daily Caffeine (cups)	Daily Sugar
Week 1	Set up tracking system	Regular routine	Regular routine	Regular routine	Regular routine	Regular routine
Week 2	Freezer cleanout	4,000	5	3,000	2	
Week 3	Pantry cleanout	5,000	10 (2–3 days per week)	2,500	1½	
Week 4	Fridge cleanout Switch snacks to Plan	6,000	15 (2–3 days per week)	2,000	1	

MONTH 2: Switch meals to the Plan one week at a time; reduce then eliminate sugar

Week	Assignments	Daily Steps	Daily Active Minutes	Daily Sodium (mg)	Daily Caffeine (cups)	Daily Sugar
Week 5	Switch breakfast to Plan	7,000	20 (2–3 days per week)	1,500	½	1 snack per day
Week 6	Switch lunch to Plan	8,000	25 (2–3 days per week)	1,200–1,500	0	1 snack per week
Week 7	Switch dinner to Plan	9,000	30 (2–3 days per week)	1,000–1,500		0
Week 8	Special order at restaurant	10,000				

MONTH 3: Add self-care and mind/body activities

Week	Assignments	Daily Steps	Daily Active Minutes	Daily Sodium (mg)	Daily Caffeine (cups)	Daily Sugar
Week 9	· Make an appointment for bodywork					
Week 10	· Buy or record a guided meditation and listen to it at least once					
Week 11	· Try a priming exercise · Take 15 minutes to write about how you're feeling about having to give up your favorite foods; wallow and move on	10,000	30 (2–3 days per week)	1,000–1,500	0	0
Week 12	· Talk to a friend and ask for 1–2 things they can do to help you					

MONTH 4: Detox your body and environment

Week	Assignments	Daily Steps	Daily Active Minutes	Daily Sodium (mg)	Daily Caffeine (cups)	Daily Sugar
Week 13	· Try dry brushing · Go barefoot on the grass or at the beach · Make 1 room in your home healthier for you · Make 1 aspect of your work environment healthier for you	10,000	30 (2–3 days per week)	1,000–1,500	0	0
Week 14						
Week 15						
Week 16						

MONTH 5: Planning to fail

Week	Assignments	Daily Steps	Daily Active Minutes	Daily Sodium (mg)	Daily Caffeine (cups)	Daily Sugar
Week 17	· Restaurant recon · Plan 1 thing that will help you through the next holiday gathering · Plan for an upcoming vacation · Think of ways you can be more supportive of yourself if you were to "fail" on the Plan	10,000	30 (2–3 days per week)	1,000–1,500	0	0
Week 18						
Week 19						
Week 20						

MONTH 6: Sleep and movement

Week	Assignments	Daily Steps	Daily Active Minutes	Daily Sodium (mg)	Daily Caffeine (cups)	Daily Sugar
Week 21	· Make your bedroom a sleep haven · Try listening to white noise or a guided sleep meditation for a few nights · Think about what you really love to do that's active rather than what you think you "should" do. Plan those activities · Focus on lots of little movements (not "working out")	10,000	30 (2–3 days per week)	1,000–1,500	0	0
Week 22						
Week 23						
Week 24						

Month 7 and on: Start trigger testing and reintroducing foods

Week	Assignments	Daily Steps	Daily Active Minutes	Daily Sodium (mg)	Daily Caffeine (cups)	Daily Sugar
Week 25	· Make your list of foods you want to test · Restart tracking if you have stopped for a while · Follow the trigger testing guidelines and experiment · If you aren't seeing great improvement in your migraine pattern, consider going lower-carb over a few weeks	10,000	30 (2–3 days per week)	1,000–1,500	0	0
Week 26						
Week 27						
Week 28						

resources

<hr>

American Headache and Migraine Association. An online patient organization supported by the American Headache Society, with MD-approved informational resources. www.ahma .memberclicks.net.

American Headache Society. A professional society of headache doctors and researchers providing scientific resources for health care professionals; helpful for patients who want to educate themselves on the latest studies. www.AmericanHeadacheSociety.org.

Brain Maker: The Power of Gut Microbes to Heal and Protect Your Brain—For Life. Written by David Perlmutter, MD, one of the world's top neurologists who is deeply committed to nutrition, this book covers the connection between gut and brain health.

Cook Eat Paleo. Excellent starting point for following a low-carb Paleo lifestyle, featuring simple recipes with unprocessed ingredients, written by Lisa Wells. www.CookEatPaleo.com.

Counterclockwise: Mindful Health and the Power of Possibility. In this book, Ellen J. Langer, PhD, includes fascinating accounts of her research into the power of priming and becoming a health learner, not a patient.

Dawn C. Buse, PhD. Dawn Buse is a psychologist at the renowned Montefiore Headache Center, who uses guided meditations extensively with her migraine patients. Her site provides many free guided meditations. www.DawnBuse.com

Heal Your Headache: The 1-2-3 Program for Taking Charge of Your Pain. This book by David Buchholz, MD, was the dietary starting point for my Plan. It includes 12 trigger-free recipes.

Living Candida-Free: Conquer the Hidden Epidemic that's Making You Sick. If you've had problems with yeast infections, try this well-researched approach by Ricki Heller, PhD.

It Starts with Food: Discover the Whole30 and Change Your Life in Unexpected Ways. Want to see how your body feels on Paleo? This all-or-nothing 30-day approach by Dallas and Melissa Hartwig has worked for hundreds of thousands of people.

MegaHeart. Website featuring salt-free resources and hundreds of recipes written by Donald Gazzaniga and his wife, Maureen. Gazzaniga reversed his heart failure by following a salt-free diet, and many followers of the site report great improvement in Meniere's symptoms by following a salt-free diet. www.MegaHeart.com.

Melissa Joulwan. The author of the best-selling Paleo cookbooks *Well-Fed* and *Well-Fed2* offers hundreds of low-carb recipes, including homemade chicken stock and olive oil mayonnaise on her user-friendly website. www.MelJoulwan.com.

Migraine. A for-profit website for migraine patients operated by Health Central. Features top migraine bloggers, an annual reader survey, and many patient information resources. www.Migraine.com.

MigraineReliefPlan.com. Free downloads, migraine-friendly recipes, and resources.

MyFitnessPal. A free app and website that allows you to track your nutrition intake. It provides an enormous database, frequent updates, and the ability to enter your own recipes into the database. It also provides syncing with fitness trackers like Fitbit. www.MyFitnessPal.com.

My Stroke of Insight: A Brain Scientist's Personal Journey. Rich suggestions from Jill Bolte-Taylor, PhD, for living playfully and mindfully, woven into a deeply inspiring stroke recovery story.

National Headache Foundation. Provides educational resources for patients and caregivers. www.headaches.org.

Passionate Nutrition: A Guide to Using Food as Medicine from a Nutritionist Who Healed Herself from the Inside Out. Read this book by Jennifer Adler if you have a difficult relationship between food and your body that you'd like to heal.

Peace Is Every Step: The Path of Mindfulness in Everyday Life. A lovely set of short essays by Thich Nhat Hanh to introduce you to the practice of mindful living, from a world-renowned Vietnamese monk and spiritual teacher.

Sodium Girl. Written by Jessica Goldman Foung, who reversed her kidney disease by following a healthful, salt-free diet. She is the author of *Sodium Girl's Limitless Low-Sodium Cookbook* and *Low-So Good.* www.SodiumGirl.com.

The Good Gut: Taking Control of Your Weight, Your Mood, and Your Long-Term Health. Take a deep dive into gut health with Justin and Erica Sonnenburg, PhDs—two of the top researchers in the field—made readable and enjoyable. Includes a family-friendly seven-day menu.

The Keeler Migraine Method: A Groundbreaking, Individualized Treatment Program from the Renowned Headache Clinic. A lifestyle-based approach to migraine treatment by Robert Cowan, MD, of Stanford Medical School.

The Kitchen Counter Cooking School: How a Few Simple Lessons Transformed Nine Culinary Novices into Fearless Home Cooks. Scared to cook, or think you hate to cook? Read Kathleen Flinn's engaging book and see if you don't feel differently.

The Migraine Trust. Describes itself as a patient-focused, research-based charity in the United Kingdom. They provide research funding, patient support, and online resources, and they actively advocate for migraine patients. www.MigraineTrust.org.

The Wahls Protocol: How I Beat Progressive MS Using Paleo Principles and Functional Medicine. Terry Wahls, MD, shares her groundbreaking personal story of reversing her progressive multiple sclerosis using three phases of the Paleo diet, including her MCT-ketogenic diet, packed with optimal nutrition.

The Willpower Instinct: How Self-Control Works, Why It Matters, and What You Can Do to Get More of It. If you're struggling with willpower, this is the book for you. Author Kelly McGonigal, PhD, is the Stanford University instructor of "The Science of Willpower" course.

The Woman's Guide to Managing Migraine: Understanding the Hormone Connection to Find Hope and Wellness. This book by Susan Hutchinson, MD, provides detailed information on how migraine and hormones interact over the whole of a woman's life, including pregnancy, breastfeeding, and menopause. If you suffer from menstrual migraine, this is worth a read.

Why We Get Fat: And What to Do About It. This book by Gary Taubes explains why exercise doesn't equal weight loss, the truth about sugar and carbohydrates, and how to fix the obesity epidemic.

Yoga for Pain Relief: Simple Practices to Calm Your Mind and Heal Your Chronic Pain. Deep relaxation and gentle exercises from Kelly McGonigal, PhD, a Stanford psychologist and former chronic pain sufferer.

You Are Not Your Pain: Using Mindfulness to Relieve Pain, Reduce Stress, and Restore Well-Being. An eight-week program from Vidyamala Burch and Danny Penman with guided meditations that help chronic pain sufferers shift their focus and live more happily.

Note: Recipes found in any of the previously mentioned books or websites may contain migraine triggers.

endnotes

—— ··· ——

1   Gary Collins, "An interview with Gary Taubes," *Paleo Magazine*, April/May 2014, 53–55.

2   Timothy C. Hain, MD, "Etiology (cause) of Meniere's syndrome," Dizziness-and-balance.com, http://www.dizziness-and-balance.com/disorders/menieres/men_eti.html, accessed May 19, 2016.

3   "Migraine Attack: The Four Phases," American Headache Society Committee on Headache Education (ACHE), http://www.achenet.org/resources/migraine_attack_the_four_phases/, accessed June 28, 2016.

4   C. Ayata, "Spreading depression: from serendipity to targeted therapy in migraine prophylaxis," *Cephalalgia* 29 (2009): 1097–1114. *Cortical spreading depression* is a wave of neurotransmitter activity that spreads across the brain during aura, temporarily and very briefly depressing brain function. Cortical spreading depression is unrelated to feelings of depression.

5   Rip Esselstyn, *The Engine 2 Diet: The Texas Firefighter's 28-Day Save-Your-Life Plan That Lowers Cholesterol and Burns Away the Pounds*, (New York: Wellness Central-Hachette Book Group, 2009).

6   A variety of tests are used to diagnose balance disorders. http://www.enteaspoonec.com/balance/.

7   https://reddit.com/r/Menieres/.

8   https://www.myfitnesspal.com/.

9   http://www.SodiumGirl.com/.

10 http://www.Megahcart.com/.

11 Jessica Goldman Foung, *Sodium Girl's Limitless Low-Sodium Cookbook: How to Lose the Salt and Eat the Foods You Love* (Boston, New York: Houghton Mifflin Harcourt, 2013).

12 Donald A. Gazzaniga and Maureen A. Gazzaniga, *The No-Salt, Lowest-Sodium Cookbook: Hundreds of Favorite Recipes Created to Combat Congestive Heart Failure and Dangerous Hypertension* (New York: Thomas Dunne Books, 2001).

13 Michael B. Fowler, MD, "Salt, Hypertension, & Heart Failure" in Gazzaniga, *The No-Salt, Lowest-Sodium, Living Well Without Salt Cookbook*.

14 http://www.headaches.org/2007/10/25/low-tyramine-diet-for-migraine/, accessed July 20, 2016.

15 Video of the Epley chair: https://www.youtube.com/watch?v=AKCaWevNHIU

16 Lawrence D. Goldberg, MD, MBA, "The Cost of Migraine and Its Treatment," American Journal of Managed Care 11 (2005): 62–67, http://www.ajmc.com/journals/supplement/2005/2005-06-vol11-n2Suppl/Jun05-2069pS62-S67/, accessed May 21, 2016. Note that his estimate in 2005 was $13B-17B.

17 https://web.archive.org/web/20100720204935/http://www.headaches.org/education/Headache_Topic_Sheets/Low_Tyramine_Diet_for_Migraine

18 http://www.mc.vanderbilt.edu/documents/neurology/files/Tyramine%20Menu%20Book%2006227101.pdf, accessed June 10, 2014.

19 K.C. Brennan, MD, personal communication, August 5, 2016.

20 David Buchholz, MD, *Heal Your Headache: The 1–2–3 Program for Taking Charge of Your Pain* (New York: Workman Publishing, 2002).

21 K. Alpay, M. Ertas, E. Orhan, D. Ustay, C. Lieners, B. Baykan, "Diet restriction in migraine, based on IgG against foods: A clinical double-blind, randomised, cross-over trial," *Cephalalgia* 30, no. 7 (2010): 829–837.

22   David Perlmutter, MD, personal communication, June 16, 2016.

23   Jonathan Borkum, MD, "Migraine triggers and oxidative stress: A narrative review and synthesis," *Headache* January 2016. Doi:10.1111/head.12725.

24   Peter Goadsby, MD, "Bench and Bedside Insights into the Premonitory Phase of Migraine," American Headache Society 58th Annual Scientific Meeting, June 12, 2016.

25   Kerrie Smyres, "The Migraine Food Trigger You've Probably Never Heard Of," *Migraine.com*, July 23, 2014. http://migraine.com/blog/the-migraine-food-trigger-youve-probably-never-heard-of/, accessed January 22, 2015.

26   Daniel M. Keller, "Migraine Attacks Shortened by Diamine Oxidase Supplements," http://www.medscape.com/viewarticle/811920, October 1, 2013, accessed August 20, 2016.

27   Sarah Ballantyne, *The Paleo Approach: Reverse Autoimmune Disease and Heal Your Body* (Las Vegas: Victory Belt Publishing, 2013).

28   K.I. Shulman, S.E. Walker, S. MacKenzie, S. Knowles, "Dietary Restriction, Tyramine, and the Use of Monoamine Oxidase Inhibitors," *Journal of Clinical Psychopharmacology* 9, no. 6 (1989): 397–402.

29   D.A. Marcus, L. Scharff, D. Turk, L.M. Gourley, "A double-blind provocative study of chocolate as a trigger of headache," *Cephalalgia* 17 (1997): 855–862.

30   W.A. Fogel, A. Lewinski, J. Jochem, "Histamine in food: Is there anything to worry about?" *Biochemical Society Transactions* 35, pt 2 (2007): 349–352.

31   Buchholz, *Heal Your Headache.*

32   S.A.N. Tailor, K.I. Shulman, S.E. Walker, J. Moss, D. Gardner, "Hypertensive Episode Associated with Phenelzine and Tap Beer–A Reanalysis of the Role of Pressor Amines in Beer," *Journal of Clinical Psychopharmacology* 14, no. 1 (1994): 5–14

33   S. Novella-Rodriguez, M.T. Veciana-Nogues, M.C. Vidal-Carou, "Biogenic Amines and Polyamines in Milks and Cheeses by Ion-Pair High Performance Liquid Chromotography," *Journal of Agricultural and Food Chemistry* 48 (2000): 5117–5123.

34   S. Casal, E.L. Mendes, M.R. Alves, R.C. Alves, M. Beatriz, P.P. Oliveira, M.A. Ferreira, "Free and Conjugated Biogenic Amines in Green and Roasted Coffee Beans," *Journal of Agricultural and Food Chemistry* 52 (2004): 6188–6192.

35   D. Ly, K. Kang, J.Y. Choi, A. Ishihara, K. Back, S.G. Lee, "HPLC Analysis of Serotonin, Tryptamine, Tyramine, and the Hydroxycinnamic Acid Amides of Serotonin and Tyramine in Food Vegetables," *Journal of Medicinal Food* 11, no. 2 (2008): 385–389.

36   D.M. Gardner, K.I. Shulman, S.E. Walker, S.A.N. Tailor, "The Making of a User Friendly MAOI Diet," *Journal of Clinical Psychiatry* 57, no. 3 (March 1996): 99–104.

37   B. Blackwell, "Correspondence, 'Cold Cures' and Monoamine-oxidase Inhibitors," *The Lancet British Medical Journal* (10 May 1969): 381–382.

38   Alpay, "Diet restriction in migraine."

39   Buchholz, *Heal Your Headache.*

40   Christine Boyd, "Gluten & Migraine: Can the Gluten-Free Diet Help?" *Gluten-Free & More* (August/September 2014): 74–75.

41   Buchholz, *Heal Your Headache.*

42   B. Stolte, D. Holle, S. Naegel, H. Diener, M. Obermann, "Vestibular migraine," *Cephalalgia* 35, no. 3 (2015): 262–270.

43   H. Neuhauser, T. Lempert, "Vertigo and dizziness related to migraine: a diagnostic challenge," *Cephalalgia* 24 (2004): 83–91.

44   Josh Turknett, MD, *The Migraine Miracle: A Sugar-Free, Gluten-Free, Ancestral Diet to Reduce Inflammation and Relieve Your Headaches for Good* (Oakland: New Harbinger Publications, 2013).

45   Gary Taubes, *Good Calories, Bad Calories: Fats, Carbs, and the Controversial Science of Diet and Health* (New York: Anchor Books, 2007).

46   Mark Sisson, *The Primal Blueprint: Reprogram Your Genes for Effortless Weight Loss, Vibrant Health, and Boundless Energy* (Malibu: Primal Nutrition, 2009).

47   Terry Wahls, MD, *The Wahls Protocol: How I Beat Progressive MS Using Paleo Principles and Functional Medicine* (New York: Avery, 2014).

48   Jennifer Adler, *Passionate Nutrition: A Guide to Using Food as Medicine from a Nutritionist Who Healed Herself from the Inside Out* (Seattle: Sasquatch Books, 2014).

49   Michael B. Fowler, MD, "Salt, Hypertension, & Heart Failure" in Gazzaniga, *The No-Salt, Lowest-Sodium, Living Well Without Salt Cookbook.*

50   Donald Gazzaniga, personal communication, May 8, 2014.

51   James Clear, "How long does it actually take to build a new habit? (Backed by science)," *Huffington Post.* http://www.huffingtonpost.com/james-clear/forming-new-habits_b_5104807.html, accessed January 23, 2015.

52   "Chronic Migraine in America Study 2013," Migraine.com. http://migraine.com/chronic-migraine -in-america-2013/the-world-is-my-trigger/, accessed January 23, 2014.

53   M. Sandler, N-Y Li, N. Jarrett, V. Glover, "Dietary migraine: recent progress in the red (and white) wine story," *Cephalalgia* 15 (1995): 101–103.

54   Ballantyne, *The Paleo Approach.*

55   Buchholz, *Heal Your Headache.*

56   Diana Cullum-Dugan, RD, LDN, "When Food Is a Headache," *Environmental Nutrition* 36, no. 5 (May 2013): (1, 6)

57   E.A. Varkey, J. Cider, Carlsson et al. "Exercise and Migraine Prophylaxis: A Randomized Study Using Relaxation and Topiramate as Controls," *Cephalalgia* 31, no. 14 (2001): 1428–1438.

58   Chip Heath & Dan Heath, *Switch: How to Change Things When Change is Hard* (New York: Broadway Books, 2010).

59   Elizabeth Seng, PhD, "Headache Disorders: Caring for the Whole Person," American Headache Society 58th Annual Scientific Meeting, June 12, 2016.

60   Christiane Northrup, MD, *The Wisdom of Menopause: Creating Physical and Emotional Health During the Change* (New York: Bantam Books, 2001).

61   Heath, *Switch.*

62   Joan Borysenko, PhD, *Minding the Body, Mending the Mind* (Cambridge: Da Capo Lifelong, 2007).

63   Carol S. Dweck, *Mindset: The New Psychology of Success* (New York: Ballantine Books, 2006).

64   Ellen J. Langer, *Counterclockwise: Mindful Health and the Power of Possibility* (New York: Ballantine, 2009).

65   Borysenko, *Minding the Body, Mending the Mind.*

66   Langer, *Counterclockwise.*

67   Joanna Kempner, *Not Tonight: Migraine and the Politics of Gender and Health* (Chicago and London: The University of Chicago Press, 2014).

68   Robert Cowan, MD, "Migraine Causes and Triggers," *Migraine World Summit*, April 15, 2016. http://migraineworldsummit.com, accessed April 15, 2016.

69   Heath, *Switch.*

70   http://ndb.nal.usda.gov/

71   Ben Paynter, "Tiny Shrimp Big Business," *Eating Well*, May/June 2014.

72 C.E. Ramsden, K.R. Faurot, D. Zamora, C.M. Suchindran, B.A. MacIntosh, S. Gaylord, A. Ringel, J.R. Hibbeln, A. Feldstein, T.A. Mori, A. Barden, C. Lynch, R. Coble, E. Mas, O. Palsson, D.A. Barrow, J.D. Mann, "Targeted alteration of dietary n-3 and n-6 fatty acids for the treatment of chronic headaches: A randomized trial," *Pain* 154 (2013): 2441–2451.

73 My thanks to Nathan Phillips and Chef Tommy Gomes of Catalina Offshore Products for contributing to this section.

74 Gazzaniga, *The No-Salt, Lowest-Sodium, Living Well Without Salt Cookbook.*

75 Adler, *Passionate Nutrition.*

76 American Heart Association revised sodium guidelines, http://www.heart.org/HEARTORG/ GettingHealthy/NutritionCenter/HealthyEating/Frequently-Asked-Questions-FAQs-About -Sodium_UCM_306840_Article.jsp, accessed November 11, 2014.

77 Gerard Mullin, MD, *The Gut Balance Revolution: Boost Your Metabolism, Restore Your Inner Ecology, and Lose the Weight For Good!* (New York: Rodale, 2015).

78 Susan Hannah, Lawrence Leung, Elizabeth Dares-Dobbie, *The Complete Migraine Health, Diet Guide, and Cookbook: Practical Solutions for Managing Migraine and Headache Pain* (Toronto: Robert Rose, 2013).

79 Ballantyne, *The Paleo Approach.*

80 Katherine Harmon, "Salt Linked to Autoimmune Diseases," *Nature* (6 March 2013), *republished in Scientific American.* http://www.scientificamerican.com/article/salt-linked-to-autoimmune-diseases/. Accessed March 1, 2015.

81 M. Kleinewietfeld, A. Manzel, J. Titze, H. Kvakan, N. Yosef, R. Linker, D. Muller, D. Hafler, "Sodium chloride drives autoimmune disease by the induction of pathogenic TH17 cells," *Nature* 496 (25 April 2013): 518–522.

82 Michael B. Fowler, MD, "Salt, Hypertension, & Heart Failure" in Gazzaniga, *The No-Salt, Lowest-Sodium, Living Well Without Salt Cookbook.*

83 Ballantyne, *The Paleo Approach.*

84 Gazzaniga, *The No-Salt, Lowest-Sodium, Living Well Without Salt Cookbook.*

85 Mullin, *The Gut Balance Revolution.*

86 Ballantyne, *The Paleo Approach.*

87 Rebecca Katz, *The Healthy Mind Cookbook: Big-Flavor Recipes to Enhance Brain Function, Mood, Memory, and Mental Clarity* (Berkeley: Ten Speed Press, 2015).

88 Mark Sisson, "What Does The WHO Report Mean for Your Meat-Eating Habit?," MarksDailyApple.com, October 28, 2015. http://www.marksdailyapple.com/what-does-the-who -report-mean-for-your-meat-eating-habit/, accessed October 29, 2015.

89 Heidi Roth, "Why You Should Be Eating More Wild Pigs Right Now," Serious Eats, April 30, 2014, http://www.seriouseats.com/2014/04/why-you-should-be-eating-more-wild-pigs-right-now.html, accessed April 13, 2016.

90 Ballantyne, *The Paleo Approach.*

91 http://news.missouristate.edu/2015/11/30/chicken-soup-may-be-good-for-more-than-the-soul/, accessed December 4, 2015.

92 Dallas and Melissa Hartwig, *It Starts with Food: Discover the Whole30 and Change Your Life in Unexpected Ways* (Las Vegas: Victory Belt Publishing, 2012).

93 Carolyn Bernstein, MD, *The Migraine Brain: Your Breakthrough Guide to Fewer Headaches, Better Health* (New York: Pocket Books, 2008).

94   Jordan Gaines Lewis, "This is What Happens to Your Brain When You Stop Eating Sugar," Quartz.com, March 1, 2015. http://qz.com/353138/this-is-what-happens-to-your-brain-when-you-stop-eating-sugar/, accessed March 9, 2015.

95   David Perlmutter MD, *Grain Brain: The Surprising Truth About Wheat, Carbs, and Sugar—Your Brain's Silent Killers* (New York: Little, Brown, 2013).

96   Candace Pert, *Everything You Need to Know to Feel Go(o)d* (Carlsbad, CA: Hay House, 2006).

97   Mullin, *The Gut Balance Revolution.*

98   Ellen Ruppel Shell, "Artificial Sweeteners May Change Our Gut Bacteria in Dangerous Ways," Scientific American, March 17, 2015. http://www.scientificamerican.com/article/artificial-sweeteners-may-change-our-gut-bacteria-in-dangerous-ways/, accessed April 10, 2015.

99   Ricki Heller, *Living Candida-Free: Conquer the Hidden Epidemic that's Making You Sick* (Philadelphia: Da Capo Press, 2015).

100 B.J. Katić, W. Golden, R.K. Cady, X.H. Hu, "GERD prevalence in migraine patients and the implication for acute migraine treatment," *Journal of Headache Pain*, Feb 2009; 10(1):35-43.

101 Mark Schatzker, *The Dorito Effect: The Surprising New Truth About Food and Flavor* (New York: Simon and Schuster, 2015).

102 Justin Sonnenburg, PhD, personal communication, July 25 2016.

103 David Perlmutter MD, *Brain Maker: The Power of Gut Microbes to Heal and Protect Your Brain—For Life* (New York: Little, Brown, 2015).

104 Justin and Erica Sonnenburg, PhDs, *The Good Gut: Taking Control of Your Weight, Your Mood, and Your Long-Term Health* (New York: Penguin, 2015).

105 Sonnenburg, *The Good Gut.*

106 Perlmutter, *Brain Maker.*

107 Ibid.

108 Justin Sonnenburg, PhD, personal communication, July 25, 2016.

109 Kathleen Flinn, *The Kitchen Counter Cooking School: How a Few Simple Lessons Transformed Nine Culinary Novices into Fearless Home Cooks* (New York: Penguin, 2011).

110 "Food Waste By The Numbers," *Conscious Company*, Fall 2015.

111 "GREAT Opportunities: Your Role in the Rising Gluten-Free Marketplace," National Foundation for Celiac Awareness PDF, 2014. Study cited by The NPD Group, 2013.

112 David Schardt, "Food Allergies," Center for Science in the Public Interest, April 2001. https://www.cspinet.org/nah/04_01/, accessed February 26, 2015.

113 Thich Nhat Hahn, *Peace is Every Step: The Role of Mindfulness in Everyday Life* (New York: Bantam Books, 1991).

114 C.M. Shiflett, *Migraine Brains and Bodies: A Comprehensive Guide to Solving the Mystery of Your Migraines* (Berkeley: North Atlantic Books, 2011). Also, "Alternative Medicine Guide: Find the Right Treatment for You," *Yoga Journal*, January 6, 2016, http://www.yogajournal.com/article/health/find-right-alternative-medicine/ accessed January 18, 2016.

115 Gay Lipchik, "Biofeedback and Relaxation Training for Headaches," ACHE website, http://www.achenet.org/resources/biofeedback_and_relaxation_training_for_headaches/, accessed June 4, 2015.

116 https://sites.google.com/site/stanleyguansite/health/health-tips/breathe-deeply-to-activate-va-gus-nerve, accessed November 5, 2015.

117 Pierre Rigaux MD, "Neuro-Stimulation and Cephaly," *Migraine World Summit*, April 19, 2016. http://migraineworldsummit.com, accessed April 19, 2016.

118 Deepak Chopra, MD, *Perfect Health: The Complete Mind Body Guide* (New York: Three Rivers Press, 1991).

119   Kelly McGonigal PhD, *The Willpower Instinct: How Self-Control Works, Why It Matters, and What You Can Do to Get More of It* (New York: Avery, 2012).

120   Vidyamala Burch and Danny Penman, *You Are Not Your Pain: Using Mindfulness to Relieve Pain, Reduce Stress, and Restore Well-Being* (New York: Flatiron Books, 2013).

121   http://www.wakehealth.edu/News-Releases/2015/Mindfulness_Meditation_Trumps_Placebo_in_Pain_Reduction.htm accessed December 28, 2015.

122   For more on healing messaging, see Louise Hay, *Heal Your Body: The Mental Causes for Physical Illness and the Metaphysical Way to Overcome Them* (Carlsbad: Hay House, 1992).

123   Burch and Penman, *You Are Not Your Pain*.

124   Hartwig, *It Starts with Food*.

125   Dawn Buse, PhD, "Behavioral Approaches to Migraine," and Romie Mushtaq, MD, "Eastern and Western Approaches for Migraine," *Migraine World Summit*, April 15 & 16, 2016. http://migraineworldsummit.com, accessed April 15 & 16, 2016.

126   Robert Cowan, MD, personal communication, July 3, 2016.

127   Rebecca R. Buttaccio, PA-C, "Risk Factors, Clinical Course, and Barriers to Care in Adults and Pediatrics," presentation at The Bridge, an educational program sponsored by The American Headache Society, June 8, 2016.

128   Stewart Tepper MD, personal communication, July 1, 2016.

129   Teri Robert, *Living Well with Migraine Disease and Headaches: What Your Doctor Doesn't Tell You That You Need to Know* (New York: HarperCollins, 2005).

130   Kempner, *Not Tonight*.

131   E.A. Varkey, J. Cider, Carlsson et al. "Exercise and Migraine Prophylaxis: A Randomized Study Using Relaxation and Topiramate as Controls," *Cephalalgia* 31, no. 14 (2011): 1428–1438.

132   http://en.wikipedia.org/wiki/Skin, accessed January 26, 2015.

133   Amie Valpone, *Eating Clean: The 21-Day Plan to Detox, Fight Inflammation, and Reset Your Body* (Boston: Houghton Mifflin Harcourt, 2016).

134   Adler, *Passionate Nutrition*.

135   G. Chevalier, S.T. Sinatra, J.L. Oschman, K. Sokal, P. Sokal, "Earthing: Health Implications of Reconnecting the Human Body to the Earth's Surface Electrons," *Journal of Environmental and Public Health* (2012) Article ID 291541, 8 pages doi:10.1155/2012/291541.

136   Pedram Shojai, OMD, *The Urban Monk: Eastern Wisdom and Modern Hacks to Stop Time and Find Success, Happiness, and Peace* (New York: Rodale, 2016).

137   Jean McFadden Layton, ND, personal communication, January 26, 2015.

138   Ballantyne, *The Paleo Approach*.

139   J.P. Zock, E. Plana, D. Jarvis, J.M. Antó, H. Kromhout, S.M. Kennedy, N. Künzli, S. Villani, M. Olivieri, K. Torén, K. Radon, J. Sunyer, A. Dahlman-Hoglund, D. Norbäck, M. Kogevinas, "The Use of Household Cleaning Sprays and Adult Asthma," *American Journal of Respiratory and Critical Care Medicine* 176, no. 8 (2007): 735–741.

140   R.P. Silva-Neto, M.F.P. Peres, and M.M. Valenca, "Odorant substances that trigger headaches in migraine patients," *Cephalalgia* 34, no. 1 (2014): 14–21.

141   "Greener Laundry by the Load: Fabric Softener versus Dryer Sheets," *Scientific American*, December 10, 2008. http://www.scientificamerican.com/article/greener-laundry/, accessed June 6, 2016.

142   Theraspecs were developed by a migraine sufferer. Axon Optics sells glasses developed based on migraine-specific photo-sensitivity research by Dr. Bradley Katz. Each company's glasses filter light differently.

143 Bradley Katz, MD, PhD, "Light Sensitivity in Migraine Patients," *Migraine World Summit*, April 16, 2016. http://migraineworldsummit.com, accessed April 16, 2016.

144 Ibid.

145 *Indoor Air Facts No. 4 (revised) Sick Building Syndrome*, United States Environmental Protection Agency, February 1991. http://www.epa.gov/iaq/pdfs/sick_building_factsheet.pdf, accessed January 26, 2015.

146 Dweck, *Mindset*.

147 Heath, *Switch*.

148 Hartwig, *It Starts with Food*.

149 Ibid.

150 Elizabeth Seng, PhD, "Migraine and Cognitive Impairment: Risk Factors and Clinical Management," American Headache Society 58th Annual Scientific Meeting, June 9, 2016.

151 Valpone, *Eating Clean*.

152 McGonigal, *The Willpower Instinct*.

153 Heller, *Living Candida-Free*.

154 Gretchen Rubin, *Better Than Before: Mastering the Habits of Everyday Life* (New York: Crown, 2015).

155 Markus Dahlem, PhD, "Modeling Neurological Disease," Migraine World Summit, April 20, 2016. http://migraineworldsummit.com, accessed April 20, 2016.

156 http://www.webmd.com/sleep-disorders/excessive-sleepiness-10/10-results-sleep-loss, accessed July 3, 2014.

157 V. Aho, H.M. Ollila, et. al., "Partial Sleep Restriction Activates Immune Response-Related Gene Expression Pathways: Experimental and Epidemiological Studies in Humans," *PLOS One*, October 23, 2013, DOI: 10.1371/journal.pone.0077184. http://journals.plos.org/plosone/article?id=10.1371/journal.pone.0077184, accessed February 9, 2015.

158 Mullin, *The Gut Balance Revolution*.

159 Stephani Sutherland, "Bright Screens Could Delay Bedtime," *Scientific American*, http://www.scientificamerican.com/article/bright-screens-could-delay-bedtime/, accessed July 3, 2014.

160 Cameron Diaz, *The Body Book: The Law of Hunger, The Science of Strength, and Other Ways to Love Your Amazing Body*, (New York: HarperCollins, 2014).

161 Buy acupressure mats from Spoonkspace.com.

162 *Young People Are Sleeping With Their Phones. Their Parents Are Sleeping With People.* Huffington Post Healthy Living, August 14, 2014. http://www.huffingtonpost.com/2013/09/16/sleep-phone-tablet-bed_n_3924161.html, accessed August 15, 2014.

163 http://dallashartwig.com/moresociallessmedia/ accessed June 6, 2016.

164 Wahls, *The Wahls Protocol*.

165 Adler, *Passionate Nutrition*.

166 Northrup, *The Wisdom of Menopause*.

167 David Allen, *Getting Things Done: The Art of Stress-Free Productivity* (New York: Penguin Books, 2001).

168 Diaz, *The Body Book*.

169 Ballantyne, *The Paleo Approach*.

170 Taubes, *Good Calories, Bad Calories*. See also Gary Taubes, *Why We Get Fat: And What to Do About It* (New York: Anchor Books, 2010).

171 Adler, *Passionate Nutrition*.

172 Mullin, *The Gut Balance Revolution*.

173 Mark Hyman, MD, *Eat Fat, Get Thin: Why the Fat We Eat Is the Key to Sustained Weight Loss and Vibrant Health*, (New York: Little, Brown, 2016).

174 Taubes, *Good Calories, Bad Calories*.

175 Monica Reinagle, MS, LD/N, CNS, "How to Avoid *The Biggest Loser* Phenomenon," *Nutrition Diva Quick & Dirty Tips* podcast, May 10, 2016, http://www.quickanddirtytips.com/health-fitness /weight-loss/how-to-avoid-the-biggest-loser-phenomenon, accessed June 6, 2016.

176 Perlmutter *Grain Brain*.

177 Sisson, *The Primal Blueprint*.

178 Dale Bond, PhD, "Strategies for Countering Inactive and Sedentary Lifestyles in the Context of Migraine and Obesity: Insights from the Women's Health and Migraine (WHAM) Trial," American Headache Society 58th Annual Scientific Meeting, June 9, 2016.

179 Buchholz, *Heal Your Headache*.

180 Adler, *Passionate Nutrition*.

181 Trupti Gokani, MD, "The Gut-Brain Link: How Your Headaches Might Stem From Your Digestion," Huffington Post, November 13, 2014. http://www.huffingtonpost.com/trupti-gokani-md/the -gutbrain-link-how-you_b_6097774.html, accessed November 13, 2014. Followed up with her to receive the abstract from her paper.

182 Alpay, "Diet restriction in migraine."; personal communication with the author, June 7, 2015.

183 Ayla Withee, MS, RDN, LDN, CLT, personal communication, June 6, 2016. http://nowleap.com /the-patented-mediator-release-test-mrt/. Find a certified LEAP therapist by searching "CLT" along with your town and the word nutrition.

184 Take Care podcast from WRVO, December 6, 2015. http://wrvo.org/post/diet-debate-and-why -theres-more-common-ground-you-think, accessed February 6, 2016.

185 Kate Christensen, "Beyond Paleo: Is Eating Like a Viking the Next It Diet?" *Vogue*, December 26, 2014, http://www.vogue.com/6159767/eat-like-a-viking-nordic-diet/, accessed December 27, 2014.

186 Wahls, *The Wahls Protocol*.

187 Sally Fallon Morell, "Differences Between the Weston A. Price Foundation Diet and the Paleo Diet," *The Weston A. Price Foundation for Wise Traditions in Food, Farming, and the Healing Arts*. October 7, 2013. http://www.westonaprice.org/health-topics/differences-between-the-weston-a -price-foundation-diet-and-the-paleo-diet/, accessed September 15, 2014.

188 Ben Paynter, "Tiny Shrimp Big Business," *Eating Well*, May/June 2014.

189 "Arsenic in Your Rice: The Latest," *Consumer Reports*, January 2015, pp. 41-42.

190 Ballantyne, *The Paleo Approach*.

191 "The benefits of soaking nuts and seeds," *Food Matters*. October 13, 2009: http://foodmatters.tv /articles-1/the-benefits-of-soaking-nuts-and-seeds, accessed February 4, 2015.

192 Wahls, *The Wahls Protocol*.

193 Joan Borysenko, PhD, *The Plant-Plus Diet Solution: Personalized Nutrition for Life* (Carlsbad, CA: Hay House, 2014).

194 Adler, *Passionate Nutrition*.

195 Schatzker, *The Dorito Effect*.

196 M.C. Morris, C.C. Tangney, Y. Wang, F.M. Sacks, D.A. Bennett, N.T. Aggarwal, "MIND diet associated with reduced incidence of Alzheimer's disease," *Alzheimer's & Dementia* 11 (2015): 1007–1014.

197 Schatzker, *The Dorito Effect*.

198 Center for Science in the Public Interest, *Sweet Nothings: Safe . . . or Scary? The Inside Scoop on Sugar Substitutes* (2014): 7.

199 Salynn Boyles, "Artificial Sweeteners May Raise Diabetes Risk," *MedPage Today*, September 22, 2014. http://www.medpagetoday.com/Endocrinology/GeneralEndocrinology/47777, accessed February 4, 2015.

200 Alec Mian PhD, "How to Find Your Migraine Protectors," *Migraine World Summit*, April 18, 2016. http://migraineworldsummit.com, accessed April 18, 2016. Find the app at https://curelator.com/.

201 Calculating protein intake: keto-calculator.ankerl.com

202 http://reddit.com/keto

203 Wahls, *The Wahls Protocol*.

204 F. Maggioni, M. Margoni, G. Zanchin, "Ketogenic diet in migraine treatment: A brief but ancient history," *Cephalalgia*, 31(10) 1150–1151.

205 Turknett, *The Migraine Miracle*.

206 M. Maalouf, J.M. Rho, M.P. Mattson, "The neuroprotective properties of calorie restriction, the ketogenic diet, and ketone bodies," *Brain Research Reviews*. 2009 Mar; 59(2):293-315. doi: 10.1016 /j.brainresrev.2008.09.002. Epub 2008 Sep 25.

207 Ballantyne, *The Paleo Approach*.

208 A. Patel, P.L. Pyzik, Z. Turner, et. al. "Long-term outcomes of children treated with the ketogenic diet in the past", *Epilepsia*. 2010 Jul;51(7):1277-82. doi: 10.1111/j.1528-1167.2009.02488.x. Epub 2010 Feb 1.

209 Turknett, *The Migraine Miracle*.

210 Adler, *Passionate Nutrition*.

211 Hartwig, *It Starts with Food*.

212 http://www.livestrong.com/article/24160-health-benefits-tart-cherry-juice/, accessed on November 23, 2015.

recipe index

—— ••• ——

Recipe	Page	Vegan/ Vegetarian	Dairy-Free	Egg-Free	Grain-free
Bacon Salad Dressing	266		DF		GF
Beet–Strawberry Smoothie	187	V	DF	EF	GF
Berry Cobbler	248	V	DF	EF	
Berry Sauce	250	V	DF	EF	GF
Berry Trifle	253	V	DF		
Blueberry–Oat Waffles	198	V	DF	EF	
Breakfast Hash	281	V	DF	EF	GF
Carob Squares	251	V	DF		GF
Cherry Clafoutis	252	V	DF		
Chicken Cacciatore	226		DF	EF	GF
Chicken or Turkey Salad	211		DF		GF
Chile Pepper Sauce	267	V	DF	EF	GF
Chopped Salad	287	V	DF	EF	GF
Cilantro Mayonnaise	268	V	DF		GF
Coconut Whipped Cream	254	V	DF	EF	GF
Creamy Not-ella Carob Butter	188	V	DF	EF	GF
Creamy Soup	288	V	DF	EF	GF
Crepes	200	V	DF		
Cucumber–Basil Water	258	V	DF	EF	GF
Denver Omelet	201		DF		GF
Egg Mini-Quiches	202	V	DF		GF
Farmers' Market Chilled Tomato-Basil Soup	212	V	DF	EF	GF
Firehouse Turkey Chili	213	V	DF	EF	GF
Fish Baked in Parchment Packets	228		DF	EF	GF
French Toast	203	V	DF		
Frittata	280	V	DF		GF

Recipe	Page	Vegan/ Vegetarian	Dairy-Free	Egg-Free	Grain-free
Granola	205	V	DF	EF	
Grilled Peaches with Cardamom—Maple Cream Sauce	256	V	DF	EF	GF
Hemp Milk	255	V	DF	EF	GF
Herbed Cheese Spread	189	V		EF	GF
Italian Dressing	269	V	DF	EF	GF
Make Your Own Bacon	197		DF	EF	GF
Maple Sesame Glazed Chicken	225		DF	EF	GF
Meatloaf	230		DF		GF
Migas	206	V	DF		
Pasta with Vegetables	282	V	DF	EF	
Pasta with Vodka Chickpea Sauce	232	V	DF	EF	GF
Patties	283		DF		
Peach–Mango Power Smoothie	194	V	DF	EF	GF
Peachy Pulled Pork	234		DF	EF	GF
Pear Upside-Down Cake	260	V	DF	EF	
Pizza	284	V	DF	EF	
Pomegranate Marinade for Beef or Chicken	270	V	DF	EF	GF
Pork Sausage Patties	208		DF	EF	GF
Provençal Chickpea Salad	218	V	DF	EF	GF
Quiche	285	V	DF		
Quick Alfredo Style Pasta Sauce	271	V		EF	GF
Ranch Dressing	272	V	DF	EF	GF
Rice Bowl	286	V	DF	EF	
Rice Pudding	262	V	DF	EF	
Roasted Chile Pepper Hummus	190	V	DF	EF	GF
Roasted Veggie Quinoa Casserole	236	V	DF	EF	
Salmon–Potato Cakes	237		DF		GF
Salmon, Asparagus, and Thyme Omelet	209		DF		GF
Salsa Verde	274	V	DF	EF	GF

Recipe	Page	Vegan/ Vegetarian	Dairy-Free	Egg-Free	Grain-free
Scallop Corn Chowder	238		DF	EF	GF
Scalloped Potatoes with Roasted Chiles	242	V	DF	EF	GF
Seedy Carrot Crackers	192	V	DF	EF	GF
Sloppy Joes	216		DF	EF	GF
Smoky Butternut Squash Soup	219	V	DF	EF	GF
Smoky Mustard Sauce	273	V	DF		GF
Spice Rub for Chicken and Fish	276	V	DF	EF	GF
Spice-Rubbed Seared Pork Chops with Oven-Baked Sweet Potatoes and Cranberry–Pear Sauce	240		DF	EF	GF
Spicy Fish Tacos	214		DF		GF
Spicy Kale and Split Pea Soup	220	V	DF	EF	GF
Spicy Kale and Swiss Chard Sauté	243	V	DF	EF	GF
Steak and Roasted Vegetable Salad	244	V	DF	EF	GF
Strawberry–Mint Water	259	V	DF	EF	GF
Sunflower Seed Butter	195	V	DF	EF	GF
Tart Cherry Marinade for Beef or Pork	277	V	DF	EF	GF
Three Bean and Potato Salad	222	V	DF	EF	GF
Tomato–Herb Salad Dressing	278	V	DF		GF
Tuna or Salmon Salad	223		DF		GF
Vanilla Ricotta Cream	263	V		EF	GF
Veggie Frittata	204	V	DF		GF
Watermelon–Mint Granita	264	V	DF	EF	GF
Wild Rice and Carrots	246	V	DF	EF	

index

Gelatin, grass-fed, 69, 164
Getting Things Done (Allen),
    148–149
Glutamates, 22
Gluten-free bread, as freezer
    staple, 50
Gluten-free diets, 26
Gluten-free foods, 57
Good Calories, Bad Calories
    (Taubes), 149–150, 162
Grain Brain (Perlmutter), 22, 26, 173
Grains
    in ancestral diet, 166
    approved and excluded, 33
    testing as trigger food, 161
Granola, 205
Grapes, in Chicken or Turkey
    Salad, 211
Green onions, how and when to
    freeze, 87
Grieving, for loss of previous diet,
    115
Grilled Peaches with Cardamom–
    Maple Cream Sauce, 256–257
Growth mindset, 129–130
Guided meditation, 110–112, 145
Gut-brain axis, 26, 80

H
Hair care, 12
Hand lotion ingredients, 121
Hartwig, Dallas and Melissa,
    131–132, 146
Hash, 281
Headache, defined, 4
HeadSpace app, 110
Heal Your Headache (Buchholz), 25,
    156–157
Heath, Chip and Dan, 48, 114, 131
Hebert, Michele, 110
Heller, Ricki, 139
Hemp seeds
    Beet–Strawberry Smoothie, 187
    Creamy Not-ella Carob Butter,
        188
    Hemp Milk, 255
    Peach–Mango Power Smoothie,
        194
Herbs, spices, and condiments
    about: approved and excluded,
        35; using extra, 88

Cilantro Mayonnaise, 268
    Herbed Cheese Spread, 189
High-fat, lower-carb diets, 150–151
Histamine
    in canned fish, 51
    as migraine trigger, 21–22
Home, detoxing of, 124–126
Hummus, Roasted Chile Pepper,
    190–191
HVAC systems, 127
Hyman, Dr. Mark, 26, 150, 165, 173,
    174–175

I
IBS, 78
Indian restaurants, avoiding of, 102
*Inner Practices of Yoga—Self-Healing,
    The* (Hebert), 110
Insomnia. *See* Sleep (month 6)
Italian Dressing, 269
Italian restaurants, tips for eating
    in, 95

J
Japanese restaurants, tips for, 95
Jarisch-Herxheimer reaction, 75
Jarred goods, as pantry staple, 55
Jicama, how and when to freeze, 87

K
Kabat-Zinn, Jon, 110
Kaiser Permanente podcasts, 110
Kale
    about: how and when to freeze,
        86
    Roasted Veggie Quinoa
        Casserole, 236
    Spicy Kale and Split Pea Soup,
        220–221
    Spicy Kale and Swiss Chard
        Sauté, 243
Katz, Dr. Bradley, 127
Katz, Dr. David, 162
Ketogenic diet, 172–175
Kitchen, detoxing of, 124–125
Kitchen Counter Cooking School, The
    (Flinn), 91

L
Langer, Ellen, 45–46, 114
Laundry, detoxing of, 126
Leaky gut syndrome, 21, 80–81
LEAP (Lifestyle Eating and
    Performance) test, 161
LED bulbs, warm versus cool
    spectrum and, 126
Leeks, how and when to freeze, 87
Leftovers, recipes using, 279–288
Lettuce, storing of, 87
Lighting, detoxing of
    in home, 126
    in office, 127
Liverwurst, 69
Living Candida-Free (Heller), 139
Living room, detoxing of, 125
Low-carb diets, 149–151, 175. *See also*
    Ketogenic diet
Low-sodium diets, 11–13, 19, 26–27, 59
Low-tyramine diet, 15, 16–17, 18–19,
    23
"Low-VOC" (volatile organic
    compound) materials, 125
Lunch, transition to approved
    (week 6), 30, 76–78
Lunch recipes, 210–223

M
Magnesium supplement, taking
    before bedtime, 148
Make Your Own Bacon, 197
Mangoes, Peach–Mango Power
    Smoothie, 194
Maple Sesame Glazed Chicken, 225
Marinades
    Pomegranate, 270
    Tart Cherry, 277
Mayonnaise, 88
    Cilantro Mayonnaise, 268
McGonigal, Dr. Kelly, 138
MCT ketogenic diet, 173, 175
Meatloaf, 230–231
Meats
    in ancestral diet, 163–164
    as refrigerator staples, 65
    see also specific meats
Mediator release testing (MRT), 161
Medication overuse headaches
    (MOH), 5, 118–120
Medications, detoxing and, 118–120

about the author

———— ••• ————

STEPHANIE WEAVER, MPH, CWHC, is an author, blogger, and certified wellness and health coach. She has a master's degree of public health in nutrition education from the University of Illinois. Find more than 350 gluten-free recipes on her blog Recipe Renovator, suitable for many special diets including migraine. Weaver writes for *The Huffington Post*, and her recipes have been featured online by *Cosmopolitan*, *Bon Appétit*, *Cooking Light*, and *Parade*. She lives in San Diego with her husband, Bob, and their golden retriever, Daisy.